Quick Reference Dictionary FOR Physical Therapy

Second Edition

EDITED BY

JENNIFER M. BOTTOMLEY, PhD², MS, PT

Geriatric Rehabilitation Program Consultant

Wayland, Massachusetts

D0149079

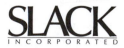

INCORPORATED

An innovative information, education, and management company
6900 Grove Road • Thorofare, NJ 08086

Care has been taken to ensure that drug selection, dosages, and treatments are in accordance with currently accepted/recommended practice. Due to continuing research, changes in government policy and regulations, and various effects of drug reactions and interactions, it is recommended that the reader review all materials and literature provided for each drug use, especially those that are new or not frequently used.

The work SLACK Incorporated publishes is peer reviewed. Prior to publication, recognized leaders in the field, educators, and clinicians provide important feedback on the concept and content that we publish. We welcome feedback on this work.

Quick reference dictionary for physical therapy / edited by Jennifer Bottomley.-- 2nd ed.

p. ; cm.

Includes bibliographical references.

ISBN 1-55642-580-5 (alk. paper)

1. Physical therapy--Dictionaries.

[DNLM: 1. Physical Therapy Techniques--Dictionary--English. W 13 Q62 2003] I. Bottomley, Jennifer M.

RM696.5 .Q53 2003

615.8'2'03--dc21

2002155834

Printed in the United States of America.

Published by: SLACK Incorporated
                       6900 Grove Road
                       Thorofare, NJ 08086 USA
                       Telephone: 856-848-1000
                       Fax: 856-853-5991
                       www.slackbooks.com

Contact SLACK Incorporated for more information about other books in this field or about the availability of our books from distributors outside the United States.

For permission to reprint material in another publication, contact SLACK Incorporated. Authorization to photocopy items for internal, personal, or academic use is granted by SLACK Incorporated provided that the appropriate fee is paid directly to Copyright Clearance Center. Prior to photocopying items, please contact the Copyright Clearance Center at 222 Rosewood Drive, Danvers, MA 01923 USA; phone: 978-750-8400; website: www.copyright.com; email: info@copyright.com

Last digit is print number: 10   9   8   7   6   5   4   3   2   1

DEDICATION

This book is dedicated to each and every student I've had the opportunity of teaching throughout my professional journey thus far and to those that I'll have the good fortune of meeting in the future.

CONTENTS

ACKNOWLEDGMENTS

This seemed like a challenging task of will to undertake and to which to adhere, but thanks to the support of my significant other, inspiration of my educators and mentors, assistance and guidance of my colleagues, inspiration of my patients/clients, and my own perseverance, the revisions of the first edition of the *Quick Reference Dictionary for Physical Therapy* toward the completion of the second edition has been accomplished.

Special thanks to all of the educators I have had the opportunity to learn from along my professional path. I offer this book to you in reflection for all you have given and for the many young professional lives you have touched through your teaching. Many of the sections of this book are drawn directly from my own undergraduate course notes and flash cards I created for study that, 25 years later, I still have and cherish as guides in my practice of physical therapy. I'd like to acknowledge with particular thanks Mary Jane Meng, MS, PT; Janet C. Lemke, MS, PT; the late, yet dearly remembered Joan K. Werner, PhD; Gertrude A. Freeman, MS, PT; and Mary Jane Nelson, BS, PT... those mentors and educators who lit the original fire that, from an ember, still burns in me today.

My gratitude is warmly extended to Amy E. Drummond, Editorial Director; John H. Bond, Vice President; Peter N. Slack, President & CEO; Carrie N. Kotlar, Acquisitions Editor; April Billick, Senior Project Editor; and Lauren Plummer, Managing Editor, for their support and encouragement throughout this endeavor.

My heartfelt gratitude and thanks to my true companion, Jennifer M. Buchwald, for her sustaining love and patience during the many hours consumed toward the completion of this work.

ABOUT THE EDITOR

Jennifer M. Bottomley, PhD[2], MS, PT, has a Bachelor's degree in PhysicalTtherapy from the University of Wisconsin, Madison and an advanced Master's degree in Physical Therapy from the MGH Institute of Health Professionals, Boston, Mass. She has a combined intercollegiate Doctoral degree in Gerontology and Health Science and Service Administration and a second PhD from The Union Institute in Health Science in Administration, Legislation, and Policy Management with a specialty in gerontology. She has practiced since 1974 in acute care, home care, outpatient clinics, nursing homes, and long-term care facilities. Currently, she works as an independent consultant setting up rehabilitation services in nursing homes and outpatient, home, and community settings in the Northeast and Pacific Northwest and serves on advisory boards for the Office of the Surgeon General and the Office on Women's Health in the Department of Health and Human Services. Jennifer is the current president of the American Physical Therapy Association (APTA) section on geriatrics and has served two terms as the vice president, two terms as the treasurer, and one term on the board of directors for that section. She is also the current editor of *GeriNotes* for the APTA's section on geriatrics. She has spearheaded national efforts through the AARP and Gray Panther's on education and physical conditioning to prevent crime, abuse, and fraud against the elderly. She has also orchestrated free screening and intervention projects for the Homeless Elderly of Massachusetts and has obtained Health Care Financing Administration grants to provide free screening and care for low income elders in 14 Central Massachusetts cities and towns. Jennifer is a nationally renowned speaker and educator. She has done clinical research in the areas of nutrition and exercise, foot care in the elderly, wound care, diabetes and peripheral vascular disease interventions, balance and falls in the Alzheimer's population, T'ai Chi as an alternative exercise form, and social policy development (inclusive of the managed care perspective) for the elderly. She has authored numerous chapters and articles in the area of geriatrics, is the presenter on six videotapes with the University of Maryland VideoPress on functional evaluation of the Alzheimer's patient and functional assessment in rheumatoid arthritis, and a four-tape series on exercise in the elderly. She has coauthored a geriatric text with Carole B. Lewis entitled, *Geriatric Rehabilitation: A Clinical Approach, Second Edition.*

PREFACE

Haven't you always wished that all of the information you've learned in your physical therapy education could be easily accessed from one source? Educating physical therapy professionals requires the acquisition of volumes of knowledge and skills in a relatively short period of time. The quantity of knowledge required for the practice of high quality physical therapy, though learned and stored, is often difficult to retrieve. It is with this in mind that the *Quick Reference Dictionary for Physical Therapy, Second Edition* has been created.

This dictionary starts with a dictionary of commonly utilized words and their definitions. Though not an exhaustive list from A to Z, the intent is to provide quick reference for vocabulary that is often encountered on a day-to-day basis as a clinician and as a student. In the real world, many of the words we use are abbreviated. The appendices that follow the body of the dictionary provide lists of frequently used and standardized acronyms and abbreviations for words (Appendix 2), medical roots from which many words are derived (Appendix 3), commonly used acronyms for evaluative tests and measures (Appendix 4), and acronyms for organizations important to the practice of physical therapy (Appendix 5).

It is important that we as physical therapy professionals maintain the highest standards of practice in the most ethical and skillful manner possible and that what we do is well documented. With the permission of the American Physical Therapy Association, the *Code of Ethics*, the *Guide for Professional Conduct*, the *Standards of Ethical Conduct for the Physical Therapist Assistant*, the *Guide for Conduct of the Affiliate Member*, the *Standards of Practice*, *Guidelines for Physical Therapy Documentation*, and the Mission and Goals Statements have been reproduced for easy reference in Appendices 6 to 12, respectively.

Our historical roots and the evolution of our profession are founded in the efforts of some remarkable practitioners in physical therapy. Historical practitioners influential in the genesis of physical therapy and our past and present presidential leadership are provided in Appendices 13 and 14, respectively. The references provided in Appendix 13 are invaluable resources from which to gain further information on the growth and advancement of the profession of physical therapy since its inception.

Often, it is difficult to access information on state licensure requirements and the variations in state practice acts. In Appendix 15, a comprehensive and current list of addresses and contact information of state licensure boards, state chapter physical therapy associations, and components of the American Physical Therapy Association is given. Additionally, Internet addresses, contact information, and legislative identification numbers for obtaining access to state practice acts are provided under each of the respective state listings.

There is a wealth of information available in every area of health care thanks to the Internet. Appendix 16, though hardly comprehensive or exhaustive, provides world wide web sites in rehabilitation that will link you to almost every conceivable piece of information that a physical therapist might need or seek for answering clinical, educational, research, legislative, and policy questions related to the practice of physical therapy.

Appendix 17 provides the definitions of impairment, disability, and handicap as established and accepted by the World Health Organization. Appendix 18 defines commonly encountered diseases and pathologies. Appendix 19 describes frequently utilized tests and measures in physical therapy. This is followed by generally accepted physical therapy interventions (Appendix 20). These appendices were created using the *Guide to Physical Therapist Practice of the American Physical Therapy Association* as a pilot to assure consistency in terminology and guarantee that all of the diseases and pathologies, tests and measures, and interventions outlined in the *Guide* were defined in this dictionary.

The next group of appendices is comprised of commonly used frames of reference for measures and information that is often needed in the clinical setting. Normal measures for range of motion of the joints are listed in Appendix 21. A comprehensive list of normal ranges for laboratory values is provided in Appendix 22. Appendix 23 gives a brief description of fractures and standard classification categories for fracture types. Reflexes and reactions of the central nervous system are presented in an easy-to-read table format in Appendix 24 The metabolic equivalent (MET) values for activity and exercise are listed in Appendix 25. Appendix 26 describes the cranial nerves and tests for cranial nerve integrity. The bones of the body are pictorially represented in Appendix 27. Appendix 28 is broken into parts A and B. Part 28A is a pictorial representation of the muscles of the body, while part 28B lists each muscle in table format and provides each muscle's origin and insertion, action, innervation, and blood supply.

Appendices 29 to 31 respectively offer weights and measures, the metric system, and English to metric conversion values. Commonly encountered symbols used as short cuts for documentation are listed in Appendix 32.

Prescription drugs are delineated by disease and disorder in Appendix 33 and recommended daily allowances of nutrients, vitamins, and minerals are provided by age groups and gender in Appendix 34.

As documentation is vital for reimbursement, reimbursement terms and guidelines for physical therapy claims review are provided in Appendix 35.

More and more, we are seeing the use of complementary and alternative therapies in the field of rehabilitation medicine. Appendix 36 defines these therapies for the clinician as patients/clients may seek alternative care as possible adjuncts to traditional care, and it is important that we are familiar with these complementary approaches.

A listing for possible resources and networking possibilities is provided in Appendix 37 by category or diagnosis. In order to advocate for our patients/clients, these organizations provide invaluable educational information and resources for assisting our patients/clients in managing their impairments, disabilities, or handicaps.

Appendix 38 provides a directory to the organizations of the American Physical Therapy Association. Mission and goals of each organization are described and contact information is offered.

The *Quick Reference Dictionary for Physical Therapy, Second Edition* has been designed to be user-friendly. In using this dictionary, if you are looking for a specific piece of information, think in terms of the "category" that it might fall under, and chances are there is an appendix that will answer your question. For example, if you are looking for the definition of a diagnosis or pathology that is not in the body of the dictionary, look in Appendix 18. As with any dictionary, there are always additional terms to add, or areas that you might like to see included in subsequent editions of the *Quick Reference Dictionary for Physical Therapy*. Blank pages for your own additions have been provided, and this author would greatly appreciate your comments on content, suggestions for additions or omissions, corrections, and constructive input that might enhance future updates of this book and keep this dictionary a dynamic and valuable resource.

Jennifer M. Bottomley, PhD[2], MS, PT

A

abduction (ABD): Movement of a body part (usually the limbs) away from the midline of the body.

abnormal: Not normal, average, typical, or usual; an irregularity.

abruptio placentae: Premature separation of the placenta from the uterine wall after 20 weeks of gestation.

abscess: A swollen, inflamed area of body tissue in which there is a localized collection of pus.

absence: An epileptic seizure characterized by abrupt loss of consciousness for a few seconds, followed by a rapid, complete recovery.

absolute endurance: Muscular endurance when force of contraction is tested over time until fatigue of the muscle occurs. Ability of muscle to sustain force or to repeatedly generate force to the point of fatigue.

absorption: Process by which a substance is made available to body fluids for distribution.

abstract thinking: Ability to derive meaning from an event or experience beyond the tangible aspects of the event itself.

acceleration: Increase in the speed or velocity of an object or reaction.

accessibility: Degree to which an exterior or interior environment is available for use in relation to an individual's physical and/or psychological abilities.

accessory movement: Involuntary arthrokinematic movements that are necessary for full normal osteokinematic movement. Two noted types are component movement and joint play.

accessory movers: Muscles capable of performing a motion; they assist prime movers.

accommodation: Process of adapting or adjusting one object or set of objects to another object or set of objects.

accreditation: Process used to evaluate educational programs against a set of standards that represents the knowledge, skills, and attitudes needed for competent practice.

accuracy of response: Percentage of errors and correct responses recorded.

achalasia: Failure of a circular sphincter or other muscle to relax and open (eg, cardiac sphincter between the esophagus and the stomach).

achromatopsia: Color blindness.

acquired amputation: Person is born with all limbs, but a limb is removed in part or total after injury or accident.

acquired deformities/disorders: Diseases, deformities, or dysfunctions that are not genetic but produced by influences originating outside of the organism.

acrocyanosis: Symmetric mottled cyanosis of the hands and feet associated with coldness and sweating. It is a vasospastic disorder accentuated by cold or emotion and relieved by warmth.

acromion process: Outer projection of the spine of the scapula; considered to be the highest part of the shoulder, it connects laterally to the clavicle.

active assistive range of motion (AAROM): Amount of motion at a given joint achieved by the person using his or her own muscle strength with assistance.

active labor: The second phase of the first stage of labor during which the cervix dilates from 4 to 8 cm.

active listening: Skills that allow a person to hear, understand, and indicate that the message has been communicated.

active play therapy: Therapy in which the therapist uses toys and particular play to advance a child's treatment or development.

active range of motion (AROM): Amount of motion at a given joint achieved by the person using his or her own muscle strength.

active stretch: Stretch produced by internal muscular force.

activin: Hormone releasing factor that assists production of follicular stimulating hormone (FSH) at the pituitary.

activities of daily living (ADL): The self-care, communication, and mobility skills (eg, bed mobility, transfers, ambulation, dressing, grooming, bathing, eating, and toileting) required for independence in everyday living.

activity: The nature and extent of functioning at the level of the person. Productive action required for the development, maturation, and use of sensory, motor, social, psychological, and cognitive functions.

activity analysis: Breaking down the activity into components to determine the human functions needed to complete the activity.

activity theory of aging: Psychosocial theory of aging suggesting that successful aging occurs when the older person continues to participate in the satisfying activities of his or her earlier adulthood.

activity tolerance: The ability to sustain engagement in an activity over a period of time.

acuity: Ability of the sensory organ to receive information. Keenness as of thought or vision.

acupressure: Use of touch at specific points along the meridians of the body to release the tensions that cause various physical symptoms. Based on the principles of acupuncture.

acupuncture: Chinese practice of inserting needles into specific points along the meridians of the body to relieve pain and induce anesthesia. It is used for preventive and therapeutic purposes.

acute: Of short and intense duration. A very serious, critical period of short duration in illness. Intensification of need or urgent.

adaptation: Satisfactory adjustment of individuals within their environment over time. Successful adaptation equates with quality of life.

adaptive devices: A variety of implements or equipment used to aide patients/clients in performing movements, tasks, or activities. Adaptive devices include raised toilet seats, seating systems, environmental controls, and other devices.

adaptive response: An appropriate response to an environmental demand.

additive activities profile test (ADAPT): Self-administered test that relates activities of daily living to physical fitness.

adduction (ADD): Movement toward the midline of the body.

adductor pads: Pads at the sides of a wheelchair that hold the hips and legs toward the midline of the body.

adenohypophysis: The anterior lobe of the pituitary gland.

adherence: Consistent behavior that is accomplished through an internalization of learning and enhanced by independent coping and problem-solving skills.

adhesion: Soft tissue restrictions and scarring resulting from injury and inflammation. The product when two or more structures become attached, united, or stuck together.

adhesive capsulitis: Inflammation of the joint capsule that causes limitations of mobility or immobility of the joint.

adjunct rotation: Osteokinematically, any spin that is not a conjunct rotation (ie, resulting from gravity, muscle action, or other external forces).

adjustment reaction disorder: Disorder characterized by a reduced ability to function and adapt in response to a stressful life event. The disorder begins shortly after the event, and normal functioning is expected to return when the particular stressor is removed.

administration: Management of institutional activities.

Administration on Aging: U. S. federal agency designated to carry out the provisions of the Older Americans Act of 1965.

administrative controls: Decisions made by management intended to reduce the duration, frequency, and severity of exposure to existing workplace hazards. It leaves the hazards at the workplace but attempts to diminish the effects on the worker (eg, job rotation or job enlargement).

adrenal gland: A pair of endocrine organs lying immediately above the kidney, consisting of an inner medulla, which produces epinephrine and norepinephrine, and an outer cortex, which produces a variety of steroid hormones.

adrenocorticotrophic hormone (ACTH): A hormone released by the adenohypophysis that stimulates the adrenal cortex to secrete its entire spectrum of hormones.

advanced directives: Living wills and care instruction in which a competent adult expresses his or her wishes regarding medical management in the event of a serious illness.

adverse effects: Undesired consequences.

advocacy: Actively supporting a cause, an idea, or a policy (eg, speaking in favor); recommending accommodations under the Americans with Disabilities Act.

aerobe: A micro-organism that lives and grows in the presence of free oxygen.

aerobic activity/conditioning/exercise: Any physical exercise or activity that requires additional effort by the heart and lungs to meet the increased demand for oxygen by the skeletal muscles. The performance of therapeutic exercise and activities to increase endurance.

aerobic capacity: A measure of the ability to perform work or participate in activity over time using the body's oxygen uptake, delivery, and energy release mechanisms.

aerobic metabolism: Energy production utilizing oxygen.

aerobic power: Maximal oxygen consumption; the maximal volume of oxygen consumed per unit of time.

aerobic training/exercise: Exercise of sufficient intensity, duration, and frequency that improves the efficiency of oxygen consumption during activity or work. Endurance-type exercise that relies on oxidative metabolism as the major source of energy production.

aesthesiometer: Tool used to apply and test two-point discrimination stimuli.

affect: Emotion or feeling conveyed in a person's face or body; the subjective experiencing of a feeling or emotion. To influence or produce a change in.

affection: Disease.

affective disorder: Marked disturbances of mood; typically characterized by disproportionately elevated mood (ie, mania), extremely depressed mood (ie, depression), or swings between the two (ie, bipolar disorder/manic depressive disorder).

affective state: The emotional or mental state of an individual, which can range from unconscious to very agitated; sometimes referred to as *behavioral state*.

afferent: Conducting toward a structure.

afferent neuron: A nerve cell that sends nerve impulses from sensory receptors to the central nervous system.

afterbirth: Amniotic membranes and placenta expelled from the uterus during the third stage of labor.

afterpains: Contractions of the uterus after the fetus and placenta are delivered.

age-appropriate activities: Activities and materials that are consistent with those used by nondisabled age mates in the same culture.

ageism: Prejudice that one age is better than another.

age stratification model: Influential model in human development based on society's behavioral expectations, as expressed through age-specific statutes and roles to which societal participants are expected to conform.

agglutination: Act of blood cells clumping together.

agility: Ease of movement.

aging: Passage of years in a person's life; the process of growing older.

aging in place: Where older adults remain in their own homes, retirement housing, or other familiar surroundings as they grow old.

agnosia: Inability to comprehend sensory information due to central nervous system damage.

agonist: Muscle that is capable of providing the power so a bone can move.

agoraphobia: An abnormal fear of being in an open space.

agraphia: Inability to write caused by impairment of central nervous system processing (not by paralysis).

airplane splint: A shoulder splint that stabilizes and maintains the shoulder in approximately 90 degrees of horizontal abduction.

airway clearance techniques: A broad group of activities used to manage or prevent consequences of acute and chronic lung diseases and impairment, including those associated with surgery.

akathisia: Motor restlessness.

alcoholism: A chronic disease characterized by an uncontrollable urge to consume alcoholic beverages excessively to the point that it interferes with normal life activities.

aldosterone: A steroid hormone produced by the adrenal cortex glands. It is the chief regulator of sodium, potassium, and chloride metabolism, thus controlling the body's water and electrolyte balances.

alexia: Condition of being unable to read.

allantois: The diverticulum from the hindgut of the embryo that appears around the 16th day of development, forming part of the umbilical cord and placenta.

allele: Alternative form of a gene coded for a particular trait.

allied health: Broad field of study encompassing diverse health professionals with special training in such fields as occupational therapy, physical therapy, respiratory therapy, speech pathology, and health information services, as well as laboratory, radiology, and dietetic services. It does not include physicians, nurses, dentists, or podiatrists.

alopecia: Absence or loss of hair; baldness.

alpha error (or Type 1 error): When the null hypothesis is rejected, the probability of being wrong or the probability of rejecting it when it should have been accepted.

alpha-fetoprotein: Nonhormonal plasma constituent in amniotic fluid that is used as a determinant of neural tube defects.

alternative delivery system (ADS): Generic term for new systems (eg, managed care) seen as alternatives to traditional fee-for-service indemnity health insurance plans.

alternative therapies: Interventions to provide holistic approaches to the management of diseases and illnesses, such as acupuncture, massage, or nutrition.

altruism: Unselfish concern for the welfare of others.

alveolar: A general term used in anatomical nomenclature to designate a small sac-like dilatation, such as the sockets in the mandible and maxilla in which the roots of the teeth are held or the small outpocketings of the alveolar sacs in the lungs, through whose walls gaseous exchange takes place.

amaurosis fugax: Temporary, partial, or total blindness often resulting from transient occlusion of the retinal arteries. May be a symptom of impending cerebrovascular accident.

ambulate: To walk from place to place.

ambulatory care: Care delivered on an outpatient basis.

amenorrhea: Absence of monthly menstruation.

American Journal of Physical Therapy: The official journal of the American Physical Therapy Association. It provides literature on physical therapy research, education, and practice.

American National Standards Institute (ANSI): Clearinghouse and coordinating body for voluntary standards activity on the national level.

American Physical Therapy Association (APTA): The American professional society that represents the field of physical therapy and those who practice within that field. It monitors the quality of physical therapy services through determining guidelines for physical therapy training programs; setting standards for practice; and supporting regulations, legislation, and research. It also publishes several publications, such as the *American Journal of Physical Therapy*, *PT Magazine*, and *PT Bulletin*.

American Sign Language (ASL): Nonverbal method of communication using the hands and fingers to represent letters, numbers, and concepts.

American Society of Hand Therapists (ASHT): Established in 1978, the ASHT is concerned with hand rehabilitation education and research among practitioners in this area. The *Journal of Hand Therapy* is a publication resulting from the work of the ASHT.

amnesia: Dissociative disorder characterized by memory loss during a certain time period or of personal identity.

amniocentesis: A low-risk prenatal diagnostic procedure of collecting amniotic fluid and fetal cells for examination through the use of a needle inserted into the abdominal wall and uterus to determine the fetal age and genetic characteristics after 4 months of gestation.

amnion: Innermost membrane enclosing the developing fetus and the fluid in which the fetus is bathed (ie, amniotic fluid).

amplitude: The maximal height of a waveform, either from the baseline or peak to peak.

amputation: Partial or complete removal of a limb; may be congenital or acquired (traumatic or surgical).

anaerobe: A micro-organism that grows in the absence of free oxygen.

anaerobic exercise/activity: Exercise or activity without oxygen; oxygen intake cannot keep up with level of exercise/activity, so oxygen debt occurs.

anakusis: Total hearing loss; deafness.

analgesia: Absence of pain sensitivity; patient may experience stimulus but it is not noxious.

analgesic: Drug for reducing pain. Some mild analgesics are nonsteroidal anti-inflammatory drugs (eg, ibuprofen), and some analgesics are narcotics (eg, morphine).

analog: Continuous information system (eg, a clock with dials that move continuously on a continuum, as opposed to a digital clock).

analogue: Contrived situation created in order to elicit specific client behaviors and allow for their observation. Representing numerical values by physical quantities so as to allow the manipulation of numerical data over a continuous range of values.

analysis: An examination of the nature of something for the purpose of prediction or comparison.

analysis of covariance (ANCOVA): Controlling the effects of any variable(s) known to correlate with the dependent variable.

analysis of variance (or F ratio or ANOVA): Establishing whether or not a significant difference exists among the means of samples.

anaphylactic shock: Condition in which the flow of blood throughout the body becomes suddenly inadequate due to dilation of the blood vessels as a result of allergic reaction.

anaplasia: Reverting of a specialized cell to its primitive or embryonic state. Synonym: dedifferentiation.

anastomosis: Surgical formation of a passage between two open vessels.

anatomical position: Standing erect, arms at the sides, with palms facing forward.

anatomy: Area of study concerned with the internal and external structures of the body and how these structures interrelate.

ANCOVA (analysis of covariance): Abbreviation for the method of controlling the effects of any variable(s) known to correlate with the dependent variable.

andragogy: Art and science of helping adults learn.

androgens: Substances that produce or stimulate the development of male characteristics.

anemia: A condition in which there is a reduction of the number or volume of red blood corpuscles or the total amount of hemoglobin in the bloodstream, resulting in paleness and generalized weakness.

anencephaly: Birth defect that characteristically leaves the child with little or no brain mass.

anesthesia: Absence of sensibility to stimuli with or without loss of consciousness.

anesthetic: Drug that reduces or eliminates sensation. It can affect the whole body (eg, nitrous oxide, a general anesthetic) or a particular part of the body (eg, Xylocaine, a local anesthetic).

aneurysm: A sac formed by local enlargement of a weakened wall of an artery, a vein, or the heart and caused by disease, anatomical anomaly, or injury.

angina pectoris: Chest pain due to insufficient flow of blood to the heart muscle.

angiography: Injection of a radioactive material so that the blood vessels can be visualized.

angioneurotic edema: Edema of an extremity due to any neurosis affecting primarily the blood vessels resulting from a disorder of the vasomotor system, such as angiospasm, angioparesis, or angioparalysis.

anhedonia: Inability to enjoy what is ordinarily pleasurable.

ankle-arm index: A numerical comparison of the systolic blood pressures in the arm and ankle obtained by dividing the ankle pressure by the arm pressure. Values below 1.0 indicate varying degrees of ischemia.

ankle/foot orthosis (AFO): An external device that controls the foot and ankle and can facilitate knee positioning and muscle response.

ankylosis: Condition of the joints in which they become stiffened and nonfunctional. Abnormal immobility and consolidation of a joint.

anomaly: Pronounced departure from the norm.

anomia: Loss of ability to name objects or to recognize or recall names; can be receptive or expressive.

anosognosia: Inability to perceive a deficit, especially paralysis on one side of the body, possibly caused by a lesion in the parietal lobe of the brain.

ANOVA (analysis of variance): Abbreviation for the statistical method used in research to compare sample populations.

anoxemia: Absence or deficiency of oxygen in the blood.

anoxia/anoxic: Absence or deficiency of oxygen in the tissues. Can cause tissue death; synonymous with hypoxia.

antagonist: Muscle that resists the action of a prime mover (agonist).

antalgic: A compensatory behavior attempting to avoid or lessen pain, usually applied to gait or movement.

antenatal: During pregnancy.

antepartum: The period from conception to birth (also called *prenatal*).

anterior: Toward the front of the body.

anterior fontanel: Region of the head that is found as a membrane-covered portion on the top of the head, generally closing by the time a child reaches 18 months. Synonym: the soft spot.

anterior horn cell: Motor neuron located anteriorly that is similar in shape to a pointed projection, such as the paired processes on the head of various animals.

anteversion: Turning forward or inclining forward as a whole without bending; usually applied to the positional relationship between the head of the femur and its shaft.

anthropometric: Human body measurements, such as height, weight, girth, and body fat composition.

antibacterial: An agent that inhibits the growth of bacteria.

antibiotic: Chemical substance that has the ability to inhibit or kill foreign organisms in the body.

antibody: A protein belonging to a class of proteins called *immunoglobulins*. A molecule produced by the immune system of the body in response to an antigen and which has the particular property of combining specifically with the antigen that induced its formation. Antibodies are produced by plasma cells to counteract specific antigens (infectious agents like viruses, bacteria, etc). The antibodies combine with the antigen they are created to fight, often causing the death of that infectious agent.

anticoagulant: A substance that prevents or retards blood clotting.

antigen: A substance foreign to the body. An antigen stimulates the formation of antibodies to combat its presence.

anti-inflammatory: Counteracting or suppressing inflammation.

antimicrobial: Designed to destroy or inhibit the growth of bacterial, fungal, or viral organisms.

antineoplastic agents: Substances, procedures, or measures used in treating cancer, administered with the purpose of inhibiting the production of malignant cells.

antioxidant: A substance that slows the oxidation of hydrocarbon, oils, fats, etc and helps to check deterioration of tissues.

antisepsis: The prevention of sepsis by the inhibition or destruction of the causative organism.

antisocial personality disorder: Personality disorder resulting in a chronic pattern of disregard for socially acceptable behavior, impulsiveness, irresponsibility, and lack of remorseful feelings. Synonyms: sociopathy, psychopathy, or antisocial reaction.

antral: Relating to a body cavity.

anuria: Absence of urine excretion.

anxiety: Characterized by an overwhelming sense of apprehension; the expectation that something bad is happening or will happen; class of mental disorders characterized by chronic and debilitating anxiety (eg, generalized anxiety disorder, panic disorder, phobias, and post-traumatic stress disorder).

anxiolytic: Anxiety-reducing drugs; formerly called *tranquilizers*.

aortic aneurysm: Aneurysm of the aorta.

aortic heart disease: A disease affecting the main artery of the body, carrying blood from the left ventricle of the heart to the main arteries of the body.

aphakia: Absence of the crystalline lens of the eye.

aphasia: Absence of cognitive language processing ability that results in deficits in speech, writing, or sign communication. It can be receptive, expressive, or both.

aphonia: Inability to produce speech sounds from the larynx.

apnea: Temporary cessation of breathing.

aponeurosis: Fibrous or membranous tissue that connects a muscle to the part that the muscle moves.

appendicular skeleton: Bones forming the limbs, pectoral girdle, and pelvic girdle of the body.

apprenticeship: Learning process in which novices advance their skills and understanding through active participation with a more skilled person.

apraxia: Inability to motor plan, execute purposeful movement, manipulate objects, or use objects appropriately.

apraxia of speech: Disruption of speech motor planning.

aquatherapy: The use of water as a therapeutic measure (eg, hydrotherapy, whirlpools, pools for exercise).

arc: Any line wholly on a surface between two chosen points other than a chord.

architectural barrier: Structural impediment to the approach, mobility, and functional use of an interior or exterior environment.

areola: Darkened area around the nipple.

arm sling: Orthosis used to provide support to the proximal upper extremity.

arousal: Internal state of the individual characterized by increased responsiveness to environmental stimuli.

arrhythmia: Variation from the normal rhythm, especially of the heartbeat.

arterial: Pertaining to one or more arteries; vessels that carry oxygenated blood to the tissue.

arterial compliance: The property of healthy arterial walls to expand and contract with blood flow pulsations.

arterial embolism/thrombosis: The obstruction of an arterial blood vessel by an embolus too large to pass through it or a thrombosis caused by the coagulation and fibrosis of blood at a particular site.

arterial insufficiency: Inadequate blood supply in the arterial system usually caused by stenosis or occlusion proximal to the inadequately supplied area.

arterioles: The smallest arterial vessels (0.2 mm diameter) resulting from repeated branching of the arteries. They are composed of smooth muscle only and conduct blood from the arteries to the capillaries.

arteriosclerosis: Thickening, hardening, and a loss of elasticity of the walls of the arteries.

arteriovenous: Designating arteries or veins or arterioles and venules.

arteriovenous fistula: An abnormal passage between the artery and the vein caused by an abscess at the junction of these vessels.

arteriovenous oxygen difference: The difference between the oxygen content of blood in the arterial system and the amount in the mixed venous blood.

arteritis: Inflammation of an artery.

arthritis: Inflammation of the joints that may be chronic or acute.

arthro-: Pertaining to joints.

arthroclasia: Artificial breaking of an ankylosed joint to provide movement.

arthrography: Injection of dye or air into a joint cavity to image the contours of the joint.

arthrokinematic: Describing the motion of a joint without regard to the forces producing that motion or resulting from it; describing the structure and shape of joint surfaces. Pertaining to the more intimate mechanisms of joints, regarding the movement of one articular surface upon another (ie, roll, glide).

arthrokinesiology: The study of the structure and function of skeletal joints.

arthropathy: Disease of a joint.

arthroplasty: Surgical replacement; formation or reformation of a joint; surgical reconstruction of a joint.

arthroscopy: Procedure in which visual equipment can be inserted into a joint so that its internal parts can be viewed.

articular cartilage: The tough, elastic tissue that separates the bones in a joint.

articulation: The joining or juncture between two or more bones. The process of moving a joint through all or part of its range of motion.

artifact: An artificial or extraneous feature introduced into an observation that may simulate a relevant feature of that observation.

asbestosis: Lung disease caused by inhaling particles of asbestos.

ASCII (American Standard Code for Information Interchange): Standardized coding scheme that uses numeric values to represent letters, numbers, symbols, etc. ASCII is widely used in coding information for computers (eg, the letter A is 65 in ASCII).

ascites: Accumulation of fluid in the abdomen.

aseptic: Free from infection or septic material; sterile.

aspermia: Lack of or failure to ejaculate semen.

asphyxia: Condition of insufficient oxygen.

aspirate: To inhale vomitus, mucus, or food into the respiratory tract.

aspiration: Inhaling fluids or solid substances into the lungs.

assessment: Process by which data are gathered, hypotheses formulated, and decisions made for further action; a subsection of the problem-oriented medical record. The measurement or quantification of a variable or the placement of a value on something (not to be confused with examination or evaluation).

assimilation: Expansion of data within a given category or subcategory of a schema by incorporation of new information within the existing representational structure without requiring any reorganization or modification of prior knowledge.

assisted-living facility: Medium- to large-sized facilities that offer housing, meals, and personal care, plus extras such as housekeeping, transportation, and recreation. Small-sized facilities are known as *board and care homes*.

assistive devices: A variety of implements or equipment used to aid patients/clients in performing tasks or movements. Assistive devices include crutches, canes, walkers, wheelchairs, power devices, long-handled reachers, and static and dynamic splints.

assistive living setting: A type of living situation in which persons live in community housing with attendant care provided for those parts of the day or those activities where assistance is required.

assistive technology: Any item, piece of equipment, or product system, whether acquired commercially off the shelf, modified, or customized, that is used to increase, maintain, or improve functional capabilities of individuals with disabilities.

assistive technology service: Any service that assists an individual with a disability in the selection, acquisition, or use of an assistive technology device.

associated reactions: Involuntary movements or reflexive increase of tone of the affected side of a person with hemiplegia or other central nervous system involvement.

association learning: Form of learning in which particular items or ideas are connected.

associative intrusions: Inappropriate associations that interfere with normal thought processes.

associative network theory of memory: Theory that related memories are stored in networks and that the stimulation of a network will result in the recall of the memories in that network.

associative play: Play in which each child is participating in a separate activity but with the cooperation and assistance of the others.

assumption: Proposition or supposition; a statement that links or relates two or more concepts to one another.

astereognosis: Inability to discriminate the shape, texture, weight, and size of objects.

asthenia: Chronic lack of energy and strength.

asthma: Respiratory disease in which the muscles of the bronchial tubes tighten and give off excessive secretions. This combination causes obstruction of the airway and results in wheezing; characterized by recurring episodes.

asymmetrical: Lack of symmetry.

asymptomatic: Showing or causing no symptoms.

ataxia: Poor balance and awkward movement.

atelectasis: Collapse or airless condition of the lung.

atheroma: A deposit of fatty (or other) substances in the inner lining of the artery wall.

atherosclerosis: Deposits of fatty substance in arteries, veins, and the lymphatic system.

athetosis: Type of cerebral palsy that involves involuntary purposeless movements that fall into one of two classes: nontension involves contorted movements and tension involves blocked movements and flailing.

atonic: Absence of muscle tone.

atopic dermatitis: A clinical hypersensitivity of the skin.

atrioventricular block: Disruption in the flow of electrical impulse through the atrium wall of the heart leading to arrhythmias, bradycardia, or complete cardiac arrest.

atrium: One of the two upper chambers of the heart. The right atrium receives unoxygenated venous blood from the body, while the left receives oxygenated blood from the lungs.

atrophy: The decrease in size of a normally developed organ or tissue due to lack of use or deficient nutrition.

atropine: Drug that inhibits actions of the autonomic nervous system; relaxes smooth muscle; treats biliary and renal colic; and reduces secretions of the bronchial tubes, salivary glands, stomach, and intestines.

attachment: Deep affective bond between individuals or a feeling that binds one to a thing, cause, ideal, etc.

attendant care: Services that provide individuals with nonmedical, personal health, and hygiene care, such as preparing meals, bathing, going to the bathroom, getting in and out of bed, and walking.

attention: Ability to focus on a specific stimulus without distraction.

attention span: Focusing on a task over time. Length of time an individual is able to focus or concentrate on a task or thought.

auditory: Pertaining to the sense or organs of hearing.

auditory defensiveness: Oversensitivity to certain sounds (eg, vacuum cleaners, fire alarms).

augmentation: The normal increase in the Doppler sound of venous flow upon compression distal to the Doppler probe or release of compression proximal to the probe. Augmentation resulting from the release of distal compression or the application of proximal compression indicates valvular incompetence.

augmentative communication: Method or device that increases a person's ability to communicate (eg, nonelectronic devices, such as communication boards, or electronic devices, such as portable communication systems, that allow the user to speak and print text).

auscultation: Process of listening for sounds within the body as a method of diagnosis. A stethoscope or other instruments may be used.

autocrine: Method of intracellular hormonal communication.

autocosmic play: Idea developed by Erikson in which a child plays with his or her own body during the first year of life.

autogeneic drainage: Airway clearance through the patient's/client's own efforts (eg, coughing).

autogeneic facilitation: Ability to stimulate one's own muscle to contract.

autogeneic inhibition: Ability to inhibit action in one's own muscle.

autoimmunity: Condition in which the body has developed a sensitivity to some of its own tissues.

autolysis: Disintegration or liquefaction of tissue or cells by the body's own mechanisms.

automatic processes: Processes that occur without much attentional effort.

automatization: When a learned motor skill is done with little conscious thought.

autonomic nervous system: Part of the nervous system concerned with the control of involuntary bodily functions.

autonomic postural responses: Refers to a set of muscle responses characterized by latencies of approximately 100 to 150 ms, which are longer than monosynaptic reflexes but shorter than voluntary muscle responses. They occur in response to balance disturbance and are important in postural control.

autonomy: State of independence and self-control.

autosomal dominant: Genetic trait carried on the autosome. When one of a pair of chromosomes contains the abnormal gene, a disorder appears. It is passed on from the affected parent to half of the children.

autosomal recessive: Genetic trait carried on the autosome. Both asymptomatic parents must carry the trait for a disorder to appear.

autosome: Any chromosome other than the X and Y (sex) chromosomes.

avocational: Leisure pursuits.

avoidance: Psychological coping strategy in which the source of stress is ignored or avoided.

avoidance learning: Form of learning through stimuli avoidance and cause and effect (eg, negative reinforcement).

avolition: Absence of interest or will to undertake activities.

axial skeleton: Bones forming the longitudinal axis of the body; consists of the skull, vertebral column, thorax, and sternum.

axilla: Area located dorsal to the humerus and glenohumeral joint. It is the site where the cords of the brachial plexus pass through in order to innervate the muscles of the arm, superficial back, and superficial thoracic region.

axiology: Branch of philosophy concerned with the study of values related to ethics, aesthetics, or religion.

axis: A line, real or imaginary, running through the center of the body; the line about which a part revolves.

axon: Long part of a nerve cell that sends information away from the cell, across a synapse, to the dendrites of another cell.

axonotmesis: Interruption of the axon with subsequent wallerian degeneration; connective tissues of the nerve, including the Schwann cell basement membrane, remain intact.

azotemia: Presence of nitrogenous bodies, especially urea, in the blood.

B cell: A type of lymphocyte capable of producing an antibody. The B cell is a white cell that is able to detect the presence of foreign agents. Once exposed to an antigen on the agent, it differentiates into plasma cells to produce antibodies.

baby boom generation: People born between the years of 1946 and 1964.

back disorder/injury: Injury to or disease of the lower lumbar, lumbosacral, or sacroiliac region of the back.

back labor: Pain arising from pressure on the lumbar and sacral nerve roots; experienced in some women as the baby's head descends in the birth canal.

back school: A structured educational program about low back problems, usually offered to a group of patients/clients.

bacterial diseases: Diseases resulting from infection by bacteria.

bacterial pneumonia: Inflammation caused by a bacterial infection in the lungs.

bactericidal: Able to kill bacteria. An agent that destroys bacteria.

bacteriostatic: An agent that is capable of inhibiting the growth or multiplication of bacteria.

balance: The ability to maintain a functional posture through motor actions that distribute weight evenly around the body's center of gravity, both statically (eg, while standing) and dynamically (eg, while walking).

balance billing: Procedure for billing the patient for the balance of amounts not covered by insurance. This can be done only with certain insurers for which the provider does not accept assignment.

barbiturate: Sedative that can cause both physiological and psychological dependence. Trade/generic names: Seconal/secobarbital, Nembutal/pentobarbital.

barriers: The physical impediments that keep patients/clients from functioning optimally in their surroundings, including safety hazards (eg, throw rugs, slippery surfaces), access problems (eg, narrow doors, high steps), and home or office design difficulties (eg, excessive distance to negotiate, multistory environment). The point of restriction of a given movement.

basal ganglia: A collection of nuclei at the base of the cortex, including the caudate nucleus, putamen, globus pallidus and functionally including the substantia nigra and subthalamic nucleus.

baseline: The known value or quantity representing the normal background level against which a response to intervention can be measured.

base-of-support: The body surfaces, such as the plantar surface of the feet, around which the center of gravity is maintained via postural responses.

basic ADL: Activities of daily living tasks that pertain to self-care, mobility, and communication.

battery: Assessment approach or instrument with several parts.

behavioral modification: The process of reinforcing desirable responses; food, praise, and tokens may be used.

behavioral setting: Milieu in which the specific environment dictates the kinds of behaviors that occur there, independent of the particular individuals who inhabit the setting at the moment.

behavioral theory: Developmental theory that suggests that learning is a relationship between certain stimuli and their subsequent responses. This learning theory sees the individual as a result of present and past environments. Behaviorists believe that learning occurs through the processes of classical or operant conditioning.

behaviorism: Theory of behavior and intervention that holds that behavior is learned, that behaviors that are reinforced tend to recur, and those that are not reinforced tend to disappear.

belly: Midsection of a muscle (usually produces a bulge) between its two ends.

benchmark: Standard against which something else is judged.

beneficence: The quality of being kind or doing good; a charitable act or generous gift. Doing good resulting in benefit to others.

benefit: Sum of money that an insurance policy pays for covered services under the terms of the policy.

benefit period: Time during which an insurance policy provides payments for covered benefits.

bereavement: Normal grief or depression commonly associated with the death of a loved one.

beta error (or Type 2 error): When the null hypothesis is accepted, the probability of being wrong or the probability of accepting it when it should have been rejected.

bifurcation: The site of division into two branches, as in an artery. Often, the area of atherosclerotic deposits.

bilateral: Pertaining to or affecting both sides of the body.

bilateral integration: The ability to perform purposeful movement that requires interaction between both sides of the body in a smooth and refined manner.

bilingual: A person who speaks two languages fluently.

bill mark-up: Process in which a legislative committee in the United States amends a bill by deleting, modifying, or adding to the bill according to the wishes of lobbyists, the public, or its own inclinations.

binocular: Pertaining to both eyes.

bioethics: Application of ethics to health care.

biofeedback: A training technique that enables an individual to gain some element of voluntary control over muscular or autonomic nervous system functions using a device that produces auditory or visual stimuli.

biological age: Definition of age that focuses on the functional age of biological and physiological processes rather than on calendar time.

biomechanical approach: This approach concerns cardiopulmonary, integumentary, musculoskeletal, and nervous (except brain) system impairments. Increased endurance, joint range of motion, strength, and reduced edema are the goals of the biomechanical approach.

biomechanics: Study of anatomy, physiology, and physics as applied to the human body.

biopsychological assessment: Evaluation used to determine how the central nervous system influences behavior and to understand the relationship between physical state and thoughts, emotions, and behavior.

biorhythm: Biological or cyclical occurrence or phenomenon (eg, sleep cycle, menstrual cycle, or respiratory cycle).

bipolar disorder: Disorder characterized by an unstable self-image, abrupt mood swings, and poor impulse control.

birth asphyxia: Stopping of the pulse and loss of consciousness as a result of too little oxygen and too much carbon dioxide in the blood, leading to suffocation during the birthing process.

birth trauma: Injury during delivery of an infant.

bite reflex: Swift biting pathological reflex action produced by oral stimulation.

blanching: Becoming white with pressure; maximum pallor.

blastema: Immature substance from which cells and tissues are created.

blepharorrhaphy: Suturing of an eyelid.

blister: Epidermal loss considered second degree due to a burn.

blood borne pathogen: Infectious disease spread by contact with blood (eg, AIDS, hepatitis B).

blood pressure (BP): Pressure of the blood against the walls of the blood vessels. Normal in young adults is 120 mmHg during systole and 70 mmHg during diastole.

Blue Cross/Blue Shield Association (BC/BS): Nationwide federation of local, nonprofit insurance organizations that contracts with hospitals and other health care providers to make payments for health care services to their subscribers.

boarding homes or board and care homes: Smaller sized housing for older adults offering supervised housing, meals, and personal care, plus housekeeping, transportation, and recreational activities.

body image: Subjective picture people have of their physical appearance.

body mechanics: The interrelationships of the muscles and joints as they maintain or adjust posture in response to environmental forces.

body righting reflex: Neuromuscular response aimed at restoring the body to its normal upright position when it is displaced.

body scheme: The perception of one's physical self through proprioceptive and interoceptive sensations.

bone graft: Transplantation of bone.

bone marrow: Tissue filling the porous medullary cavity of the diaphysis of bones.

bone scan: Radiographic scan that evaluates skeletal involvement related to connective tissue disease.

borborygmus: Rumbling and gurgling sound made by the movement of gas in the intestines.

borderline personality: Disorder characterized by abrupt shifts in mood, lack of coherent sense of self, and unpredictable, impulsive behavior.

botulism: Fatal toxemia caused by ingestion of botulinum neurotoxin, which causes muscle weakness and paralysis.

boutonnière deformity: Abnormality that results from interruption of the ulnar and medial nerves at the wrist; it causes metacarpal phalangeal joint hyperextension and interphalangeal joint flexion.

bowstringing: Spanning the shortest distance between two joints.

brachial plexus: Network of nerves that originates as roots C5, C6, C7, C8, and T1 and terminates as nerves that innervate the upper extremity.

bradycardia: Slowness of heartbeat (eg, less than 60 beats/minute).

bradykinesia: Slowness of body movement and speech.

Braille: Standardized system for communicating in writing with persons who are blind. Grade II Braille is standard literary Braille.

brain death: Irreversible destruction of the cortex and brainstem. Ways to determine are lack of responsiveness, apnea, absence of reflexes, dilation of pupils, flatline electroencephalogram, and absence of cerebral blood flow for a given period of time.

brain lateralization: Refers to the differentiation of function with the brain's two hemispheres. The left hemisphere controls the right side of the body, as well as spoken and written language, numerical and scientific skills, and reasoning. The right hemisphere controls the left side of the body and influences musical and artistic awareness, space and pattern perception, insight, imagination, and generating mental images to compare spatial relationships.

brain scan: Nuclear medicine diagnostic procedure used to detect tumors, cerebrovascular accidents, or other lesions in the brain.

brain tumor: Abnormal growth of cells within the cranium that may cause headaches, altered consciousness, seizures, vomiting, visual problems, cranial nerve abnormalities, personality changes, dementia, and sensory and motor deficits.

Braxton Hicks contractions: Intermittent contractions of the uterus during pregnancy.

break test: Form of muscle testing in which the therapist produces force against a muscle that is isometrically contracted at its greatest mechanical advantage. This test is used to determine the strength of that muscle.

breech: Describes the position of the fetus in which anything but the head is presented first.

bronchiectasis: A chronic dilatation of the bronchi or bronchioles marked by fetid breath and paroxysmal coughing, with expectoration of mucopurulent matter.

bronchiolectasis: Dilation of the bronchioles.

bronchopneumonia: Inflammation of the bronchi accompanied by inflamed patches in the nearby lobules of the lungs. Also termed *bronchiolitis*.

bronchopulmonary dysplasia: A disordered growth or faulty development of bronchial and lung tissue.

bruit: Soft blowing sound heard upon auscultation. Caused by turbulence as a result of deposits in the arterial lumen that alter normal hemodynamics.

bruxism: Grinding of teeth.

budget neutrality: Provision of the Omnibus Budget Reconciliation Act of 1989, the legislation creating the Medicare Resource-Based Relative Value System payment system, that requires that expenditures resulting from changes in medical practice or payment methodology neither increase nor decrease from what they would have been under a continuation of the customary, prevailing, and reasonable charge system.

bullous dermatosis: A large blister or cutaneous vesicle filled with serous fluid.

bunion: A swelling of the bursa mucosa of the first metatarsal head with callusing of the overlying skin and lateral migration of the great toe.

burn: A lesion caused by the contact of heat.

burnout: State of mental fatigue that results in the inability to generate energy from one's occupational performance areas.

bursa: Sac that contains synovial fluid. Bursae are located in superficial fascia, in areas where movement takes place and aid in decreasing friction.

bursectomy: Excision of bursae.

bursitis: Inflammation of a bursa resulting from injury, infection, or rheumatoid synovitis. It produces pain and tenderness and may restrict movement at a nearby joint.

bypass: A surgically created detour between two points in a physiologic pathway, often to circumvent obstructions. Similar to a shunt.

C **cachectic:** Marked state of poor health and malnutrition secondary to disease, treatment, or poor nutrient intake.

calcification: The deposition of calcium salts in body tissues. A calcified substance or structure.

calibration: Determination of what the output of a measuring instrument means and then compared with known values.

callosities: Hardened, thickened places on the skin.

candidiasis: Infection by fungi of the genus candida, most commonly involving the skin, oral mucosa, respiratory tract, and vagina.

cane: Stick or short staff used to assist one during walking; it can have a narrow or broad base depending on the amount of support needed.

cannulation: The process of inserting an artificial tube into a part of the body, such as an artery.

capacitance: Elastic capacity of vessels and organs of the body.

capacity: One's best, includes present abilities as well as the potential to develop new abilities.

capillaries: Extremely narrow vessels forming a network between the arterioles and the veins. The walls are composed of a single layer of cells through which oxygen and nutritive materials pass out to the tissues, and carbon dioxide and waste products are admitted from the tissues into the blood stream (osmosis).

capitation: Method of payment for health services in which a provider receives a fixed, prepaid, per capita amount for each person enrolled in the health plan for whom the provider has responsibility for all necessary health care services.

capsular pattern: A proportional limitation of motion, characteristic for each joint, secondary to a lesion of the synovial membrane and/or the fibrous capsule.

capsular restriction: Limitation of mobility and range due to tightness or rigidity of the joint capsule.

carboxyhemoglobin: A compound formed from hemoglobin on exposure to carbon monoxide, with formation of a covalent bond with oxygen and without change of the charge of the ferrous state.

carbuncle: A painful bacterial infection deep beneath the skin having a network of pus-filled boils.

carcinogen: Any substance or agent that produces or increases the incidence of cancer.

carcinoma: Any of the several kinds of cancerous growths deriving from epithelial cells.

cardiac arrest: Cessation of effective heart action.

cardiac arrhythmia: Irregularity in the rhythm of the heartbeat.

cardiac contusion: Bruising of the heart due to direct trauma or injury to the myocardium.

cardiac output: Volume of blood pumped from the heart per unit of time. Cardiac output is the product of heart rate and stroke volume.

cardiac tamponade: Acute compression of the heart due to effusion of the fluid into the pericardium or the collection of blood in the pericardium from rupture of the heart or a coronary vessel.

cardiomyopathy: A subacute or chronic disorder of heart muscle of unknown or obscure etiology, often with associated endocardial, and sometimes with pericardial involvement, but not atherosclerotic in origin.

cardiopulmonary: Pertaining to the heart and lungs.

cardiopulmonary resuscitation (CPR): Procedure instituted immediately upon cardiac arrest that seeks to restore heart and lung function. These measures may include defibrillation, external cardiac compression, and mouth-to-mouth resuscitation.

cardiorrhaphy: Suture of the heart muscle.

cardiotonic: Drug that promotes the force and efficiency of the heart.

cardiovascular (CV): Pertaining to heart and blood vessels.

cardiovascular insufficiency: Inability of the cardiovascular system to perform at a level necessary for basic homeostasis of the body.

cardiovascular pump: Structures responsible for maintaining cardiac output, including the cardiac muscle, valves, arterial smooth muscle, and venous smooth muscle.

cardiovascular pump dysfunction: Abnormalities of the cardiac muscles, valves, conduction, or circulation that interrupt or interfere with cardiac output or circulation.

cardioversion: The use of electrical current to convert irregular rhythms or no rhythms to an active, regular, rhythmical heartbeat.

caregiver: One who provides care and support to a person.

carotid body: A small oval mass of cells and nerve endings located in the carotid sinus. These cells respond to chemical changes in the blood by altering the rate of respiration and other bodily changes.

carotid endarterectomy: Excision of the thickened, atheromatous tunica intima of the carotid artery.

carotid sinus: A slight dilatation at the point of carotid bifurcation. This sinus contains cells and nerve endings that respond to a change in blood pressure by altering heart rate.

carpals: Bones of the wrist; there are eight carpal bones in each wrist.

carrier: Private contractor to Health Care Financing Administration that administers claims processing and payment for Medicare B services (eg, Medicare).

cascade effect: Ability of the blood to clot via multiple factors.

cascade system: Theoretical prototype used as a conceptual framework for providing educational services for children with disabilities. Children are placed into the class that best fits their needs and is as close as possible to an everyday classroom.

case management: The use of a legally mandated case manager to oversee the coordination of services for a client. This manager, whose roles may include helper, teacher, planner, and advocate, assists in facilitating the needs of a client and his or her family.

case manager: Individual who assumes responsibility for coordination and follow-up on a given client case.

cataplexy: Sudden episode of loss of muscle function.

cataract: Abnormal progressive condition of the lens of the eye characterized by loss of transparency.

catastrophic health insurance: A type of health insurance that provides protection against the high cost of treating severe or lengthy illnesses or disabilities.

catatonia: Motor abnormality usually characterized by immobility or rigidity in which no organic base has been identified.

catecholamines: Active proteins epinephrine and norepinephrine.

categorization: The ability to classify; to describe by naming or labeling.

cathartic: Drug that relieves constipation and promotes defecation for diagnostic and operative procedures.

catheter: A thin tube of woven plastic or other material to which blood will not adhere. Inserted into a vein or artery. Also inserted into the urethra for collection of urine.

cauda equina: Spinal nerves descending in the spinal column below the level of L2.

caudal: Away from the head or toward the lower part of a structure.

causalgia: A condition of severe burning pain usually caused by a peripheral nerve injury.

cause and effect: When something occurs as a result of a motion or activity.

cauterization: Coagulation of blood by the application of chemicals or heat. Electrocautery is often used in surgery to reduce blood loss.

cell migration: Movement of cells in the wound repair process.

cellulitis: An inflammation of connective tissue, especially subcutaneous tissue. Inflammation of tissue around a lesion characterized by redness, swelling, and tenderness. Signifies infection.

center of gravity: Point at which the downward force created by mass and gravity is equivalent or balanced on either side of a fulcrum.

central nervous system (CNS): Consists of all the neurons of the brain, brainstem, and spinal cord.

central tendency: The typical, middle, or central scores in a distribution.

central venous pressure (CVP): The pressure representative of the filling pressure of the right ventricle, measured peripherally or centrally, corrected for hydrostatic pressure between the heart and point of measurement. Used to monitor fluid replacement.

centrifugal control: The brain's ability to regulate its own input.

centrifuge: Machine that separates components of blood for further testing through high-speed, rotational movement.

cephalad: Toward the head or upper portion of a part or structure. Synonym: superior.

cephalocaudal pattern: Sequence in which the greatest growth always occurs at the top (ie, the head) with physical growth in size, weight, and feature differentiation, gradually working its way down from top to bottom.

cephalopelvic disproportion: A condition in which the infant's head is unable to fit through the pelvic outlet and is an indication for cesarean delivery.

cerclage: A purse string ring suture placed around an incompetent cervix at the level of the os at 12 to 14 weeks of gestation to prevent premature delivery from an incompetent cervix.

cerebellar ataxia: Disorder of the brain that results in total or partial inability to coordinate voluntary bodily movements, as in walking.

cerebellar degeneration: Deterioration or loss of function or structure of brain tissue.

cerebral angioplasty: Injection of dye into the cerebral vascular system to observe its function.

cerebral atrophy: Deterioration of the cerebral tissue.

cerebral contusion: Bruising of brain tissue.

cerebral cyst: A sac-like structure filled with fluid or diseased matter in the tissue of the brain.

cerebral degeneration: Deterioration or loss of function or structure in the cerebral region of the brain.

cerebral embolism: The obstruction of a blood vessel by an embolus in the brain.

cerebral laceration: Torn or mangled cerebral tissue.

cerebrovascular: Pertaining to blood vessels and circulation in the brain.

cerebrovascular insufficiency: A lack of oxygen in the brain due to restriction or blockage of cerebral vessels.

certification: Process developed to ensure that each practitioner has the knowledge, skills, and attitudes required for competent professional practice. The process was developed to ensure that each practitioner has the knowledge, skills, and attitudes required for competent professional service in an area of specialization (eg, geriatrics, pediatrics, cardiopulmonary, orthopedics, neurology).

certified hand therapist (CHT): Individual who has been certified by the Hand Therapy Certification Commission to practice in the area of hand rehabilitation.

cervical spondylosis: Dissolution of the cervical vertebrae.

cervical vertebrae: Seven small neck bones between the skull and thoracic vertebrae; they support the head and allow movement.

cervicalgia: Any disorder causing pain in the cervical region.

cervix: The neck of the uterus, which leads into the vagina and thins and dilates during labor.

cesarean section: Delivery of a child by abdominal surgery.

CHAMPUS (Civilian Health and Medical Program of the Uniformed Services): Program paid for by the Department of Defense that pays for care that civilian health providers deliver to retired members and dependents of active and retired military personnel. This program does not charge premiums but has cost-sharing provisions.

characteristic behavior: Behavior typical of one's performance under everyday conditions.

checklist: Type of assessment approach in which a list of abilities, tasks, or interests is presented and those items meeting a designated criterion are checked. An interest checklist, for example, might list a number of activities in varied categories and ask the respondent to check those that are viewed as most interesting.

chemotherapy: The use of drugs or pharmacologic agents that have a specific and toxic effect on a disease-causing pathogen.

chest pain: Angina resulting from ischemia of the heart tissue.

chest physical therapy (physiotherapy): The use of vibration, shaking, or tapping techniques in various postural drainage positions to facilitate the expectoration of secretions in the lungs. Breathing techniques. *See* Appendix 20.

Cheyne-Stokes respiration: Breathing characterized by rhythmic waxing and waning and a fluctuation in the depth of breathing. May result in periods of apnea, especially seen in coma resulting from affection of the nervous system.

chickenpox: An acute, communicable disease caused by a virus and marked by slight fever and an eruption of macular vesicles that appear as a rash.

chilblains: A localized itching and painful erythema on the skin, which is a disease of the small blood vessels of the skin and may result in ulceration and necrosis.

child abuse: Intentional physical or psychological injury inflicted upon children by caretaker(s).

child development play programs: Hospital play programs for children who have a long-term hospital stay that include curricula ordinarily found in preschool or elementary school classrooms.

child neglect: Inadequate social, emotional, or physical nurturing of children.

chi square (χ^2): A statistical test used to establish whether or not frequency differences have occurred on the basis of chance.

chloasma-mask of pregnancy: Pigmentation appearing on the forehead and cheeks of some pregnant women.

chloroform: Colorless, heavy liquid formerly used as a general anesthetic.

cholecystectomy: Removal of the gallbladder.

cholecystitis: Inflammation of the gallbladder.

choledocholithotomy: Incision into the bile duct for removal of gallstones.

cholestasis: Suppression or arrest of bile flow.

chondrocyte: Cartilage cell embedded in lacunae within the matrix of cartilage connective tissue.

chondromalacia: Softening of the articular cartilages.

chord: The shortest line (path) between any two points on a surface.

chorea: Abrupt irregular movements of short duration involving the fingers, hands, arms, face, tongue, or head.

chorion: The outermost membrane that encases the fetus.

chorionic villus biopsy: Biopsy of the chorionic villus that determines chromosomal and metabolic abnormalities of the fetus from 9 to 11 weeks of gestation.

choreoathetosis: Type of cerebral palsy characterized by uncontrollable, jerky, irregular twisting movements of the arms and legs.

chromosome: Threadlike structure made up of genes; there are 46 chromosomes in the nucleus of each cell of a human.

chronic: Of long duration or frequent recurrence.

chronic bronchitis: Chronic inflammation of the bronchial tubes. A long-continued form, often with a more or less marked tendency to recurrence after stages of quiescence. Diagnosis is made when a chronic cough for up to 3 months in 2 consecutive years is present.

chronic disorders: Characterized by slow onset and long duration; rarely develop in early adulthood, increase in middle adulthood, and become common in late adulthood.

chronic respiratory disease: Lung disease resulting from constrictive or obstructive conditions of the airways.

chronological: An individual's age; definition of age that relies on the amount of calendar time that has passed since birth.

chronotropic: Affecting the time or rate, applied especially to nerves whose stimulation or agents whose administration affects the rate of contraction of the heart.

chylothorax: The presence of effused chyle (pockets of milky fluid) in the thoracic cavity.

CINAHL (Cumulative Index to Nursing and Allied Health Literature): Provides access to virtually all major English language nursing journal publications from the American Nursing Association and the National League for Nursing and primary journals from 13 allied health professions, including physical therapy.

cicatrix: Scar; the fibrous tissue replacing normal tissue destroyed by injury or disease.

circulation: Movement in a regular or circuitous course, as the movement of blood through the heart and blood vessels.

circumcision: The surgical removal of foreskin from the male penis.

circumduction: Movement in which the distal end of a bone moves in a circle while the proximal end remains stable, acting like a pivot.

circumferential-pressure splints: Splint in which there is no middle reciprocal force present; forces involved in this type of splint are equally distributed on the opposing surfaces involved.

claim: Request to an insurer for payment of benefits under an insurance policy.

claim adjudication: Determination of payment on a claim based on the type of contract, type of coverage, and present use.

class: Group containing members who share certain attributes, such as economic status, social identifications, or cultural identity.

class I lever system: Lever system in which the fulcrum is between the force and the resistance (eg, seesaw). The mechanical advantage can be less than, more than, or equal to one.

class II lever system: Lever system in which the resistance is between the fulcrum and the force. The mechanical advantage is always greater than one.

class III lever system: Lever system in which the force is between the fulcrum and the resistance. The mechanical advantage is always less than one.

classical conditioning: Method of eliciting specific responses through the use of stimuli that occur within a period of time that permits an association to be made between them. Also called *Pavlovian conditioning*, after the Russian scientist who made the technique famous.

classification: Arrangement according to some systematic division into classes or groups.

Classification of Jobs According to Worker Trait Factors (COJ): Lists the worker trait factors (eg, environmental conditions, aptitudes) for those job titles listed in the *Dictionary of Occupational Titles* (*DOT*). Used in conjunction with the *DOT*.

claudication: Lameness, limping; usually caused by poor circulation of blood to the leg muscles. Intermittent claudication is a complex of symptoms characterized by absence of pain or discomfort in a limb at rest or the commencement of pain, tension, and weakness with walking, which intensifies with continued walking and is relieved by rest. Usually seen in occlusive arterial diseases of the limbs.

clavicle: Bone that acts as a brace to hold the upper arm free from the thorax to allow free movement and serves as a place for muscle attachment. Synonym: collarbone.

cleansing breath: The breath taken at the beginning and end of a labor contraction to signal the support person to begin and end each breathing technique.

clients: Individuals who are not necessarily sick or injured but who can benefit from a physical therapist's consultation, professional advice, or services. Clients are also businesses, school systems, and others to whom physical therapists offer services.

client-centered rehabilitation: Therapeutic orientation in which the therapist guides and supports the client in problem solving and goal achievement.

climacteric: Major turning point in a female's life from ability to reproduce to a state of nonreproductivity. Transitional phase of life leading to menopause.

clinical guidelines: Systematically developed statements to assist practitioner and patient decisions about appropriate health care for specific clinical circumstances (eg, *Guide to Physical Therapy Practice*).

clinical reasoning: Thinking that directs and guides clinical decision making; reflective thinking.

clinical trial: Studies using human subjects.

clinical utility: Factors, such as clarity of instruction, cost, and facileness in using the assessment, that determine the amount of the assessment's utility.

clitoris: Small, round-shaped organ at the anterior part of the vulva.

clonus: Spasmodic alternation of contraction and relaxation of muscles.

closed-chain movements: The distal end of a kinematic chain is fixed or stabilized, and the proximal end (ie, origin) moves (eg, push-ups). Also called *closed kinetic chain* usually involving multiple joints.

closed question: Question that asks for a specific response (eg, one that may be answered with "yes" or "no").

closed reduction: Situation in which a broken bone can be manipulated into its natural position without surgery. External manipulation.

close-packed position: The point in a joint's range of motion at which maximal stability exists due to the stretch placed on periarticular structures. A position in which joint surfaces are fully congruent and/or the periarticular structures are maximally taut. Surface contact is maximal, and the surfaces are tightly compressed. The joint surfaces cannot be separated by distractive forces.

close supervision: Contact that is daily, direct, and given on the work premises.

clubbing: A proliferative change in the soft tissues about the terminal phalanges of the fingers or toes with no osseous changes.

clubfoot: Birth defect in which the soles of the feet face medially and the toes point inferiorly; occurs in about one out of 1,000 births and may be caused genetically or by the folding of the foot up against the chest during fetal development. Synonym: talipes.

clubhand: Medical condition seen in children in which the hand is radically displaced; the radius bone may be partially formed or may be absent.

cluster trait sample: Assesses a number of traits inherent in a job or various jobs, such as dexterity, strength, endurance, range of motion, and speed.

coagulation: The process of blood clot formation.

coagulopathy: A pathological defect in coagulation of the blood.

coarctation: Literally a pressing together. In practice, a narrowing of a vessel, usually congenital in origin.

coccyodynia: Painful coccyx usually resulting from an injury whereby sitting is difficult.

cocontraction: Simultaneous contraction of agonist and antagonistic muscle groups that act to stabilize joints.

codeine: Highly addictive narcotic derived from the opium family.

code of ethics: Statement that a certain group follows; sets the guidelines so that a high standard of behavior is maintained.

codependence: Condition in which substance dependence is subtly supported by the codependent who meets some need through the continued dependence of the individual.

coefficient of contingency (C): A statistical test used on nominal data to determine correlation.

coefficient of determination (r2): Determining what proportion of information about y is contained in x.

cognition: Mental processes that include thinking, perceiving, feeling, recognizing, remembering, problem solving, knowing, sensing, learning, judging, and metacognition. The act or process of knowing, including both awareness and judgment.

cognitive development: Process of thinking and knowing in the broadest sense, including perception, memory, and judgment.

cognitive disability: Physiologic or biochemical impairment in information-processing capacities that produces observable and measurable limitations in routine task behavior.

cognitive domains: Levels of performance abilities delineated in a hierarchy related to knowing and understanding.

cognitive learning: Form of learning that encompasses the forming of mental plans of events and objects.

cognitive stages in development: Jean Piaget's theory proposing that children's biological development is related to their environment, which enables children to progress through discreet, age-related stages in forming cognitions.

cognitive theory: Theory that focuses on intelligence, reasoning, learning, problem solving, memory, information processing, and thinking as the tools that individuals use to understand environmental stimuli.

cogwheel rigidity: During passive range of motion, a series of catches in the resistance.

cohesiveness: Growth of interpersonal harmony and intimacy within a group.

cohort effects: Effects that are due to an individual's time of birth or generation but not to actual age.

coinsurance: Component of a health insurance plan that requires the insurer and client each pay a percentage of covered costs.

collagen: Main supportive protein of skin, tendon, bone, cartilage, and connective tissue.

collective variable: Fewest number of dimensions that describes a unit of behavior.

Colles' wrist fracture: Transverse fracture of the distal end of the radius (just above the wrist).

colloid osmotic pressure: The pressure exerted by substances capable of influencing osmosis of water across membranes.

colonized: Presence of bacteria that cause no local or systemic signs or symptoms.

color agnosia: The inability to recognize colors.

colostrum: Watery-like milk secreted from a woman's breasts during pregnancy and during the first few days postpartum.

coma: Abnormally deep unconsciousness with the absence of voluntary response to stimuli.

commitment: Degree of importance attached to an event by an individual based on his or her beliefs and values. The degree of commitment is an important element in motivation.

commitment procedures: Legal process by which persons are institutionalized.

community-based rehabilitation (CBR): Rehabilitation implemented through the combined efforts of people with disabilities, their families, communities, and the appropriate health, education, vocational, and social services.

community forum: A needs assessment technique that invites residents/members of the target population to discuss their concerns at open "town hall" type meetings.

community rehabilitation programs: Structured daily social alternatives, including daily, evening, and weekend programs, as well as prevocational and vocational skills development. They provide supported employment, work adjustment, and job placement and also include leisure programs.

community/work integration or reintegration: The process of assuming or resuming roles in the community or at work.

comorbidity: Characterized by the presence of symptoms of more than one ailment (eg, depression and anxiety).

competence: Achievement of skill equal to the demands of the environment; also a legal term referring to the soundness of one's mind.

competition: Rivalry for objects, resources, facilities, or position in an organization.

compliance: Subservient behavior that implies following orders or directions without self-direction or choice. Also related to respiratory mechanics with change in respiratory volume over pressure gradient. Refers to the elasticity and expandability of the lungs.

component: Fundamental unit; in relation to activities, refers to processes, tools, materials, and purposefulness.

component movements: A type of accessory movement that is directly associated with the production of osteokinematic movement (ie, the inferior glide and superior roll of the humeral head on the glenoid fossa associated with elevation of the humerus).

comprehensive battery: Battery of tests that measure different components of cognitive functioning and perceptual and motor functioning.

comprehensive child life play program: Intervention that allows children and their parents to use play as a means of anxiety reduction, emotional expression, and social and cognitive development during a child's prolonged hospital stay.

compression therapy: Treatment using devices or techniques that decrease the density of a part of the body through the application of pressure.

compulsion: A repetitive, distressing act that is performed to relieve obsession-related fear.

computer-assisted tomography (CAT): Scanning procedure that combines x-rays with computer technology to show cross-sectional views of internal body structures.

computerized assessment: Assessment that includes the administration, scoring, and interpretation of test results done by a sophisticated computer program.

conative hypothesis: Theory that autistic children choose not to play and interact with other children rather than their being unintellectual.

concave-convex rule: The principle that expresses the relationship between the osteokinematics and arthrokinematics of a given movement. The articulating convex surface of a joint is always greater in surface area than that of its adjoining concave surface.

consensus: A common center or agreement.

concentration: The ability to maintain attention for longer periods of time in order to keep thoughts directed toward completing a given task.

concentric contraction: Muscular contraction during which the muscle fibers shorten in an attempt to overcome resistance.

concept: Mental image, abstract idea, or general notion.

concrete-operational stage: Term coined by Jean Piaget to denote development of a group of skills acquired in middle childhood, including decentration, class inclusion, and taking another's perspective. In this stage, such mental operations can only be applied to "concrete" objects.

concussion: Resulting from impact with an object (usually to the brain).

conditioning: Learning process that alters behavior through reinforcements or associating a reflex with a particular stimulus to trigger a desired response. Also a cardiovascular effect related to exercise and the overall improvement of functional endurance.

conduction: Conveying energy (eg, heat, sound, or electricity).

conference committee: Committee of legislators with one purpose of working out compromises between different versions of a bill.

confidentiality: Maintenance of secrecy regarding information confided by a client.

conflict of interest: Situation in which a person may have hidden or other interests that conflict or are inconsistent with providing services to a client or agency.

congenital: Present or existing at birth.

congenital amputation: Condition in which a child is born without part or all of a limb or limbs.

congenital anomalies/disorders: Structural abnormalities resulting from birth defects or genetic disorders.

congenital defects: Abnormalities or deformations of the skull or vertebrae in which there is a failure to enclose the neural structures or a complete absence of different parts of the brain itself.

congregate housing: Housing for unrelated individuals, often older persons, usually sponsored by government or nonprofit organizations.

congregate meal site: Place located in a central setting where meals are provided to a group of older persons, such as a senior center, housing site, or church.

conjunctivitis: Inflammation of the conjunctiva of the eye.

conjunct rotation: Osteokinematically, the involuntary spin that accompanies all impure (arcuate) swings and diadochal (a succession of two movements at an angle to each other) pure cardinal swings.

connective tissue: Structural material of the body that connects tissues and links anatomical structures together.

consent: Agree to participate.

conservation: Cognitive skill that requires the realization that a quantity of a substance remains constant regardless of changes in form.

constrictive pericarditis: Inflammation of the pericardium that results in constriction. The pericardium is covered with fibrinous deposits.

construct: Conceptual structure used in science for thinking about the factors underlying observed phenomena.

constructional apraxia: The inability to reproduce geometric designs and figures.

construct validity: In research, the extent to which a test measures the construct (mental representation) variables that it was designed to identify.

consultation: Process of assisting a client, an agency, or other provider by identifying and analyzing issues, providing information and advice, and developing strategies for current and future actions.

consumer price index (CPI): Published by the U. S. Department of Labor, a measure of increases in the price of a market basket of goods and services by region of the country.

contact dermatitis: Inflammatory response of the skin due to contact with a toxic or costic agent (eg, chemical, poison ivy).

contamination: The soiling by contact or introduction of organisms into a wound.

context: Refers to the social, physical, and psychological milieu of a situation.

continuing education: Educational programming that provides opportunities for certification or training to improve an individual's knowledge and practices.

continuity theory of aging: Psychosocial theory of aging that focuses on the integration of the older person's past experiences, inner psyche, and the changes that occur with aging in such a way as to preserve the individual's sense of self.

continuous passive motion machine (CPM): Device used to passively move a joint through the full range of movement available early in the postoperative period following joint surgery to prevent loss of range of motion.

contract: Agreement, usually written, between practitioner and agency that specifies the services to be provided and the responsibilities of each party.

contractile protein: A substance produced to remove waste at an intra- and extracellular level.

contractility: Capacity for becoming short in response to a suitable stimulus.

contraction: The tightening of a muscle to create stabilization or movement. Also, the pulling together of wound edges in the healing process. The development of tension within a muscle or muscle group with or without changes in its overall length.

contractions: Shortening and tightening of the uterine muscle fibers during and after labor.

contracture: Static shortening of muscle and connective tissue that limits range of motion at a joint.

contraindication: Condition that deems a particular type of treatment undesirable or improper.

contralateral: Pertaining to, situated on, or affecting the opposite side.

contrast bath: The immersion of an extremity in alternating hot and cold water.

contrecoup injury: Usually more extensive damage on the opposite side of the brain from the point of impact during a strike to the head.

contributory insurance: Type of group insurance in which the employee pays for all or part of the premium and the employer or union pays the remainder.

control group: Comparison group in research.

control stage: Second stage of group development; it includes a leadership struggle on group and individual levels.

contusion: A bruise.

convergence: The ability of the brain to respond only after receiving input from multiple sources.

convergent problem solving: Developing one correct solution by the forming of separate pieces of information.

conversion disorder: Disorder characterized by the presence of physical symptoms or deficits that cannot be explained by medical findings.

convulsion: Paroxysms of involuntary muscular contractions and relaxation; spasm.

cooperative play: Goal-set form of play that involves two or more children striving for that goal.

coordinated care: Term that the Health Care Financing Administration often uses more or less generically for managed care plans, particularly if they are gatekeepers.

coordination: Property of movement characterized by the smooth and harmonious action of groups of muscles working together to produce a desired motion.

co-payment: Specified amount of money per visit or unit of time that the client pays, while the insurer pays the rest of the claim.

copious: Large amounts. Used when referring to respiratory secretions during chest physical therapy.

corporal potentiality: The ability to screen out vestibular and postural information at conscious levels in order to engage the cortex in higher order cognitive tasks.

corpus luteum: Endocrine body that produces progesterone and develops in the ovary at the site of the ruptured ovarian follicle.

correlation coefficient: The relationship among two or more variables.

cortically programmed movements: Movements that are based on input from structure in the cortex (motor strip or basal ganglia).

corticorubrospinal pathway: Descending pathway that serves limb control; from the motor cortex through the red nucleus in the brainstem and onto the spinal cord.

corticospinal pathway: Oversees the finely tuned movements of the body by controlling finely tuned movements of the hands; this pathway travels from the motor cortex to the spinal neurons that serve the hand muscles.

cortisone: Hormone produced in the cortex of the adrenal gland that aids in the regulation of the metabolism of fats, carbohydrates, sodium, potassium, and proteins.

cosmesis: A concern in rehabilitation, especially regarding surgical operations or burns, for the appearance of the patient/client.

cost benefit analysis: Process used to evaluate the economic efficiency of new policies and programs by comparing an outcome and the costs required to achieve it.

cost containment: Approach to health care that emphasizes reduced costs.

cost effectiveness: Extent to which funds spent to improve health and well-being reduce overall cost of care.

cost sharing: Requirement in health insurance plans for the client to pay part of the cost of care.

counterculture: Subculture that rejects important values of the dominant society.

coup injury: Brain contusions and lacerations beneath the point of impact when the head is struck.

coxa valgus: The angle of the neck of the femur to the shaft is greater than 120 degrees angled outward.

crackle: Abnormal, short, sharp, respiratory sound heard upon auscultation. Superficial crepitation heard in the early stages of acute fibrinous pleurisy.

cramp: A painful muscle contraction brought on by involuntary use of that muscle or muscle group.

cranial nerve: Nerve extending from the brain.

crater: Tissue defect extending at least to the subcutaneous layer seen in wounds.

credentialing: Process that gives title or approval to a person or program, such as certification, registration, or accreditation.

creep: A measure of the deformation in a material as a result of a constant load applied over a specific time interval.

crepitus: Dry, crackling sound or sensation, such as made by the ends of two bones grating together.

cretinism: Condition in which an individual is small, unusual looking, and has severe mental retardation as a result of the lack of thyroid hormone.

criterion: Particular standard, level of performance, or expected outcome.

criterion-referenced tests: Goal of these tests is to evaluate specific skills or knowledge where the criterion is full mastery of them.

criterion validity: Test that measures and predicts the specific behaviors required to function in, meet the standards of, and be successful in daily life.

critical inquiry: Important investigation or examination.

critical path: Optimal sequencing and timing of diagnosis or procedure-based intervention.

critical period: Fixed time period very early in development during which certain behaviors optimally emerge.

cross-addiction: Addiction to a variety of chemical substances.

cross-linking: Theory that aging is caused by a random interaction among proteins that produce molecules that make the body stiffer.

cross-sectional research: Nonexperimental research sometimes used to gather data on possible growth trends in a population.

crowning: Indicates the presenting part of the infant visible at the vaginal opening; sometimes refers to the time at which the widest diameter of the presenting part is passing through the vaginal opening.

crusted: Dried secretions found in wound care.

cryotherapy: Therapeutic application of cold (eg, ice).

cryptomenorrhea: Monthly signs of menstruation without blood flow.

crystal arthropathies: Diseases of the joints that result in crystallization, such as gout and pseudogout.

cue: Subjective and objective input that serves as a signal to do something. A secondary stimulus that guides behavior.

cueing: Hints or suggestions that facilitate the appropriate response.

cuirass: A covering for the chest.

culture: Patterns of behavior learned through the socialization process, including anything acquired by humans as members of society (eg, knowledge, values, beliefs, laws, morals, customs, speech patterns, economic production patterns). The system of meanings and customs shared by some identifiable group or subgroup and transmitted from one generation of that group to the next.

curb cut: Short ramp cutting through a curb.

curvature of the spine: Structural deformity of the spine resulting in scoliosis, kyphoscoliosis, lordosis, or kyphosis.

custom: Habitual practice that is adhered to by members of the same group or geographical region.

cyanosis: Blue discoloration of the skin and mucous membranes due to excessive concentration of reduced hemoglobin in the blood.

cyclodialysis: Formation of an opening between the anterior chamber and the suprachoroidal space for draining the aqueous humor.

cyst: Closed sac or pouch with a definite wall that contains fluid, semifluid, or solid material.

cystocele: Downward and forward displacement of the bladder toward the vaginal opening, often related to weakness or traumatized muscles from childbirth.

cytokine: A soluble factor produced by myriad cells involved in communication between immune cells. Many cytokines are growth factors.

cytomegalovirus (CMV): One of a group of highly host-specific viruses that infect man, monkeys, or rodents, with the production of unique large cells bearing intranuclear inclusions.

cytostatic: The ability to inhibit cellular growth.

cytotoxic: The ability to kill cells.

D database: Collection of data organized in information fields in electronic format.

daytime splint: Splint used during the daytime, which must be designed in such a way that it may be removed several times a day so that the client can prevent joint stiffening by moving the joint(s) to the full range of motion.

death rates: Number of deaths occurring within a specific population during a particular time period, usually in terms of 1000 persons per year.

debility: Weakness or feebleness of the body.

debridement: Excision of contused and necrotic tissue from the surface of a wound; **autolytic d.** self-debridement (ie, removal of contused or necrotic tissue through the action of enzymes in the tissues); **sharp d.** debridement using a sharp instrument.

debris: Remains of broken down or damaged cells or tissue.

decidua: Mucous membrane lining the uterus (or endometrium) that changes in preparation for pregnancy and is sloughed off during menstruation and during postpartum.

decision making: The process of making decisions (eg, the choice of certain preferred courses of action over others).

declarative memory: The registration, retention, and recall of past experiences, sensations, ideas, thoughts, and knowledge through the hippocampal nuclear structures or the amygdala that result in long-term memory.

deconditioning: The physiologic changes in systemic function following prolonged periods of rest and inactivity.

decorticate rigidity: Exaggerated extensor tone of the lower extremities and flexor tone of the upper extremities resulting in abnormal posture due to damage to the brainstem.

decortication: Removal of portions of the cortical substance of a structure or organ, as of the brain, kidney, lung, etc.

decubitus ulcer: Open sore due to lowered circulation in a body part. Usually secondary to prolonged pressure at a bony prominence.

dedifferentiation: *See* anaplasia.

deductible: Amount of loss or expense that an insured or covered individual must incur before an insurer assumes any liability for all or part of the remaining cost of covered services.

deductive reasoning: A serial strategy in which conclusions are drawn on the basis of premises that are assumed to be true.

deep vein thrombosis: A blood clot in a deep vein.

defense mechanisms: Unconscious processes that keep anxiety producing information out of conscious awareness (eg, compensation, denial, rationalization, sublimation, and projection).

defibrillation: The stoppage of fibrillation of the heart. The separation of the fibers of a tissue by blunt dissection.

defibrillator: An apparatus used to counteract fibrillation by application of electric impulses to the heart.

defibrination syndrome: A syndrome resulting from a deprival of fibrin.

deficiency: The quality or state of being deficient, absence of something essential, incompleteness, lacking, a shortage.

deficiency disease: A disease caused by a dietary lack of vitamins, minerals, etc or by an inability to metabolize them.

deficit: Inadequate behavior or task performance. A lack or deficiency; **developmental d.** the difference between expected and actual performance in an aspect of development (eg, motor, communication, social).

deglutition: The act of swallowing.

degrees: In reference to the measurement of range of motion, the amount of movement from the beginning to the end of the action.

degrees of freedom: The options or directions available for movement from a given point.

dehydration: Absence of water. Removal of water from the body or a tissue. A condition that results from undue loss of water.

deinstitutionalization: Patients who have been hospitalized for an extended period of time, usually years, are transferred to a community setting.

delay of gratification: Postponement of the satisfaction of one's needs.

delirium: Characterized by confused mental state with changes in attention, hallucinations, delusions, and incoherence.

delirium tremens (DT): Condition caused by acute alcohol withdrawal, characterized by trembling and visual hallucinations; may lead to convulsions.

delusion: Inaccurate, illogical beliefs that remain fixed in one's mind despite having no basis in reality.

delusional disorder: Psychosis characterized by the presence of persistent delusions often involving paranoid themes in an individual whose behavior otherwise appears quite normal.

demarcation: Line of separation between viable and nonviable tissue.

dementia: State of deterioration of personality and intellectual abilities, including memory, problem-solving skills, language use, and thinking, that interferes with daily functioning.

demography: Scientific study of human populations particularly in relation to size, distribution, and characteristics of group members.

demyelinating disease: Disease that destroys or damages the myelin sheath of the nerves.

demyelination: The destruction of myelin, the white lipid covering of the nerve cell axons. The loss of myelin decreases conduction velocity of the neural impulse and destroys the "white matter" of the brain and spinal cord.

dentofacial anomalies: Relating to abnormalities of the oral cavity and surrounding facial musculature and joints.

dendrite: Short processes found on the end of a nerve cell that send or receive information from another neurotransmitter.

dendritic growth: New evidence indicating growth (rather than the common descriptions of decline) in the brains of the elderly.

denude: Loss of epidermis.

Department of Health and Human Services (DHHS): Department within the U. S. government that is responsible for administering health and social welfare programs.

dependence: Need to be influenced, nurtured, or controlled; relying on others for support.

dependent: Person who can be claimed on insurance.

depolarization: The process or act of neutralizing polarity, such as in a heartbeat.

depression: Characterized by an overwhelming sense of sadness that may be brought on by an event or series of events, but lasts far longer than a reasonable time.

depth perception: The ability to determine the relative distance between self and objects and figures observed.

derangement: To upset the arrangement, order, or function of a system. Clinically, it describes various affections—either intra-articular, extra-articular, or both—often caused by trauma or abnormal use that interfere with the function of a joint.

dermal: Related to the skin or derma. Synonym: skin.

dermatome: Area on the surface of the skin that is served by one spinal segment.

dermatomyositis: Systemic connective tissue disease characterized by inflammatory and degenerative changes in the skin, leading to symmetric weakness and some atrophy.

dermis: The inner layer of skin in which hair follicles and sweat glands originate; involved in grade II to IV pressure sores.

descriptive ethics: Ethics used to describe the moral systems of a culture.

descriptive statistics: An abbreviated description and summary of data.

desensitization: To deprive or lessen sensitivity.

desquamation: Process by which old layers of skin cells (epidermis) are shed.

detectable warning: Standardized surface feature built in or applied to walking surfaces of other elements to give warning of hazards on a circulation path.

detrusor muscle: The muscular component of the bladder wall.

developmental: Pertaining to gradual growth or expansion, especially from a lower to a higher state of complexity. Pertaining to development.

developmental assessment: Evaluation of a child with disorders that should be repeated every 2 months until the child reaches age 2.

developmental delay: The failure to reach expected age-specific performance in one or more areas of development (eg, motor, sensory-perceptual). Wide range of childhood disorders and environmental situations in which a child is unable to accomplish the developmental tasks typical of his or her chronological age.

developmental disabilities: A physical or mental handicap or combination of the two that becomes evident before age 22, is likely to continue indefinitely, and results in significant functional limitation in major areas of life.

developmental skills: Skills that are developed in childhood, such as language or motor skills.

deviance: Behavior that is in contrast to acceptable standards within a community or culture.

dexterity: Skill in using the hands or body, usually requiring both fine and gross motor coordination. Synonym: agility.

diabetic retinopathy: Complication of diabetes in which small aneurysms form on renal capillaries.

diadochal: A succession of two movements at an angle to each other.

diagnosis (Dx): Technical identification of a disease or condition by scientific evaluation of history, physical signs, symptoms, laboratory tests, and procedures.

diagnosis related groups (DRG): Classifications of illnesses and injuries that are used as the basis for prospective payments to hospitals under Medicare and other insurers.

diagnostic interview: Interview used by a professional to classify the nature of dysfunction in a person under care.

dialect: Variation of a language; particular to a certain geographical region.

dialysis: The process of separating crystalloids and colloids in a solution by the difference in their rates of diffusion through a semipermeable membrane; crystalloids pass through readily, colloids very slowly or not at all.

diameter: Measurements of the pelvic inlet and fetal head. Biparietal diameter is the largest transverse diameter of the fetal skull at term.

diaphoresis: Perspiration, especially profuse perspiration.

diaphragmatic breathing: The use of the diaphragm to draw air into the bases of the lungs.

diaphragmatic hernia: A hernia in the diaphragm.

diastole: Period of time between contractions of the atria or the ventricles during which blood enters the relaxed chambers from the systemic circulation and lungs; significant in blood pressure readings.

Dictionary of Occupational Titles **(DOT):** Text that provides information about the jobs that exist in the U. S. economy. It has an alphabetized list of all occupational job titles, a brief description of those jobs in the United States, a listing of those job titles arranged by industry, and an analysis of the requirements placed on the worker performing the job.

diffuse: Spread out or dispersed. Not concentrated.

diffusion: The process of becoming diffused or widely spread. Dialysis through a membrane.

digital: Discrete form of information (eg, a clock that displays only digits at any given moment, as opposed to analog).

dignity: Importance of valuing the inherent worth and uniqueness of each person.

dilation (dilatation): The stretching and enlarging of the cervical opening to 10 cm to allow birth of the infant.

dilation and curettage (D & C): Widening of the cervical canal with a dilator and the scraping of the uterine endometrium with a curette.

diminutive: Suffix added to a medical term to indicate a smaller size, number, or quantity of that term.

diplegia: Involvement of two extremities.

diplopia: Double vision.

direct service: Treatment or other services provided directly to one or more clients by a practitioner.

disability: The inability to engage in age-specific, gender-related, and sex-specific roles in a particular social context and physical environment. Any restriction or lack (resulting from an injury) of ability to perform an activity in a manner or within the range considered normal for a human being.

disability behavior: Ways in which people respond to bodily indications and conditions that they come to view as abnormal; how people monitor themselves, define and interpret symptoms, take remedial action, and use sources of help.

discharge: The process of discontinuing interventions included in a single episode of care, occurring when the anticipated goals and desired outcomes have been met. Other indicators for discharge: The patient/client declines to continue care, the patient/client is unable to continue to progress toward goals because of medical or psychosocial complications, or the physical therapist determines that the patient/client will no longer benefit from physical therapy.

discharge planning: To enhance continuity of care, plans are made to prepare the client for moving from one setting to another, usually a multidisciplinary process.

disclosure: In dealing with informed consent, the client has to be informed of what he or she is going to do for a study in which he or she participates.

discontinuation: The process of ending physical therapy services that have been provided during an episode of care.

disc prolapse: Displacement of intervertebral disc tissue from its normal position between vertebral bodies; also referred to as slipped, herniated, or protruded disc.

discrimination: The act of making distinctions based on differences in areas such as culture, race, gender, or religion.

disease: Deviation from the norm of measurable biological variables as defined by the biomedical system; refers to abnormalities of structure and function in body organs and systems.

disengagement theory of aging: Psychosocial theory of aging suggesting that successful aging occurs when both the elderly individual and society gradually withdraw from one another, ultimately leading to death.

disinhibition: The inability to suppress a lower brain center or motor behavior, such as a reflex. It indicates damage to higher structures of the brain.

dislocation: Displacement of bone from a joint with tearing of ligaments, tendons, and articular capsules. Symptoms include loss of joint motion, pain, swelling, temporary paralysis, and occasional shock.

disorder: Disruption or interference with normal functions or established systems.

disorientation: Inability to make accurate judgments about people, places, and things.

disruption: To disrupt or interrupt the orderly course of events.

distal: In terms of anatomical position, located further from the trunk.

distractibility: Level at which competing sensory input are able to draw attention away from tasks at hand.

distraction: Linear separation of joint surfaces without rupture of the binding ligaments and without displacement.

distress: The state of being in pain, uncomfortable, or suffering. Any affliction that is distressing.

distribution: Refers to manner through which a drug is transported by the circulating body fluids to the sites of action.

disuse atrophy: The wasting degeneration of muscle tissue that occurs as a result of inactivity or immobility.

diuresis: Increased secretion of urine.

divergence: The brain's ability to send information from one source to many parts of the central nervous system simultaneously.

diversity: Quality of being different or having variety.

documentation: Process of recording and reporting the information gathered and intervention performed on a client. It ensures that the client receives adequate services and that the provider is reimbursed for them.

doll's eyes: When the head is turned in one direction, the eyes look in the opposite direction; this indicates damage to the higher brain centers.

domain: Specific occupational performance area of work (including education), self-care, self-maintenance, play, and leisure.

dormant: Time period when a disease remains inactive.

dorsal: In terms of anatomical position, located toward the back.

dorsal column tracts: Afferent ipsilateral ascending tracts for fine discriminative touch, vibratory sense, and kinesthesia.

dorsal splint: Splint applied to the dorsal aspect of the hand to prevent full extension of the wrist or any of the finger joints.

dorsosacral position: *See* lithotomy position.

dorsum: The back or analogous to the back.

double-blind study: Strategy used in research that attempts to reduce one form of experimental error.

dressing stick: Long rod with a clothes hook attached to one end used to pull on clothing.

drug half-life: The time required for half the drug remaining in the body to be eliminated.

dual diagnosis: Presence of more than one diagnosis at the same time, most often a combination of a substance use disorder and some other condition, but may include any situation in which comorbidity exists.

ductus arteriosus: The channel between the pulmonary artery and aorta in the fetus, usually closing soon after birth.

durable medical equipment: Equipment covered by the Medicare program for patient use. Equipment must meet specific criteria and may be rented or purchased.

durable medical equipment, prosthetics, orthotics, and supplies (DMEPOS): Medically necessary equipment and supplies (eg, oxygen equipment, wheelchairs, braces, or splints) that a health care provider prescribes for a patient's home use.

durable power of attorney: Legal instrument authorizing one to act as another's agent for specific purposes and/or length of time.

duration recording: Researcher's use of a device that keeps track of time and measures how long a given behavior lasts.

dynametry: Measurement of the degree of muscle power.

dynamic equilibrium: The ability to make adjustments to the center of gravity with a changing base-of-support.

dynamic flexibility: Amount of resistance of a joint(s) to motion.

dynamics: Study of objects in motion.

dynamic spatial reconstructor: Piece of equipment that transmits x-rays throughout the body to produce a full-sized, three-dimensional image of an organ in motion on a television monitor.

dynamic splint: Orthosis that allows controlled movement at various joints; tension is applied to encourage particular movements.

dynamic strength: Force of a muscular contraction in which joint angle changes.

dynamic systems theory: Theory concerning movement organization that was derived from the study of chaotic systems. It theorizes that the order and the pattern of movement performed to accomplish a goal come from the interaction of multiple, nonhierarchical subsystems.

dynamometer: Device used to measure force produced from muscular contraction.

dynamometry: Measurement of the degree of muscle power.

dysarthria: Group of speech disorders resulting from disturbances in muscular control.

dyscalculia: Learning disability in which there is a problem mastering the basic arithmetic skills (eg, addition, subtraction, multiplication, and division), and their application to daily living.

dysdiadochokinesia: The inability to perform rapid alternating movements.

dysesthesia: Sensation of "pins and needles" such as that experienced when one's extremity "goes to sleep." Manifested by unpleasant or painful touch perception.

dysfunction: Complete or partial impairment of function.

dysfunctional hierarchy: Levels of dysfunction, including impairment, disability, and handicap.

dysgraphia: Imperfect ability to process and produce written language.

dyskinesia: Impairment of voluntary motion.

dyslexia: Impairment of the brain's ability to translate images received from the eyes into understandable language.

dysmenorrhea: Pain experienced during menstrual periods.

dysmetria: Condition seen in cerebellar disorders in which the patient overshoots a target because of an inability to control movement.

dyspareunia: Occurrence of pain during sexual intercourse.

dyspepsia: Poor digestion.

dysphagia: The inability to swallow.

dysplasia: Abnormal development in number, size, or organization of cells or tissue.

dyspnea: The inability to breathe; difficulty breathing.

dyspraxia: Difficulty or inability to perform a planned motor activity when the muscles used in this activity are not paralyzed.

dysreflexia: A life-threatening, uninhibited, sympathetic response of the nervous system to a noxious stimulus that is experienced by an individual with a spinal cord injury at T7 or above.

dysrhythmia: Disturbance in rhythm in speech, brain waves, or cardiac irregularity.

dyssomnia: Sleep disorder.

dystocia: A difficult childbirth; a fetal dystocia is difficult labor due to abnormalities of the fetus relative to size or position; a maternal dystocia is difficult labor due to abnormalities of the birth canal or uterine inertia.

dystonia/dystonic: Distorted positioning of the limbs, neck, or trunk that is held for a few seconds and then released.

E

early childhood education: School or other educational program for children ages 3 to 5 years.

early intervention: Multidisciplinary, comprehensive, coordinated, community-based system for young children with developmental vulnerability or delay from birth to age 3 years and their families. Services are designed to enhance child development, minimize potential delays, remediate existing problems, prevent further deterioration, and promote adaptive family functioning.

eccentric contraction: Muscular contraction during which the muscle generates tension while lengthening. Eccentric exercise occurs mainly in stabilizing the body against gravity.

echodensities: Ultrasound changes that can be evidence of brain tissue damage.

echolalia: Uncontrollable repetitive verbalization of words that do not fit the situation.

echopraxia: Repetitive movement that does not fit the situation.

eclampsia toxemia: An acute toxic condition of pregnancy and puerperal women with symptoms of coma, seizures, high blood pressure, renal dysfunction, and proteinuria.

ectoderm: Layer of cells that develop from the inner cell mass of the blastocyst. This layer eventually develops into the outer surface of the skin, nails, part of teeth, lens of the eye, the inner ear, and central nervous system.

ectopia: Displacement or malposition.

ectropion: Eversion of the edge of the eyelid.

eczema: An inflammatory skin disease characterized by lesions varying greatly in character, with vesiculation, infiltration, watery discharge, and the development of scales and crusts.

edema: Accumulation of large amounts of fluid in the tissues of the body.

education: The process of training and developing knowledge, skill, mind, and character. Formal schooling at an educational institution.

educational approaches: Interventions that make use of factual learning/teaching to change behaviors.

educational evaluator: Teacher who reports results of tests of academic, developmental, and readiness levels in number concepts as well as the sequence of listening, speaking, reading, and writing.

effacement: Thinning and shortening of the cervix occurring before or during dilation and expressed in percentages of 0% to 100%.

effectiveness: Degree to which the desired result is produced.

efferent: Conducting away from a structure, such as a nerve or a blood vessel.

efferent neuron: Includes motor neurons.

efficacy: Having the desired influence or outcome.

effusion: Escape of fluid into a joint or cavity.

egophony: A bleating quality of voice observed in auscultation in certain cases of lung consolidation.

egress, means of: Continuous and unobstructed path of travel from any point in a building or structure to a public way and consisting of three separate and distinct parts: the exit access, the exit, and the exit discharge. A means of egress comprises the vertical and horizontal means of travel and shall include intervening room spaces, doorways, hallways, corridors, passageways, balconies, ramps, stairs, enclosures, lobbies, horizontal exits, courts, and yards.

ejection fraction: Percentage of blood emptied from the ventricles at the end of a contraction.

elastic stiffness: The amount of tissue force produced when a tissue is deformed and held at a given length.

elastic traction: Splinting method often used to correct joint deformity. Materials used include rubber bands, elastic thread, and springs, which are now available in varying degrees of strength.

electrical potential: The amount of electrical energy residing in specific tissues.

electrical stimulation: Intervention through the application of electricity.

electrocardiogram (EKG): A graphic recording of the electrical activity of the heart.

electrocautery: Cauterization by means of a wire loop or needle heated by direct current.

electroencephalography: Study of the electrical activity of the brain.

electrogoniometer: Electronic device that measures the position of a joint or joints to which it is applied.

electrolytes: Mineral salts that conduct electricity in the body when in solution.

electromyography (EMG): The examining and recording of the electrical activity of a muscle.

electronic fetal monitoring: The monitoring of the fetus and uterine contractions through internal and external pressure and sound transducers during labor.

electrophysiologic testing: The process of examining and recording the electrical responses of the body.

electrophoresis: The movement of charged particles through a medium as a result of changes in electrical potential.

electrotherapeutic modalities: A broad group of agents that use electricity to produce a therapeutic effect.

electrotherapy: The use of electrical stimulation modalities in treatment.

elder: Term used to refer to individuals in the later years of the life span, arbitrarily set between the age 65 to 70 and beyond.

elder abuse: Intentional physical or psychological injury inflicted upon older adults by caretakers.

embolism: Sudden blocking of an artery by a clot of foreign material (ie, embolus) brought to the site of lodging via the blood stream.

embryo: The fetus from conception to 8 weeks of gestation.

embryonic period: Prenatal period of development that occurs from 2 to 8 weeks after conception. During this period, cell differentiation intensifies, support systems for the cells form, and organs appear.

embryotomy: Extraction of a dead fetus by dismemberment.

emetic: Drug that promotes vomiting.

empathy: While maintaining one's sense of self, the ability to recognize and share the emotions and state of mind of another person.

emphysema: An abnormal swelling of the lung tissue due to the permanent loss of elasticity or the destruction of the alveoli, which seriously impairs respiration.

empirical base: Knowledge based upon the observations and experience of master clinicians.

employee assistance program (EAP): Mental health services offered to workers through confidential counseling at work and outside referrals to appropriate professionals. EAPs attempt to treat employees in their current work and living settings. EAPs were originally established to decrease corporate costs resulting from such problems as alcoholism and drug abuse among workers.

empowerment: To enable.

enactive representation: Motoric encoding of information about the world (eg, child thinks "rattle" and shakes hand).

encephalitis: Disease characterized by inflammation of the parenchyma of the brain and its surrounding meninges; usually caused by a virus.

encephalopathy: Any disease that effects the tissues of the brain and its surrounding meninges.

encoding (cognitive): Processes or strategies used to initially store information in memory.

endarterectomy: The surgical removal of endarterium and atheromatous material from an arterial segment that has become stenosed.

endarterium: The innermost layer of the arterial wall; also called *the intima*.

end feel: Sensation imparted to the hands of the clinician at the end point of range of motion.

end-diastolic volume: The amount of filling of the ventricles of the heart during diastole.

endocarditis: Inflammation of the endocardium; a disease generally associated with acute febrile or rheumatic diseases and marked by dyspnea, rapid heart action, and peculiar systolic murmurs.

endocardium: The thin endothelial membrane lining the cavities of the heart.

endocrine: Designating or any gland producing one or more hormones, such as the thyroid and its hormone thyroxine.

endogenous: Growing from within. Developing or originating within the organism.

endometriosis: Abnormal proliferation of the uterine mucous membrane into the pelvic cavity.

endothelial: Pertaining to the epithelial cells that line the heart cavities, blood vessels, lymph vessels, and serous cavities of the body.

end-systolic volume: The amount of blood remaining in each ventricle after each heartbeat.

endurance: The ability of a muscle to sustain forces or to repeatedly generate forces.

endurance testing: Used to determine the capacity of an individual to sustain the energy output needed to fulfill a task.

energy conservation techniques: Applying procedures that save energy; may include activity restriction, work simplification, time management, and organizing the environment to simplify tasks.

endotracheal: Within or through the trachea. Performed by passage through the lumen of the trachea (eg, endotracheal tube).

enfolded activity: Performing multiple activities in a given time frame.

engagement: Signifies that the fetus has firm head-down position within the mother's pelvis and is no longer floating above the bony pelvis.

engineering controls: Changes to the workstation, equipment, or tools to eliminate hazards at the sources.

enteral: Administration of a pharmacologic agent directly into the gastrointestinal tract by oral, rectal, or nasogastric routes.

enteric: Pertaining to the intestines.

enterocele: Herniation of the intestine below the cervix associated with congenital weakness or obstetric trauma.

enthesopathy: Any inflammation of a joint.

entropion: Inversion of the edge of the eyelid.

entry level: Individual with less than 1 year of work experience.

enucleation: Removal of an organ or other mass from its supporting tissues.

enuresis: The inability to control urine, usually bedwetting.

environment: External social and physical conditions or factors that have the potential to influence an individual.

environmental approaches: Interventions based on changing the environment (eg, changing support systems, modifying job or home).

environmental assessment: Process of identifying, describing, and measuring factors external to the individual that can influence performance or the outcome of treatment. These can include space and associated objects, cultural influences, social relationships, and system available resources.

environmental barrier: Any type of obstacle that interferes with a person's ability to achieve optimal occupational performance.

environmental contingencies: Factors in the environment that influence the patient's performance during an evaluation.

environmental control unit (ECU): Device that allows those with limited physical ability to operate other electronic devices by remote control.

environmental fit: The process of matching the individual's capacity with opportunities for action in the physical, social, and cultural environments.

environmental support: Any environmental element that facilitates an individual's ability to attain his or her optimum occupational performance.

enzyme: A protein functioning as a biochemical catalyst, necessary for most major body functions. Biochemical substances that are capable of breaking down necrotic tissue.

epicardium: The layer of the pericardium that is in contact with the heart.

epicritic sensation: The ability to localize and discern fine differences in touch, pain, and temperature.

epidemiology: A study of the relationships of the various factors determining the frequency and distribution of diseases in a human environment. Science concerned with factors, causes, and remediation as related to the distribution of disease, injury, and other health-related events.

epidermis: The outer cellular layer of skin.

epidural: Anesthesia injected into the epidural space of the spine, which can produce loss of sensation from the abdomen to the toes.

epigenesis: Elements of each developmental stage are represented in all developmental stages.

epilepsy: Group of disorders caused by temporary sudden changes in the electrical activity of the brain that results in convulsive seizures or changes in the level of consciousness or motor activity.

epinephrine: A hormone secreted by the adrenal medulla in response to splanchnic stimulation and stored in the chromaffin granules, being released predominantly in response to hypoglycemia. It increases blood pressure, stimulates heart muscle, accelerates the heart rate, and increases cardiac output.

episiotomy: Refers to an incision through the perineum that allows for less pressure on the fetal head during delivery.

episode of care: All patient/client management activities provided, directed, or supervised by the physical therapist from initial contact through discharge.

episodic memory: Memory for personal episodes or events that have some temporal reference.

epispadias: Congenital opening of the urethra on the dorsum of the penis or opening by separation of the labia minora and a fissure of the clitoris.

epistaxis: Nosebleed.

epistemology: Dimension of philosophy that is concerned with the questions of truth by investigating the origin, nature, methods, and limits of human knowledge.

epithelialization: Regeneration of the epidermis across a wound surface.

Epstein-Barr virus (EBV): The virus that causes infectious mononucleosis. It is spread by respiratory tract secretions (eg, saliva, mucus).

equality: Requires that all individuals be perceived as having the same fundamental rights and opportunities.

equilibrium reaction: Reaction that occurs when the body adapts and posture is maintained, and when there is a change of the supporting surface; any of several reflexes that enables the body to recover balance.

equinovarus: Deformity of the foot in which the foot is pointing downward and inward; clubfoot.

equipment: Device that usually cannot be held in the hand and is electrical or mechanical (eg, table, electrical saw, or stove); devices can be specifically designed to assist function or compensate for absent function or they can be labor-saving and convenience gadgets.

ergometer: Device that can measure work done.

ergometry: Measurement of work.

ergonomics: Field of study that examines and optimizes the interaction between the human worker and the nonhuman work environment. The relationship among the worker, the work that is done, the tasks and activities inherent in that work, and the environment in which the work if performed. Ergonomics uses scientific and engineering principles to improve the safety, efficiency, and quality of movement involved in work.

ergonomic work site analysis: Analysis that categorizes jobs on the basis of the qualifications and physical demands they require in order to ensure that a person is capable of performing a given job safely.

eructation: Producing gas from the stomach, often with a characteristic sound; belching.

erythema: First-degree reddening of the skin due to a burn or injury.

erythrocyte: Red blood cell that contains hemoglobin, an oxygen-carrying pigment responsible for the red color of blood.

eschar: Thick, leathery necrotic tissue; devitalized tissue; a slough produced by burning or by a corrosive application.

essential fat: Stored body fat that is necessary for normal physiologic function and found in bone marrow, the nervous system, and all body organs.

essential functions: Fundamental, not marginal, job duties. In deciding whether a function is essential, the following questions are considered: Are employees in the position required to perform the function? Will removing that function fundamentally change the job?

essential hypertension: High blood pressure that is idiopathic, self-existing, and has no obvious external cause. Intrinsic hypertension.

Escherichia coli **(E. coli):** A species of organisms constituting the greater part of the intestinal flora. In excess, it causes urinary tract infections and epidemic diarrheal disease.

estrogen: The female hormone that is responsible for maintenance of female sex characteristics and is formed in the ovary, placenta, testis, and adrenal cortex.

ethical dilemma: Conflict of moral choices with no satisfactory solution that is often caused by attempting to balance two or more undesirable alternatives with no overriding principle to tell an individual what to do.

ethical jurisdiction: Right or authority to interpret the system of values imposed by a group. In the profession of physical therapy, the American Physical Therapy Association, National Board for Certification of Physical Therapy, and state regulatory boards have jurisdiction.

ethical relativism: View that each person's values should be considered equally valid.

ethical research practice: Refers to the investigator's obligation to respect the individual's freedom to decline to participate in research or to discontinue participation at any time.

ethics: System of moral principles or standards that govern personal and professional conduct.

ethnic: Member of, or pertaining to, groups of people with a common racial, national, linguistic, religious, or cultural history.

ethnicity: Component of culture that is derived from membership in a racial, religious, national, or linguistic group or subgroup, usually through birth.

ethnocentrism: Process of judging different cultures or ethnic groups only on the basis of one's own culture or experiences.

ethnogerontology: Study of ethnicity in an aging context.

ethologic theory: Branch of developmental theory that emphasizes innate, instinctual qualities of behavior that predispose individuals to behave in certain patterns.

ethology: The systemic study of the formation of the core characteristics of being human.

etiology: Dealing with the causes of disease.

etiquette: Particular behaviors that are observed by a certain society as being acceptable.

euthanasia: The deliberate ending of life of a person suffering from an incurable disease; has been broadened to include the withholding of extraordinary measures to sustain life, allowing a person to die.

evaluation: Process of obtaining and interpreting data necessary for treatment; a dynamic process in which the physical therapist makes clinical judgments based on data gathered during the examination.

eversion: Turning outward.

evidence-based practice: Practice founded on research that supports its effectiveness.

evisceration: Removal of the contents of a cavity.

exacerbation: Increase in the severity of a disease or any of its symptoms.

examination: The process of obtaining a history, performing relevant systems reviews, and selecting and administering specific tests and measures.

excoriation: Linear scratches on the skin.

excretion: Process through which metabolites of drugs (and active drug itself) are eliminated from the body through urine and feces, evaporation from skin, exhalation from lungs, and secretion into saliva.

excursion: A range of movement regularly repeated in performance of a function.

exercise therapy: Manages musculoskeletal disorders by restoring strength to weakened muscles, restoring mobility or increased range of motion, correcting postural faults, preventing joint deformity, and improving joint stability.

exertional angina: Paroxysmal thoracic pain due most often to anoxia of the myocardium precipitated by physical exertion. Synonym: angina.

exhaustion: Depletion of energy with the consequent inability to respond to stimuli.

exocrine: Secreting outwardly (the opposite of endocrine).

exogenous: Growing by additions to the outside. Developed or originating outside the organism.

exophthalmos: Abnormal protrusion of the eyeball, which results in a marked stare.

expected outcomes: The intended results of patient/client management, with the changes in impairments, functional limitations, and disabilities and the changes in health, wellness, and fitness needs that are expected as the result of implementing the plan of care.

expectorate: To expel mucus or phlegm from the lungs; to spit.

expertise: The possession of a large body of knowledge and procedural skill that allows the solution of most domain problems effectively and efficiently.

explanatory model: Model held by an individual about an illness episode containing knowledge, thoughts, and feelings about etiology, timing, and mode of onset of an illness; the pathophysical process; the natural history and the severity of the illness; ethnoanatomy and ethnophysiology; and appropriate treatments and their rationale.

exploratory laparotomy: Incision into the abdominal cavity in order to view the condition of abdominal organs.

expressive aphasia: Language and communication are reduced with reading, writing, and speaking affected; the inability to verbalize one's own needs.

extended care facility (ECF): Facility that is an extension of hospital care; derived from Medicare legislation.

extended school year programs: Programs run during the summer months or weekends for children.

extension (EXT): Straightening a body part.

external stimulation: Factors in the area where the activity is being performed, which may enhance or impede performance.

external validity: The degree to which an experimental finding is predictable to the population at large.

exteroceptive: Receptors activated by stimuli outside of the body.

extinction: Behavioral approach to discouraging a particular behavior by ignoring it and reinforcing other more acceptable behaviors.

extracranial: Anatomic structures outside the cranial vault (skull).

extrafusal muscle: Striated muscle tissue found outside the muscle spindle.

extrapyramidal: Outside of the pyramidal tracts.

extrapyramidal signs: Motor symptoms that mimic Parkinson's disease, dyskinesia, and other lesions in the extrapyramidal tract.

extrinsic: Coming from or originating outside.

extrinsic motivation: Stimulation to achieve or perform that initiates from the environment.

exudate: Material, such as fluid, cells, or cellular debris, that has escaped from blood vessels and been deposited in tissues or on tissue surfaces, usually as a result of inflammation. An exudate, in contrast to a transudate, is characterized by a high content of protein, cells, or solid materials derived from cells; accumulation of fluids in wound. May contain serum, cellular debris, bacteria, and leukocytes.

F

FEV₁: The percentage of the vital capacity that can be expired in 1 minute.

face validity: Dimension of a test by which it appears to test what it purports to test.

fact: Truth or reality.

factor analysis: Statistical test that examines relationships of many variables and their contribution to the total set of variables.

false negative: Statistical research term indicating the rate of negative results on a diagnostic test when disease was actually present.

false positive: Statistical research term indicating the rate of positive results on a diagnostic test when no disease was actually present.

family therapy: Intervention that focuses on the context of the entire family system.

fascia: A thin layer of connective tissue covering, supporting, or connecting the muscles or inner organs of the body.

fasciculation: A small local contraction of muscles, visible through the skin, representing a spontaneous discharge of a number of fibers innervated by a single motor nerve filament.

fasciitis: Inflammation of a fascia.

fat emboli: Embolus formed by an ester of glycerol with fatty acids, which cause a clot in the circulatory system and can result in vessel obstruction.

fatigue: State of exhaustion or loss of strength and endurance; decreased ability to maintain a contraction at a given force.

Federal Register: Publication in which proposed federal U. S. rules and regulations as well as requests for proposals for grants are published.

feedback: Knowledge of the results of an individual's performance to the extent that the individual's behavior is changed or reinforced in a desirable direction.

feedback control: Refers to the postural control mechanism of automatic responses that occurs when there is a displacement of one's center of gravity that is not under voluntary control. Automatic postural responses.

feed-forward control: Refers to the postural control mechanism of automatic responses that occurs during an intentional displacement of the center of gravity, as during voluntary movement.

fee-for-service: Payment method by which a health care provider is reimbursed for each encounter or service rendered.

fee schedule: List of accepted charges or established allowances for specified medical or dental procedures.

festinating gait: Patient walks on his or her toes as pushed. Starts slowly, increases, and may continue until the patient grasps an object in order to stop (eg, in Parkinson's disease).

fetal alcohol syndrome (FAS): Low birth weight, developmental delays, and physical defects in infants caused by mothers consuming alcohol during pregnancy.

fetal distress: Decrease in fetal heart rate and the possibility of meconium-stained amniotic fluid related to jeopardized fetal oxygen supply.

fetal growth retardation: Condition of babies who are especially small for their gestational age at birth.

fetus: Describes the baby from the 8th week after conception until birth.

fibrillation: Small, local involuntary muscle contraction.

fibrin: A whitish, insoluble protein formed from fibrinogen by the action of thrombin, as in the clotting of blood. Fibrin forms the essential portion of a blood clot.

fibroblast: Chief cell of connective tissue responsible for forming the fibrous tissues of the body, such as tendons and ligaments.

fibrosis: Formation of fibrous tissue, fibroid degeneration.

fidelity: Duty to be faithful to the client and the client's best interest; includes the mandate to keep all client information confidential.

figure ground: A person's ability to distinguish shapes and objects from the background in which they exist.

fine motor coordination: Motor behaviors involving manipulative, discreet finger movements, and eye/hand coordination. Dexterity.

fine motor pattern of development: Mastery of smaller muscles (eg, fingers); takes place after gross-motor development.

finger goniometer: Instrument used to measure the range of movement of the finger joints.

first stage of labor: Initial part of labor when the cervix effaces and dilates to 10 cm; includes the early, active, and transition phases.

fiscal management: Method of controlling the economics of problems at hand. It is concerned with discovering, developing, defining, and evaluating the financial goals of a department.

fissure: Any cleft or groove.

fistula: Abnormal tube-like duct or passage from a normal cavity or tube to a free surface or another cavity.

fixator: Muscle that contracts to brace one bone, to which a mover attaches.

flaccidity: State of low tone in the muscle that produces weak and floppy limbs.

flexibility: Range of motion at a joint or in a sequence of joints.

flexion (FLEX): Act of bending a body part.

floating: Refers to the fetus floating within the uterus in the abdomen above the bony pelvis.

floppy disk: Magnetic storage medium used in a computer for electronic information of high or low density, single- or double-sided, and sizes of 3.5 and 5.25 inches.

flow: Optimal experience.

fluid goniometer: Goniometer that has a circular chamber filled with fluid that has a 360-degree scale. It is used to measure the change in the angle of a joint.

fluid intelligence: The ability to use new information.

fluidotherapy: Dry whirlpool (ie, the application of dry heat through a fluidotherapy machine).

focal epilepsy: Jerking or stiffening of many muscles on the same side of the body that crosses over to the opposite side and then continues. The person does not fully lose consciousness, but consciousness is altered.

folkways: Social customs to which people generally conform; traditional patterns of life common to a people.

follicle stimulating hormone (FSH): One of the gonadotropic hormones of the anterior pituitary, which stimulates the growth and maturation of graafian follicles in the female and spermatogenesis in the male.

foot-drop splint: Splint used to prevent the development of plantar flexion contractures.

footling breech: Position of the fetus in which presentation of a foot is the presenting part.

force: Product of mass and acceleration; a kinematic measurement that encompasses the amount of matter, velocity, and its rate of change of velocity; also strength, energy, and power.

force couple: Body being acted upon by two equal and parallel forces from opposite directions; the points of application of these forces must be on opposite sides of the object and be operating at some distance apart from one another.

force plate: An embedded plate used to measure the force that a person exerts when walking.

forceps: Locked tong-like obstetrical instruments used to aide in the delivery of the fetal presenting part.

fracture (Fx): Pertaining to broken bone(s).

fragile X syndrome: Sex-linked disorder in males that results when the bottom tip of the long arm of the X chromosome is pinched off.

frame of reference: Organization of interrelated, theoretical concepts used in practice.

frank breech: Position of the fetus in which both legs are flexed against the abdomen and the sacrum is the presenting part.

Frank-Starling mechanism: The intrinsic ability of the heart to adapt to changing volumes of inflowing blood.

freedom: Allows the individual to exercise choice and to demonstrate independence, initiative, and self-direction.

free radicals: Any molecule that contains one or more unpaired electrons. Changes in cells that result from the presence of free radicals are thought to result in aging.

fremitus: A thrill or vibration, especially one that is perceptible on palpation.

Fresnel prism: Prism applied to a person's glasses that shifts images toward the center of the visual field.

friction: Surface damage caused by skin rubbing against another surface.

frontal plane: Runs side to side, dividing the body into front and back portions.

frostbite: To injure the tissues of the body by exposure to intense cold.

fulcrum: The intermediate point of force application of a three- or four-point bending construction; entity on which a lever moves.

fulminant: Sudden; severe; occurring suddenly and with great intensity.

full-thickness skin loss: Third-degree burn or wound in which skin is completely destroyed and underlying structures (eg, muscles, vessels) can be visualized.

function: Those activities identified by an individual as essential to support physical, social, and psychological well-being and to create a personal sense of meaningful living. Performance; action.

functional assessment: Observation of motor performance and behavior to determine if a person can adequately perform the required tasks of a particular role or setting.

functional electrical stimulation (FES): Stimulation of nerves from surface electrodes in order to activate specific muscle groups for facilitating function.

functional limitation: Restriction of the ability to perform a physical action, activity, or task in an efficient, typically expected, or competent manner.

functional mobility: Moving from one position or place to another, such as in-bed mobility, wheelchair mobility, and transfers; performing functional ambulation; and transporting objects. The ability to perform functional activities and tasks without restriction.

functional muscle testing: Performance-based muscle assessment in particular positions stimulating functional tasks and activities and usually under specific test conditions.

functional position: Hand configuration predominantly used in hand splinting in the past decades for hands that required immobilization. It involves 20 to 30 degrees wrist extension, 45 degrees metacarpal joint flexion, 30 degrees proximal interphalangeal joint flexion, and 20 degrees distal interphalangeal joint flexion, with the thumb abducted.

functional reach: A simple clinical measure of functional balance that quantifies one's forward reach capacity prior to loss of balance. Measures one's ability to move center of gravity to the margins of the base-of-support.

functional reserve: Refers to the excess or redundant function that is present in virtually all physiologic systems.

fundus: The top upper portion of the uterus.

furuncle: A painful nodule formed in the skin by circumscribed inflammation of the corium and subcutaneous tissue, enclosing a central slough or "core." It is caused by bacteria, which enter through the hair follicles or sudoriparous glands.

G

gag reflex: Involuntary contraction of the pharynx and elevation of the soft palate elicited in most normal individuals by touching the pharyngeal wall or back of the tongue.

gait: The manner in which a person walks, characterized by rhythm, cadence, step, stride, and speed.

galactosemia: Recessive, inherited metabolic disorder that prevents an individual from converting galactose to glucose, which results in serious physical and mental challenges.

galvanic skin response (GSR): Change in the electrical resistance of the skin as a response to different stimuli.

ganglion: A mass of nerve cells serving as a center from which impulses are transmitted. A cystic tumor on a tendon sheath.

gangrene: Decay of tissue in a part of the body when the blood supply is obstructed by disease or injury.

gastric intubation: Forced feeding, usually through a nasogastric tube.

gastric lavage: Washing out the stomach with repeated flushings of water.

gate-control theory: The pain modulation theory developed by Melzak and Wall that proposes that presynaptic inhibition in the dorsal gray matter of the spinal cord results in blocking of pain impulses from the periphery.

gatekeeper: A primary care physician who is responsible for coordinating all services.

gender identity: A child's realization that males and females are different due to physical characteristics. Synonym: core gender identity.

generalization: Skills and performance in applying specific concepts to a variety of related solutions.

general systems theory: Conceptualizes the individual as an open system that evolves and undergoes different forms of growth, development, and change through an ongoing interaction with the external environment.

genes: Biologic unit that contains the hereditary blueprints for the development of an individual from one generation to the next.

genetic: Pertaining to reproduction or to birth of origin; hereditary traits.

geniculostriate system: Visual system pathways that transmit information for identifying the nature of objects in the environment.

genital prolapse: The falling out or slipping out of place of an internal organ, such as the uterus, rectum, vagina, or bladder.

genotype: The genetic constitution of an organism or group.

geriatric day care: Ambulatory health care facility for older adults.

geriatrics: Area of study concerned with medical care of individuals in old age. The branch of medicine that treats all problems unique to old age and aging, including the clinical problems associated with senescence and senility.

germinal period: Stage or interval of time from conception to implantation of the blastocyte to the uterus, approximately 8 to 10 days.

gerontological tripartite: Approach to the study of aging that collectively combines three phenomena of the aging process: the biological capacity for survival, the psychological capacity for adaptation, and the sociological capacity for the fulfillment of social roles.

gerontology (GER): Area of study concerned with the care, health issues, and special problems of the elderly.

gestation: Total period of time the baby is carried in the uterus, approximately 40 weeks in humans.

globin: The protein constituent of hemoglobin; also any member of a group of proteins similar to the typical globin.

glomerulus: A tuft or cluster; used in anatomical nomenclature as a general term to designate such a structure, as one composed of blood vessels or nerve fibers.

glottis: The vocal apparatus of the larynx, consisting of the true vocal cords and the opening between them (ie, rima glottides).

glucagon: A hyperglycemic-glycogenolytic factor thought to be secreted by the pancreas in response to hypoglycemia or stimulation by the growth hormone of the anterior pituitary gland.

glucocorticoid: Hormone from the adrenal cortex that raises blood sugar and reduces inflammation.

glucose: A thick, syrupy, sweet liquid generally made by incomplete hydrolysis of starch.

glucosuria: Presence of glucose in the urine. Secretion of excess sugar into the urine is often a sign of diabetes mellitus.

glycogenesis: The formation or synthesis of glycogen.

glycogenolysis: The splitting of glycogen in the body tissue.

glycoprotein: A substance produced metabolically that creates osmotic force.

Golgi tendon organ (GTO): Sensory receptors in the tendons of muscles that monitor tension of muscles.

goniometer: Instrument for measuring movement at a joint.

goniometry: Measurement of the angle of the joint or a series of joints.

gout: Painful metabolic disease that is a form of acute arthritis; characterized by inflammation of the joints, especially of those in the foot or knee.

graded activity: Activity that has been modified in one or more of a variety of ways in order to provide the appropriate therapeutic demand or challenge for a person.

grading: A scheme or categorization of treatments, movements, disease stages, and wound stages.

graft: The replacement of a defect in the body with a portion of suitable material, either organic or inorganic. Also, the material used for such replacement.

grand mal: Type of seizure in which there is a sudden loss of consciousness immediately followed by a generalized convulsion.

grand multipara: A woman who has given birth seven or more times.

granulation: The formation of a mass of tiny red granules of newly formed capillaries, as on the surface of a wound that is healing.

granulocyte: Any cell containing granules, especially a granular leukocyte. A heterogeneous class of leukocytes characterized by a multilobed nucleus and intracellular granules. Granulocytes include neutrophils, eosinophils, basophils, and mast cells.

granulocytosis: Increase in circulating granulocyte number.

graphesthesia: The ability to identify letters or designs on the basis of tactile input to the skin.

graphomotor: Pertains to movement involved in writing.

gratification: The ability to receive pleasure, either immediate (immediately upon engaging in an activity) or delayed (after completion of the activity).

gravida: A pregnant woman.

gravity: Constant force that affects almost every motor act characterized by heaviness or weight. The tendency toward the center of the earth.

gray matter: Area of the central nervous system that contains the cell bodies.

grip force: Pressure exerted on a held object or in lifting an object.

gross motor coordination: Using large muscle groups for controlled, goal-directed movements. Motor behaviors concerned with posture and locomotion.

gross motor pattern of development: Mastery of larger muscles (proximal musculature); takes place before fine motor development.

group: Plurality of individuals (three or more) who are in contact with one another, who take each other into account, and who are aware of some common goal.

group dynamics: Forces that influence the interrelationships of members and ultimately affect group outcome.

group process: Interpersonal relationship among participants in a group.

group therapy: Any intervention directed toward groups of individuals rather than an individual alone.

Guide to Physical Therapy Practice: A document prepared by the American Physical Therapy Association that represents expert consensus and contains preferred practice patterns describing common sets of management strategies used by physical therapists for selected patient/client diagnostic groups.

gustatory: Pertaining to the sense of taste.

gyral atrophy: Decreases in the gray or white matter of the brain or both.

H **HET model (Human-Environment-Technology model):** Conceptual framework designed to convey the relationship between human performance deficits and the use of technologies to address these deficits.

habilitation: Process of giving a person the resources, including specialized treatment and training, to promote improvement in activities of daily living, thereby encouraging maximum independence.

habit: Performed on an automatic, preconscious level.

habit spasm: Tic that lasts for a long period of time and develops habitually.

habituate: Process of accommodating to a stimulus through repeated diminishing exposure.

half-life: Measure of the amount of time required for 50% of a drug to be eliminated from the body. The time in which the radioactivity originally associated with an isotope will be reduced by one half through radioactive decay.

hallucinate: Sense (eg, see, hear, smell, or touch) of something that does not exist externally.

halo effect: Error based on the fact that if a person is believed to possess one positive trait, he or she may possess others as well.

handicap: Disadvantage, resulting from an impairment or disability, that limits or prevents the fulfillment of a role that is normal (depending on age, sex, and social and cultural factors) for that individual. The social disadvantage of a disability.

handicapping situation: A barrier to the performance of an activity (eg, a nonaccessible building, an attitude discrimination, a policy that denies access).

Hawthorne effect: Research error due to response differences paid to the participant by the researcher.

Hayflick's limit: Biologic limit to the number of times a cell is able to reproduce before it dies. A finite capacity for cellular division.

hazard: State that could potentially harm a person or do damage to property.

head injury (HI): Caused by direct impact to the head, most commonly from traffic accidents, falls, industrial accidents, wounds, or direct blows.

health: Physical and mental well-being with freedom from disease, pain, or defect and normalcy of physical, mental, and psychological functions.

healthcam: Camera that takes pictures of movement and is calibrated to measure the distance moved.

health care policy: A principle, plan, or course of action to manage health care in the United States as pursued by a government organization or individual.

health education: A combination of educational, organizational, economic, and environmental supports for behavior conducive to health.

health maintenance: Screening and intervention for potential health risks to prevent disease and promote health and well-being.

health maintenance organization (HMO): Prepaid organized health care delivery system.

health policy: Set of initiatives taken by a government to direct resources toward promoting, improving, and maintaining the health of its citizens.

health promotion: Programs put in place to promote the physical, mental, and social well-being of the person. Includes a focus on the individual's ability to function optimally in her or his environment and a balance in mind and body across all of an individual's life experiences.

heart disease: Any of the diseases of the heart.

heart failure: The inability of the heart to pump enough blood to maintain an adequate flow to and from the body tissues.

heart-lung machine: Performs functions of the heart and lungs during open heart surgery so these organs may be operated on.

heat therapy: Application of heat on a body part; used to relieve the symptoms of musculoskeletal disorders.

heavy work: Exerting up to 50 to 100 pounds of force occasionally, or 25 to 50 pounds of force frequently, or 10 to 20 pounds of force constantly to move objects.

helplessness: Psychological state characterized by a sense of powerlessness or the belief that one is not capable of meeting an environmental demand competently.

hemangioma: Benign tumor composed of newly formed blood vessels clustered together.

hemangiosarcoma: A malignant tumor formed of endothelial and fibroblastic tissue.

hematocrit: The volume percentage of erythrocytes in whole blood.

hematoma: Localized collection of blood in an organ or within a tissue.

hemianesthesia: Total loss of sensation to either the left or right side of the body.

hemianopsia: Blindness in one half of the field of vision in one or both eyes.

hemiparesis: Weakness of the left or right side of the body.

hemiplegia (Hemi): Condition in which half of the body is paralyzed due to anoxia during birth or as a result of an aneurysm or cerebral vascular accident.

hemodynamics: The study of the interrelationship of blood pressure, blood flow, vascular volumes, physical properties of the blood, heart rate, and ventricular function.

hemoglobin: The oxygen-carrying pigment of the erythrocytes formed by the developing erythrocyte in bone marrow.

hemolysis: The liberation of hemoglobin. The separation of the hemoglobin from the corpuscles and its appearance in the fluid in which the corpuscles are suspended.

hemolytic: Pertaining to, characterized by, or producing hemolysis.

hemophilia: Lack of clotting factors that results in a hemorrhage.

hemoptysis: Expectoration of blood due to hemorrhage in the respiratory system.

hemorrhage: The escape of large quantities of blood from a blood vessel; heavy bleeding.

hemothorax: A collection of blood in the pleural cavity.

hepatitis: Inflammation of the liver.

here-and-now experience: Immediate experience in the group is examined as a projection of the person's past and provides members with an opportunity to test new and more adaptive interpersonal skills.

hereditary: The genetic transmission of a particular quality or trait from parent to offspring.

hernia: The protrusion of all or part of an organ through a tear in the wall of the surrounding structure such as the protrusion of part of the intestine through the abdominal muscles.

herniated vertebral disc: Weakness in annulus allowing nucleus pulposus to protrude; sometimes presses against the nerve root and spinal cord, causing radicular symptoms.

heroin: Highly addictive narcotic from the opium family.

heuristic: Clinical reasoning strategies, or shortcuts, that simplify complex cognitive tasks.

hidrosis: Formation and excretion of sweat.

hierarchy: A ranking system having a series of levels running from lowest to highest.

high risk pregnancy: A pregnancy in which the mother or fetus is in danger of a compromised outcome.

hilus: A depression or pit at that part of an organ where the vessels and nerves enter.

hip/knee/ankle/foot orthosis (HKAFO): A device to control all lower extremity segments.

hippocampus: A nuclear complex forming the medial margin of the cortical mantle of the cerebral hemisphere forming part of the limbic system.

hirsutism: Excessive growth of hair in unusual places, especially in women.

histogram: Bar graph.

history (Hx): An account of past and present health status that includes the identification of complaints and provides the initial source of information about the patient/client. The history also suggests the individual's ability to benefit from physical therapy services.

holism: View of the human mind and body as being one entity.

holistic: A concept in which understanding is gained by examination of all parts working as a whole; a model or approach to health care that takes into account all internal and external influences during the process.

holophrase: Infants' one word utterances.

home health program: Health or rehabilitation services provided in a client's home.

homeostasis: Physiological system used to maintain internal processes and constancy of the internal metabolic balance despite changes in the environment.

homogamy: Notion that similar interests and values are important in forming strong, lasting personal relationships.

homogeneity of variance: Assumption that the variability within each of the sample groups should be fairly similar.

homologous: Corresponding in structure, position, and origin. Derived from an animal of the same species but of different genotype.

homonymous hemianopsia: Loss of the same side of the field of vision in both eyes usually due to optic nerve damage.

homoscedasticity: Standard deviations of the scores along the regression line is fairly equal.

horizontal plane: Runs transversely across, dividing the body into upper and lower parts. Parallel to the ground.

hormone: A chemical substance produced in the body that has a specific effect on the activity of a certain organ; applied to substances secreted by endocrine glands and transported in the blood stream to the target organ on which their effect is produced.

hospice programs: Care for terminally ill clients and emotional support for them and their families.

human: An organism that maintains and balances itself in the world of reality and actuality by being in active life and active use.

human chorionic gonadotrophin (HCG): A growth hormone that influences the gonads.

human development: Ongoing changes in the structure, thought, or behavior of a person that occur as a function of both biologic and environmental influences.

human factors engineering: Profession that investigates and optimizes function of interactions between humans and machines.

human immunodeficiency virus (HIV): The virus that causes AIDS, which is contracted through exposure to contaminated blood or bodily fluid (eg, semen or vaginal secretions).

human subject: Living individual about whom an investigator conducting research obtains data through intervention.

humerus: Long bone of the upper arm.

humoral: Pertaining to any fluid or semifluid in the body.

humoral immunity: Immune function via soluble factors found in blood and other body fluids.

hyaluronic acid: Substance that, under compressive forces, lubricates cells.

hydatidiform mole: Anomaly of the placenta, which forms a nonmalignant mass from cystic swelling of the chorionic villi; no embryo is present.

hydration: Providing adequate water.

hydrocele: Accumulation of serous fluid in a sac-like cavity, especially in the testes.

hydrocephalus: Enlargement of the head due to an increase in cerebrospinal fluid within the brain.

hydrocephaly: Condition characterized by abnormal accumulation of cerebrospinal fluid within the ventricles of the brain, which leads to enlargement of the head.

hydrophilic: Attracting moisture.

hydrophobic: Repelling moisture.

hydrostatic pressure: A pressure created in a fluid system, such as the circulatory system.

hydrostatic weighing: Underwater weighing to determine body volume; body volume is used to determine body density from which body composition can be calculated.

hydrotherapy: Intervention using water.

hydroureter: Abnormal distention of the ureter with urine due to an obstruction.

hyperalimentation: The ingestion or administration of a greater than optimal amount of nutrients.

hyperbaric oxygen: Oxygen under greater pressure than normal atmospheric pressure.

hyperbilirubinemia: Excessive amount of bilirubin in the blood.

hypercalcemia: Excessive amount of calcium in the blood.

hypercapnia: Excessive amount of carbon dioxide in the blood.

hypercholesterolemia: Excessive amount of cholesterol in the blood.

hyperemesis gravidarum: Extreme vomiting in pregnancy.

hyperemia: Presence of excess blood in the vessels; engorgement.

hyperesthesia: Increased sensitivity, often unpleasant, to cutaneous stimulation.

hyperglycemia: Abnormally increased content of sugar in the blood.

hyperkalemia: Excessive amount of potassium in the blood.

hyperlipidemia: An abnormally high concentration of lipids in the blood.

hypermetria: Distortion of target-directed voluntary movement. The limb moves beyond its target.

hypermobility: Condition of excessive motion in joints.

hypernatremia: Excessive amount of sodium in the blood.

hyperpathia: Severely exaggerated, subjective, painful response to stimuli.

hyperplasia: Increased number of cells.

hyperpnea: Abnormal increase in the depth and rate of the respiratory movements.

hypertension: Any abnormally high blood pressure or a disease of which this is the chief sign.

hyperesthesia: Abnormally increased sensitivity to stimulation.

hypertonus: Muscular state wherein muscle tension is greater than desired; spasticity. Hypertonus increases resistance to passive stretch.

hypertrophic scarring: Excessive markings left by the healing process in the skin or an internal organ.

hypertrophy: Increased cell size leading to increased tissue size. The morbid enlargement or overgrowth of an organ or part due to an increase in size of its constituent cells (eg, hypertrophic cardiomyopathy).

hyperuricemia: Excess of uric acid in the blood.

hyperventilation: Increased expiration and inspiration potentially caused by anxiety.

hyperventilation of pregnancy: Because of an increase in respiratory tidal volume during normal respiration there is an increase in the respiratory minute volume, which makes the mother feel like she is hyperventilating.

hypnotic: Drugs or conditions that produce drowsiness or sleep.

hypochondriasis: In the absence of medical evidence, a sustained conviction that one is ill or about to become ill; abnormal concern about one's health.

hypoesthesia: Diminished ability to recognize stimuli.

hypokinetic disease: Complications arising from inactivity. Synonym: disuse syndrome.

hypometria: Distortion of target-directed voluntary movement in which the limb falls short of reaching its target.

hypomobile: When motion is less than that which would normally be permitted by the structures.

hyponatremia: Decreased amount of sodium in the blood.

hypoplasia: Defective or incomplete development (eg, osteogenesis imperfecta).

hypospadias: Abnormal congenital opening of the male urethra on the undersurface of the penis.

hypotension: Abnormally low blood pressure.

hypothesis: Conclusion drawn before all the facts are known; working assumption that serves as a basis for further investigation; a plausible explanation or best guess about a situation.

hypothetico-deductive reasoning: Form of problem solving in which several possible ideas are tested in order of probability to reach a solution.

hypotonicity: Decrease in the muscle tone and stretch reflex of a muscle resulting in decreased resistance to passive stretch and hyporesponsiveness to sensory stimulation.

hypotonus: Muscular state wherein muscle tension is lower than desired; flaccidity. Hypotonus decreases resistance to passive stretch.

hypovolemia: Abnormally decreased volume of circulating fluid (ie, plasma) in the body.

hypoxia: Any state in which an inadequate amount of oxygen is available to the tissues, without respect to cause or degree. Deficiency of oxygen in the blood. *See* anoxia.

hysterectomy: Surgical removal of the uterus.

hysterical conversion: Somatoform disorder characterized by the loss of functioning of some part of the body not due to any physical disorder, but apparently due to psychological conflicts.

I **ICD code:** International Classification of Diseases codes used for billing and reimbursement purposes.

ICIDH: International Classification of Impairments, Disability, and Handicaps developed by the World Health Organization.

icing: Ice is applied in small, overlapping circles for 5 to 10 minutes until skin flushing and numbness occur.

iconic representation: Memory of the stimuli in terms of pictorial images or graphics that stand for a concept without defining it fully.

ideation: An internal process in which the nervous system gathers information from stimuli in the environment or recruits information from memory stores to formulate an idea about what to do.

ideational apraxia: The inability to formulate a plan to complete a request commanded.

identity: Gradually emerging and continually changing sense of self; used in Erik Erikson's theory of development.

identity diffusion: Eriksonian psychosocial crisis in which integration of childhood skills, goals, and roles does not occur.

ideomotor apraxia: Interference with the transmission of the appropriate impulses from the brain to the motor center; results in the inability to translate an idea into motion.

idiopathic: Designating a disease whose cause is unknown or uncertain.

illness: Experience of devalued changes in being and in social function. It primarily encompasses personal, interpersonal, and cultural reactions to sickness.

imaginative play: Activities that include make-believe games.

imbalance: Lack of balance, as in proportion, force, and functioning.

immediate recall: The ability to recall information within a short time after the information has been received.

immersion: To plunge, dip, or drop into a liquid.

immunoglobulin (Ig): Glycoprotein found in blood and other body fluids that may exert antibody activity. All antibodies are Ig molecules, but not all Ig exhibits antibody activity.

immunosuppression: A decrease in responsiveness of the immune system with an imbalance of the antigen-antibody relationship.

impairment: A loss or abnormality of psychological, physiological, or anatomical structure or function; **secondary i.** impairments that originate from other, pre-existing impairments.

impedance: Resistance to flow or movement.

impingement: To trap and compress.

impotence: Weakness, especially the inability of the male to achieve or maintain erection.

impulsive: To act without planning or reflection.

incidence: During a specified time period, the number of new cases of a certain illness or injury in a population. It is demonstrated as the number of new cases divided by the total number of people at risk.

incompetence: Failing to meet requirements; incapable; unskillful. Lacking strength and sufficient flexibility to transmit pressure, thus breaking or flowing under stress.

incompetent cervix: Cervix that prematurely dilates as pregnancy progresses.

incontinence: Inability to control excretory functions.

incubator: An apparatus for maintaining a premature infant in an environment of proper temperature and humidity.

indemnity: Standard fee-for-service insurance policies provided by employers, organizations, or individuals. Usually the most expensive type, this insurance covers service from any provider.

indemnity insurance: Type of insurance based on payments only when an illness or accident has occurred.

independence: Lack of requirement or reliance on another; adequate resources to accomplish everyday tasks.

independent practice association (IPA): Partnership, corporation, association, or other legal entity that has entered into an arrangement for provision of its services with persons who are licensed to practice medicine.

independent variable: Antecedent variable.

indirect services: Those activities, strategies, and interventions provided to agencies and others to assist them in providing direct care services.

individual education plan (IEP): Interdisciplinary plan required for special education students in the United States under the provisions of Public Law 94-142. Allows parents or guardians to examine all school records and to participate with professionals in making educational placement decisions and in developing written diagnostic-prescriptive plans for school-aged children.

individual habilitation plan (IHP): A written multidisciplinary plan of care for a developmentally disabled adult that identifies needs, strategies for meeting those needs, and the individuals involved in providing the program. This may be a part of a referral to physical therapy.

individual transition plan (ITP): Adolescents about to graduate from high school may have this plan, which focuses on preparation for vocational or educational programming immediately after high school.

inductive fallacy: Overgeneralizing on the basis of too few observations.

inductive reasoning: Generation and testing of a hypothesis on the basis of evidence to indicate its validity.

induration: Abnormal firmness of tissue with a definite margin.

industry: According to Erik Erikson and his theory of development, this is when children in elementary school focus on applying themselves in doing certain activities that are reflective of being successful in the adult world.

infancy: Time of development of a child from a few weeks after birth until the second year of life.

infantile myoclonic: Sudden, brief, involuntary muscle contractions producing head drops and flexion of extremities.

infarct: An area of coagulation necrosis in a tissue due to local anemia resulting from obstruction of circulation to the area.

infection: The state of being infected, especially by the presence in the body of bacteria, protozoa, viruses, or other parasites.

infective: To cause infection; infectious.

inference: Possible result or conclusion that could be deduced from evaluation data.

inferential (predictive) statistics: Utilizing the measurements from the sample to anticipate characteristics of the population.

inferential therapy: Form of electrotherapy that applies a large variety of low-level frequencies to deep structures in the body. It is useful in treating swelling.

inferior: In terms of anatomical position, located below the head.

inflammation: The condition into which tissues enter as a reaction to injury, including signs of pain, heat, redness, and swelling.

inflammatory: Pertaining to or characterized by inflammation.

informal social network: People who provide support but who are not connected with any formal social service agency.

informant interview: Interview in which a therapist gathers information about the client or environment from significant others.

informational support: A type of social support that informs, thereby reducing anxiety over uncertainty.

informed consent: Requirement that the person must be given adequate information about the benefits and risks of planned treatments or research before he or she agrees to the procedures.

inguinal: Pertaining to the groin.

inhibition: Arrest or restraint of a process.

injury: Physical harm or damage to a person.

innate goodness: View presented by Swiss-born French philosopher Jean-Jacques Rosseau that stressed that children are inherently good.

inpatient: Services delivered to the patient during the hospitalization.

inotropic: Affecting the force or energy of muscular contractions. Either weakening the force of contraction or increasing the force of muscular contraction.

inquiry: An investigation or examination.

insertion: Distal attachment of a muscle that exhibits most of the movement during muscular contraction.

inservice education: In-house seminars or special training sessions, either in- or outside the facility.

insight: Self-understanding. Understanding of consequences/ramification of a situation or an action.

in situ: Localized site, confined to one place (eg, cancer that has not invaded neighboring tissues).

instability: Description of a joint that has lost its structural integrity and is overtly hypermobile.

instinctual drives: Aspect of the psychodynamic theory in which Freud believes that there are two primary instinctual impulses that demand gratification: sex and aggression.

institution: Any public or private entity or agency.

institutionalization: Effects of dehumanizing and depersonalizing characteristics of the environment that result in apathy, a significant decrease in motivation and activity, and increased passivity of an individual. Also refers to confinement.

instrumental activities of daily living (IADL): Essential activities that are used to measure independent living capability and are not considered basic daily living activities or self-care tasks. Activities include shopping, cooking, home chores, heavy household chores, managing money, and structured play for infants and children. Activities that are important components of maintaining independent living.

insufficiency: Deficiency or inadequacy. The failure or inability of an organ or tissue to perform its normal function.

insurance denial: When a third party has denied payment for a service; organizations may appeal denials if they believe the criteria have not been equitably applied.

intake interview: Interview in which the therapist identifies the client's needs and his or her suitability for treatment.

integration: Unifying or bringing together; in children, the developmental ability to link successive actions instead of viewing each action as a separate, unrelated event; usually acquired by 2 years of age.

integumentary: Pertaining to or composed of skin.

intelligence: Potential or ability to acquire, retain, and use experience and knowledge to reason and problem solve.

intention tremor: Rhythmical, oscillatory movement initiated with an arm or hand.

interactive reasoning: One of three clinical reasoning styles used by physical therapists. The process involves individualizing treatment for the specific needs of the patient/client.

interdecile range: Scores including the central 80% of a distribution.

interdependence: A concept that recognizes the mutual dependencies of individuals within social groups.

interface: Program or device that links the way two or more pieces of equipment or person/machine units work together.

interferon (IFN): A class of unrelated cytokine proteins formed when cells are exposed to viruses. It is an antiviral chemical, secreted by an infected cell, that strengthens the defenses of nearby cells not yet infected.

intermediate care facilities (ICF): Facilities designed to give personal care, simple medical care, and intermittent nursing care.

intermittent positive-pressure breathing: Mechanical device that uses air pressure to inflate and deflate the lungs for breathing.

internal: Having to do with the inner nature of a thing.

internal postural control: The ability of the body to support and control its own movement without reliance on supporting structures in the environment.

internal validity: The cause and effect relationship can be identified by the results of an experiment.

International Classification of Diseases (ICD): Disease classification system developed by the World Health Organization.

interneuron: Nerve cell that links motor and sensory nerves.

internodal: The space between two nodes; the segment of a nerve fiber connecting two nodes (often called *internodal bundles* or *pathways*).

interoceptive: Receptors activated by stimuli from within visceral tissues and blood tissues.

interpolar: Situated between two poles.

interval data: Measurements that are assigned values so the order and intervals between numbers are recognized.

intervention: The purposeful and skilled interaction of the physical therapist with the patient/client, and when appropriate, with other individuals involved in care, using various methods and techniques to produce changes in the condition. The interactions and procedures used in treating and instructing patients/clients.

intervertebral disks: Pads of fibrous elastic cartilage found between the vertebrae. They cushion the vertebrae and absorb shock.

intima: Refers to the innermost surface of a vessel, especially an artery.

intracranial: Occurring within the cranium.

intrafusal muscle: Striated muscle tissue found within the muscle spindle.

intrauterine hypoxia: Stopping of the pulse and loss of consciousness as a result of too little oxygen and too much carbon dioxide in the blood, leading to suffocation during the birthing process.

intravascular: Directly into a vessel.

intrinsic motivation: Concept in human development that proposes that people develop in response to an inherent need for exploration and activity.

intubation: The insertion of a tube; especially the introduction of a tube into the larynx through the glottis, performed for the introduction of an external source of oxygen.

intussusception: Telescoping of the bowel within itself.

inventory: Assessment comprised of a list of items to which the person gives responses.

inversion: Turning inward or inside out.

involuntary movement: Movement that is not done of one's own free will; not done by choice. Unintentional, accidental, not consciously controlled movement.

involution: A rolling or turning inward over a rim, such as a toenail growing back into the soft tissue of the toe. Also a term used to describe the return of the uterus to the nonpregnant size and position following delivery of a baby.

iodine: Element important for the development and function of the thyroid gland.

iontophoresis: Introduction of ions into tissues by means of electric current.

ipsilateral: Situated on or affecting the same side.

ischemia: Reduced oxygen supply to a body organ or part. Deficiency of blood in a part due to functional constriction or actual obstruction of a blood vessel.

ischemic heart disease: Lack of blood supply to the heart.

Islets of Langerhans: Irregular structures in the pancreas composed of cells smaller than the ordinary secreting cells. These masses (islands) of cells produce an internal secretion, insulin, which is connected with the metabolism of carbohydrates, and their degeneration is one cause of diabetes.

isoenzyme: One of the multiple forms in which a protein catalyst may exist in a single species, the various forms differing chemically, physically, and/or immunologically.

isokinetic contraction: A concentric or eccentric contraction that occurs at a set speed, commonly produced when opposing a resistance that accommodates to the force produced at all points in the range of motion.

isokinetic strength: Force generated by a muscle contracting through a range of motion at a constant speed.

isometric contraction: Static muscle contraction in which the muscle generates tension but does not change length. Concentric or eccentric contractions of variable speed, commonly produced when opposing a fixed resistance throughout a range of motion.

isometric strength: Force generated by a contraction in which there is no joint movement and minimal change in muscle length.

isotonic contraction: Contraction of a muscle during which the force of resistance remains constant throughout the range of motion.

isotonic strength: Force of contraction in which a muscle moves a constant load through a range of motion.

isthmus: Narrow structure connecting two larger parts.

itinerant: Traveling from place to place.

J

Jamar grasp dynamometer: Instrument used to measure the strength of a person's grip.

jamming: A proprioceptive technique in which intermittent joint approximation is used to facilitate cocontraction around a joint by eliciting postural responses.

jaundice: A condition in which the eyeballs, the skin, and the urine become abnormally yellow as a result of increased amounts of bile pigments in the blood. Usually secondary to conditions such as hepatitis or liver failure.

jaw jerk: Closure of the mouth caused by striking the lower jaw while it hangs passively open. This reflex is rare in normal individuals.

Jewett brace: A hyperextension trunk brace that provides a single three-point force system via a sternal pad, a suprapubic pad, and a thoracolumbar pad, which restricts forward flexion in the thoracolumbar area.

job capacity evaluation: Assessment of the match between the person's capabilities and the critical demands of a specific job.

job description: Provides a written statement of a particular position in order to identify, define, and describe its parameters.

job satisfaction: Positive feelings arising from work-related tasks.

job specification: Based on a job description and used primarily in the hiring process, it states the minimum requirements needed for a position (eg, level of education, length of experience, and skills). Utilized as basis for industrial rehabilitation interventions.

joint: Junction of two or more bones.

joint capsule: Any sac or membrane enclosing the junction of the bones.

joint integrity: The intactness of the structure and shape of the joint, including its osteokinematic and arthrokinematic characteristics.

joint mobility: Functional joint play and flexibility allowing for freedom of joint movement. The capacity of the joint to be moved passively, taking into account the structure and shape of the joint surface in addition to the characteristics of the tissue surrounding the joint.

joint mobilization: A manual therapy employing mobilization techniques, which include graded passive oscillations at the joint to improve joint mobility.

joint play: A type of accessory movement in which intra-articular movement (give) occurs in response to an external force (ie, the separation of the tibia and fibula on dorsiflexion, manual distraction of the humeral head, etc).

joint protection: Application of procedures to minimize joint stress.

joint range of motion (JROM): Freedom of motion in joints. A goniometer is used to measure joint mobility on a 180-degree scale.

joint receptor: Anatomically localized in joint capsules and ligaments, they include the Golgi-type endings, Golgi-Mazzoni corpuscles, Ruffini's corpuscle, and free nerve endings. In general, they detect joint movement in the gravitational field, causing the discharge of receptors in the somatic, visual, and vestibular afferent systems to maintain posture and balance.

joints: Junctures in the body where bones articulate. The classifications are synarthrosis (ie, nonmoving), amphiarthrosis (ie, slightly moving), or diarthrosis (ie, freely moving).

judgement: The ability to use data or information to make a decision.

jump sign: A test that screens for binocular vision, which is when both eyes cannot focus on a single point or target. The patient/client focuses on an object and the therapist then covers one eye; if the uncovered eye "jumps" to refocus on the object, this is a positive jump sign.

junctional rhythm: Rapid heart rate with a characteristically inverted P wave often preceding, following, or falling within the QRS complex on an EKG. Causes are usually digitalis toxicity, acute inferior myocardial infarction, or heart failure.

justice: Notion that all cases should be treated alike and fairly in accord with general standards of right and wrong.

juvenile: Pertaining to youth or childhood diseases, such as juvenile diabetes or juvenile arthritis.

K

kalemia: The presence of potassium in the blood.

Kegel exercises: Pelvic floor strengthening exercises developed by Dr. Arnold Kegel.

keratin: A scleroprotein that is the principle constituent of epidermis, hair, nails, and the organic matrix of the enamel of the teeth.

keratitis: Inflammation of the cornea.

keratosis: Any horny growth, such as a wart or callosity.

ketone: Any compound containing a carbonyl group, CO.

ketosis: A condition characterized by an abnormally elevated concentration of ketone (acetone) bodies in the body tissues and fluids, causing an acidosis. Also referred to as *ketoacidosis*.

keyboard emulating interface: Hardware device connected to the computer or a software program installed on the computer that allows input from an alternate device to be accepted as a standard keyboard input.

keyword method: Mnemonic system that uses a part of the word to be learned to make an association that triggers the recall of the desired meaning or information.

kinematics: Area of kinesiology that is not concerned with cause but rather with measuring, describing, and recording motions.

kinesics: The study of body movements, gestures, and postures as a means of communication. Synonym: body language.

kinesiology: The study and science of motion.

kinesthesia: A person's sense of position, weight, and movement in space. The receptors for kinesthesia are located in the muscles, tendons, and joints.

kinesthetic: Sense derived from end organs located in muscles, tendons, and joints and stimulated by movement. Also called *proprioception*.

kinetic chain: A complex motor system formed by a series of joints a) open: series of joints in which the terminal one is free; b) closed: series of joints in which the terminal one meets sufficient external resistance to prohibit or restrain its free motion.

kinetics: Area of kinesiology that is concerned with cause, as well as the forces that produce, modify, or stop a motion.

knee/ankle/foot orthosis (KAFO): A device applied externally to control knee, ankle, and foot motion and position.

Kohn's pores: Openings in the interalveolar septa of the lungs.

Krebs cycle: Tricarboxylic acid cycle that results in the energy production of adenosine triphosphate.

Kurzweil reading machine: Computerized device that converts print into speech. The user places printed material over a scanner that "reads" the material aloud by means of an electronic voice.

Kussmaul's respiration: Air hunger (as seen in patients with chronic obstructive pulmonary disease).

kyphoscoliosis: Backward and lateral curvature of the spinal column, such as that seen in vertebral osteochondrosis (Scheuermann's disease).

kyphosis: Abnormal anteroposterior curving of the spine; hunchback or roundback.

L **labia:** The external folds surrounding the vagina and urethra.

labile: Changeable.

labor: Refers to the uterine contractions that produce dilation and effacement of the cervix, assisting in descent of the fetus and delivery through the vaginal opening.

labyrinthine righting reflexes: These begin at birth and continue through life. The head orients to a vertical position with the mouth horizontal when the body is tipped or tilted. Tested with the eyes closed.

lactation: Refers to the process by which milk is made in the breasts and secreted for nourishment of the infant.

lactiferous: Secreting milk.

laissez faire style: Low involvement.

laminectomy: Surgical excision of the posterior arch of the vertebra.

Landau reflex: Seen with infants at 3 months to 2 years. When lifting under the thorax in a prone position, first the head and then the back and legs will extend. If the head is put into a flexed position, the extensor tone will disappear.

lanugo: Fine hair on the body of the fetus after the fourth month in utero.

laryngospasm: Spasmodic closure of the larynx.

latent period: Time during which a disease is in existence but does not manifest itself.

latent phase: Early phase of the first stage of labor that ends when the cervix is fully effaced and 3 to 4 cm dilated.

latent stage (latency): Fourth of Freud's stages of psychosexual development, characterized by the development of the superego (ie, conscience) and by the loss of interest in sexual gratification; typically occurs from the age of 6 to 11 years in western cultural groups. Also, latency in the duration of effectiveness following cessation of treatment or intervention.

lateral: In terms of anatomical position, located away from the midline of the body.

lateral corticospinal tract (LCST): Contralateral descending motor tract. Upper motor neurons influencing lower motor neurons either directly or indirectly.

laterality: Tendency toward one side or the other (eg, right-handedness, left-handedness). Dominant side for skilled activities.

lateralization: The tendency for certain processes to be more highly developed on one side of the brain than the other. In most people, the right hemisphere develops the processes of spatial and musical thoughts, and the left hemisphere develops the areas for verbal and logical processes.

lateral shift: A clinical term denoting an apparent translatoric displacement of the trunk on the lower lumbopelvic region.

lateral trunk flexion: The ability to move the trunk from side to side without moving the legs, which is essential for maintaining balance.

launching: Process in which youths move into adulthood and leave their family of origin.

learned helplessness: Process in which the person attributes his or her lack of performance to external factors rather than lack of effort.

learned nonuse: A process that occurs after an injury, such as a cerebrovascular accident. Immediately following the injury, motor function is extremely impaired due to diaschisis (ie, cortical shock). Attempts to use the affected limb at this time fail, and the client learns that the limb is useless. Compensation with the unaffected limb begins and produces successful results (a reward behavior), and further attempts at using the involved limb continue to be unsuccessful (a punished behavior). This pattern of reinforcement results in a strong learned response of not trying to use the affected limb. Thus, the client does not realize that a return of function of the affected limb may have gradually occurred.

learning: Enduring ability of an individual to comprehend and/or competently respond to changes in information from the environment and/or from within the self. As one learns about the environment, alterations occur in the definition of the self and possible behaviors.

learning disability: Learning problem that is not due to environmental causes, mental retardation, or emotional disturbances; often associated with problems in listening, thinking, reading, writing, spelling, and mathematics.

learning environment: All the conditions (internal and external), circumstances, and influences surrounding and affecting the learning of the patient/client.

learning stations: Activities or special equipment are placed around the room for an individual to use and be evaluated on for therapeutic feedback or educational achievement.

learning theory: Theoretical base behind the behavioral frame of reference in which behavior is best learned when environmental influences are introduced.

least restrictive environment: Most normal learning environment in which a person with a disability can have his or her educational needs met.

legislative review: Review of a bill by the legislature when they perceive that an agency has misinterpreted the intent or has excessively revised existing regulations.

leg length discrepancy: Asymmetrical length of the lower extremities when one is compared to the other.

leisure: Category of activities for which freedom of choice and enjoyment are the primary motives.

length of stay (LOS): The duration of hospitalization, usually expressed in days.

lesion: Injury to the central or peripheral nervous system that may prevent the expression of some functions and/or it may allow the inappropriate, uncoordinated, uncontrolled expression of other functions.

letdown reflex: The involuntary release of milk through the nipples that occurs at the beginning of breastfeeding.

lethargy: Sluggishness or inactivity.

leukocyte: White blood cell; colorless blood corpuscles that function to protect the body against micro-organisms causing disease.

leukocytosis: An increase in circulating lymphocyte number.

leukopenia: Decreased white blood cell count.

levator syndrome: Spasm of the muscles surrounding the anus, causing severe rectal pain.

level: Even. No slope.

level of arousal: An individual's responsiveness and alertness to stimuli in the environment.

levels of processing: Durability of the memory trace is a function of the level to which the information was encoded.

lever system: System consisting of a rigid bar (lever), an axis (fulcrum), a force, and a resistance to that force. The distance between the axis and the point of application of force is known as the *force arm*; the distance between the axis and the point of application of resistance is known as the *resistance arm*.

licensure: Process established by a governmental agency to determine professional qualification.

lie of the fetus: Relationship of the long axis of the fetus to the long axis of the mother.

life cycle: From conception to death of an organism.

life expectancy: Number of years in the lifespan of an individual in a particular cultural group.

life review: Process in which one looks back at one's life experiences, evaluating, interpreting, and reinterpreting them.

life roles: Daily life experiences that occupy one's time, including roles of student, homemaker, worker (active or retired), sibling, parent, mate, child, and peer.

lifespan perspective: Makes seven basic contentions about development: it is lifelong, multidimensional, multidirectional, plastic, historically embedded, multidisciplinary, and contextual.

lifestyle: Pattern of daily activities over time that is stable and predictable, through which an individual expresses his or her self-identity.

ligament: Inelastic fibrous thickening of an articular capsule that joins one bone to its articular mate, allowing movement at the joint.

ligation: Application of a ligature (a ligature being any material used for tying a vessel or to constrict a part).

lightening: Occurs when the fetal head drops into the pelvic inlet, allowing the uterus to descend to a lower level, relieving pressure on the diaphragm and making breathing easier during the last few weeks of pregnancy.

light work: Exerting up to 20 pounds of force occasionally, up to 10 lbs of force frequently, or a negligible amount of force constantly to move objects.

Likert scale: Point system that is used to rank a particular level of skill, function, or attitude.

limbic system: Primitive central nervous system associated with emotional and visceral functions in the body. A group of brain structures that include amygdala, hippocampus, dentate gyrus, cingulate gyrus, and their interconnections with the hypothalamus, septal areas, and brainstem.

limitation: Act of being restrained or confined.

limiting charge: Statutory limit on the amount a nonparticipating health care provider can charge Medicare patients for services.

limits-of-stability: The boundary or range that is the furthest distance in any direction a person can lean away from vertical (midline) without changing the original base of support (eg, stepping, reaching, etc) or falling.

linear processing: Learning or solving a problem using a step-by-step process in which each step is dependent on what occurred before.

line of pull: Attachments of a muscle, direction of its fibers, and the location of its tendons at each joint at which the muscle crosses.

linea nigra: Pigmented line appearing on the abdomen, from the pubis to the umbilicus, in pregnant women.

lingula: A small tongue-like structure. In the cerebellum, the part of the vermis of the cerebellum, on the ventral surface, where the superior medullary velum attaches (lingula cerebelli). In the lung, a projection from the lower portion of the upper lobe of the left lung, just beneath the cardiac notch, between the cardiac impression and the inferior margin (lingula of left lung). In the lower jaw, the sharp medial boundary of the mandibular foramen to which is attached the sphenomandibular ligament (lingula mandibulae). Lastly, the lingula sphenoidalis, a ridge of bone on the lateral margin of the carotid sulcus, projecting backward between the body and great wing of the sphenoid bone.

lipofuscin: A dark, pigmented lipid found in the cytoplasm of aging neurons.

lithotomy position: Position in which the client lies on his or her back with thighs flexed upon the abdomen and the lower legs on the thighs, which are abducted.

lobectomy: Excision of a lobe, as of the lung, thyroid, brain, or liver.

localized inflammation: Swelling, redness, and increased temperature that is isolated to the injured or infected part of the body.

lochia: Discharge of blood, mucous, and tissue from the vagina after delivery, often lasting up to 6 weeks after birth, but usually referring to the bright red discharge of the first 2 weeks postpartum.

locomotion: The ability to move from place to place.

locus of control: Psychological term referring to one's orientation to the world of events. Persons with an internal locus of control believe they can influence the outcome of events. Those with an external locus of control, conversely, believe that the outcome of events is largely a matter of fate or chance (ie, that they cannot have influence over the outcome of events).

logical classification: The ability to sort objects by their defining properties occurs at the age of 5 or 6 years.

long cane: Mobility device used by individuals with visual impairments who sweep it in a wide arc in front of them.

longevity: Long life or life expectancy.

long-handled reacher: Reacher with a long handle that can aid in dressing or retrieving objects that are out of arm's reach.

longitudinal arch: Comprised of the motions of metacarpal, proximal interphalangeal, and distal interphalangeal joints of the digital ray. Splints involving these joints are said to involve the longitudinal arch. Also the arch of the foot medially.

longitudinal research: Study in which subjects are measured over the course of time to gather data on potential trends.

long-term care (LTC): Array of services needed by individuals who have lost some capacity for independence because of a chronic illness or condition.

long-term memory: Permanent memory storage for long-term information.

long-term support system: Ensuring that individuals have access to the services that are needed to support independent living.

loose associations: Thoughts shift with little or no apparent logic.

lordosis: Abnormal forward curvature of the lumbar spine; swayback.

lower motor neuron (LMN): Sensory neuron found in the anterior horn cell, nerve root, or peripheral nervous system.

low technology: Electronic or nonelectronic products or systems that have assumed a more commonplace role and accessibility in society.

low-temperature thermoplastics: Materials that are presently most often used for splinting and orthotics fabrication. These materials soften and become more pliable with heat. After these materials are cooled, they remain in the shapes to which they were molded/shaped.

lumbar rotation: Rotating the client's pelvis away from the painful side; technique to treat spinal pain.

lumbar stabilization: Exercises whose objective is to strengthen the deep spine muscles as a foundation for good trunk stability.

lumpectomy: Excision of a small primary breast tumor, leaving the rest of the breast intact.

lung: The organ of respiration.

luteinizing hormone (LH): A gonadotrophic hormone of the anterior pituitary that acts with the follicle-stimulating hormone to cause ovulation of mature follicles and secretion of estrogen by theca and granulosa cells. It is also concerned with corpus luteum formation and, in the male, stimulates the development and functional activity of interstitial cells.

lymphadenitis: Inflammation of the breast tissue, causing enlargement.

lymphadenopathy: Disease of the lymph nodes, characterized by malaise and general enlargement of the nodes.

lymphatic system: The system containing or conveying lymph.

lymphedema: Swelling of an extremity caused by obstruction of the lymphatic vessels.

lymphoblast: T lymphocytes that have been altered during a viral attack to release a variety of chemicals that encourage greater defensive activity by the immune system.

lymphocyte: A particular type of white blood cell that is involved in the immune response and produced by lymphoid tissue.

lymphoidectomy: Excision of lymphoid tissue.

lymphoma: Any of the various forms of cancers of the lymphoid tissue.

M **maceration:** Softening of tissue by soaking in fluids.

macular degeneration: Common eye condition in which the macula is effected by edema, the pigment is dispersed, and the macular area of the retina degenerates. It is the leading cause of visual impairment in persons older than 50.

macrophage: A phagocyte cell residing in tissues and derived from the monocyte.

magnetic resonance imaging (MRI): A scanning technique using magnetic fields and radio frequencies to produce a precise image of the body tissue; used for diagnosis and monitoring of disease.

malaise: A vague feeling of bodily discomfort or uneasiness, as in an early illness.

main effects: The action of two or more independent variables, each working separately.

mainstreamed: Concept in education that a child with a disability be put into a "typical" classroom for a portion or all of the school day.

maintenance: Programs for the maintenance of functional capabilities.

major depressive disorder: Mood disorder characterized by features, such as downcast mood, loss of interest in activities, insomnia, and feelings of fatigue and worthlessness, that cause impairment in daily functioning.

major medical insurance: Type of insurance designed to offset the heavy medical expenses resulting from a prolonged illness or injury.

make test: Form of muscle testing in which the therapist provides resistance against a muscle while it is moving through its range.

malposition: Faulty or abnormal position.

managed care: Integrated delivery systems. Cost containment approach that enables the payer to influence the delivery of health services prospectively (ie, before services are provided).

management: The act, art, or manner of managing, handling, controlling, or directing.

management by objectives: Managerial system that improves the productivity of an organization by setting goals of progress that can be periodically measured and using time tables and time limits to adhere to productivity goals.

management strategies: A strategic plan for managing, handling, controlling, or directing businesses or services.

mandated reporter: Person who, in the practice of his or her profession, comes in contact with children and must make a report or see that a report is made when he or she has reason to believe that a child has been abused.

mania: Excessive activity, flight of thought, and grandiosity.

manipulation: A passive therapeutic movement, usually of small amplitude and high velocity, at the end of the available range.

manipulative therapy: Passive movement technique that can be classified into either joint manipulation or mobilization. Manipulation is a sudden small thrust that is not under the patient's control, while mobilization is a passive movement technique in which the patient can control the movement.

Mann-Whitney *U*-Test: Test on rank-ordered data of the hypothesis of difference between two independent random samples. The independent t-test is its ordinal likeness.

manual therapy: A broad group of skilled hand movements used by the physical therapist to mobilize soft tissues and joints for the purpose of modulating pain, increasing range of motion, reducing or eliminating soft tissue inflammation, inducing relaxation, improving contractile and noncontractile tissue extensibility, and improving pulmonary function.

marketing: Managerial process by which individuals and groups obtain what they want by creating and exchanging products, services, or ideas with others.

mass: Amount of space an object takes up without regard to gravity; a kinematic measurement.

massage: Manipulation of the soft tissues of the body for the purpose of effecting the nervous, muscular, respiratory, and circulatory systems.

master care plan: Treatment plan that includes the list of client problems and identifies the treatment team's intervention strategies and responsibilities.

mastery: Achievement of skill to a criterion level of success.

mastication: Chewing; tearing and grinding food with the teeth while it becomes mixed with saliva.

material culture: Artifacts, industry, architecture, and other material aspects of a particular society.

maturation: Sequential unfolding of behavioral and physiological characteristics during development.

maturational theory: Developmental theory that views development as a function of innate factors, which proceed according to a maturational and developmental timetable.

mature group: Members take on all necessary roles, including leadership. The purpose is to balance task accomplishment with need satisfaction of all group members. The therapist is an equal member of this group.

maximal oxygen consumption (max VO_2, maximal oxygen uptake, aerobic capacity): The greatest volume of oxygen used by the cells of the body per unit time.

maximal voluntary ventilation (MVV): The greatest volume of air that can be exhaled in 15 seconds.

maximum heart rate (age predicted): Highest possible heart rate usually achieved during maximal exercise. Maximum heart rate decreases with age and can be estimated as 220 - age.

maximum voluntary contraction (MVC): Greatest amount of tension a muscle can generate and hold only for a moment, as in muscle testing.

McCarron-Dial system (MDS): Assessment used to determine the prevocational, vocational, and residential functioning levels of individuals with disabilities and the general population.

Meals on Wheels: Program designed to deliver hot meals to the elderly, individuals with physical disabilities, or other people who lack the resources to provide for themselves with nutritionally adequate warm meals on a daily basis.

mean (x): Arithmetic average. Measure of central tendency.

meatus: Passage or opening within the body.

mechanical advantage (MA): In kinesiology, the ratio of amount of effort expended to work performed. MA = length of force arm/length of resistance arm.

mechanical efficiency: Amount of external work performed in relation to the amount of energy required to perform the work; equal to force arm/resistance arm.

mechanical modalities: A broad group of agents that use distraction, approximation, or compression to produce a therapeutic effect.

mechanical ventilation: The use of a respirator for external support of breathing and the use of an ambu bag to mechanically inflate the lungs.

mechanics: The study of physical forces.

mechanism of labor: Describes the five positions that the fetal head assumes through the pelvis: descent, flexion, internal rotation, extension, and external restitution.

mechanistic view (reductionism): Belief that a person is passive and that his or her behavior must be controlled or shaped by the society or environment in which he or she functions. Supports that the mind and body should be viewed separately and that the human being, like a machine, can be taken apart and reassembled if its structure and function are sufficiently well understood.

meconium: Fetal bowel movements.

medial: In terms of anatomical position, located closer to the midline of the body.

medial longitudinal fasciculus (MLF): Pathway in the brainstem that connects the vestibular system with the cranial nerves that serve the eye muscles (III, IV, VI).

median (Mdn): The value or score that most closely represents the middle of a range of scores.

mediastinum: The mass of tissues and organs separating the two lungs, between the sternum in front and the vertebral column behind, and from the thoracic inlet above to the diaphragm below. It contains the heart and its large vessels, trachea, esophagus, thymus, lymph nodes, and other structures and tissues.

Medicaid: U. S. federally funded, state-operated program of medical assistance to people with low incomes, regardless of age.

medical skinfold caliper: Instrument used to measure body fat.

Medicare: U. S. federally funded health insurance program for the elderly, certain people with disabilities, and most individuals with end-stage renal disease, funded by Title VIII of the Social Security Act.

Medicare Part A: Hospital insurance program of Medicare, which covers hospital inpatient care, care in skilled nursing facilities, and home health care.

Medicare Part B: Supplemental medical insurance program of Medicare, which covers hospital outpatient care, physician fees, home health care, comprehensive outpatient rehabilitation facility fees, and other professional services.

medicine ball: Heavy exercise ball used to increase strength and coordination of a client.

medium work: Exerting up to 20 to 50 pounds of force occasionally, 10 to 25 lbs of force frequently, or greater than negligible up to 10 pounds of force constantly to move objects.

MEDLINE: National Library of Medicine computer database that covers approximately 600,000 references to biomedical journal articles published currently and in the 2 preceding years.

megabyte: 1000 kilobytes or 1,000,000 bytes of electronic information; measure of the capacity of memory, disk storage, etc.

meiosis: Sperm and ova are produced by the reduction division process. Each contain only half of the parent cell's original compliment of chromosomes (23 in humans).

melatonin: Hormone produced by the pineal gland and secreted into the bloodstream.

memory: The mental process that involves registration and encoding, consolidation and storage, and recall and retrieval of information.

memory processes: Strategies for dealing with information that is under the individual's control.

memory structure: Unvarying physical or structural components of memory.

menarche: First menstrual period of a female; usually occurs between 9 and 17 years of age.

menopause: Period of life in women marking the end of the reproductive cycle; accompanied by cessation of menstruation for 1 year, decreases in hormonal levels, and alteration of the reproductive organs.

menstruation: Periodic discharge of a bloody fluid from the uterus through the vagina occurring at more or less regular intervals from puberty to menopause.

mental retardation: Significantly subaverage general intellectual functioning concurrent with deficits in adaptive behavior and manifested during the developmental period.

mental status exam: Any diagnostic procedure used to evaluate intellectual, emotional, psychological, and personality functions.

mesoderm: Middle layer of cells that develops from the inner cell mass of the blastocyst, eventually becoming the muscles, the bones, the circulatory system, and the inner layer of the skin.

mesothelioma: A tumor developed from mesothelial tissue.

metabolic acidosis: Metabolic environment of acidity. A pathologic condition resulting from accumulation of acid or loss of base in the body and characterized by an increase in hydrogen ion concentration (decrease in pH).

metabolic alkalosis: A pathologic condition resulting from the accumulation of base or loss of acid in the body and characterized by a decrease in hydrogen ion concentration (increase in pH).

metabolic equivalent level (MET): Method used to measure endurance levels; represents the energy requirements needed to maintain metabolic functioning as well as perform varying activities. It is an abbreviation for oxygen consumption during activities. The greater the exertion, the greater the METs required for an activity.

metabolism: The sum of all physical and chemical processes by which living organized substance is produced and maintained, and also the transformation by which energy is made available for the uses of the organism. The term also describes the process by which the body inactivates drugs. Synonym: biotransformation.

metaethics: Branch of philosophy that examines similarities in ways decisions between right and wrong are made.

meta-analysis: Type of research in which previous research studies are examined to determine outcome trends.

microbacteria: A genus of micro-organism made up of gram-positive rods, found in dairy products, and characterized by relatively high resistance to heat.

microcephalous: Condition in which an atypically small skull results in brain damage and mental retardation.

microchip: Electronic device that consists of thousands of electronic circuits, such as of transistors on a small sliver or chip of plastic. Such devices are the building blocks of computers. Synonym: integrated circuit.

microcomputer: Medium-sized computer that usually serves as a central computer for many individuals. Used primarily in academic and research settings.

microneurography: A technique for the recording of action potentials from individual peripheral nerve fibers.

micturition: The act of urinating.

midwives: Attendants who assist women during labor and delivery.

migraine: Headache associated with periodic instability of the cranial arteries; may be accompanied by nausea.

milieu therapy: Treatment in which the environment is designed to provide specific levels of feedback.

mind-body relationship: The effect of the mind (and mental disorders) on the body and the effect of the body (and physical disorders) on the mind.

minimal brain damage (MBD): Superficial damage to the brain that cannot be detected using objective instruments. Such damage is usually assessed from deviations in behavior.

minimal risk: The probability and magnitude that harm and discomfort anticipated in the research are not greater in and of themselves than those ordinarily encountered in daily life or during the performance of routine physical or psychological examinations or tests.

minimal supervision: Contact provided on an as needed basis; may be less than monthly.

minority group: Group differing, especially in race, religion, or ethnic background, from the majority of a population.

minute ventilation: The volume of air inspired and exhaled in 1 minute. The highest minute ventilation achieved during exercise is also called the *maximum breathing capacity*.

miscarriage: Spontaneous delivery/abortion of a fetus.

mission statement: Statement of purpose of an agency or organization.

mitogen: A substance that stimulates cell division (ie, mitosis) in lymphocytes.

mitosis: Cell duplication and division that generates all of an individual's cells except for the sperm and ova.

mnemonics: Memory-enhancing, learning techniques that link a new concept to an established one.

mobile arm support: Frictionless arm support that is mounted to a wheelchair, table, or belt around the waist and uses gravity in an inclined plane to assist movement of the arms when the shoulder and elbow muscles are weak.

mobility sphere: Territory within which individuals regularly travel in their daily activity patterns. Its dimensions depend on distances that the person can travel by ambulation or available modes of transportation, as well as on the accessibility features of the environment.

mobilization: A passive therapeutic movement at the end of the available range of motion at variable amplitudes and speed.

modality: A broad group of agents that may include thermal, acoustic, radiant, mechanical, or electrical energy to produce physiologic changes in tissues for therapeutic purposes.

mode (Mo): Value or score in a set of scores that occurs most frequently.

model: An approach, framework, or structure that organizes knowledge to guide reasonable decision making.

modeling: Process by which a behavior is learned through observation and imitation of others.

modem: Device that enables communication between two computers via the telephone line signals.

modernization theory: Theory that looks at how a society is organized as a basis for how older adults are treated.

modulation: A variation in levels of excitation and inhibition over sensory and motor neural pools.

molecular pharmacology: The study of interaction of drugs and subcellular entities.

molding: The shaping of the fetal head by the overlapping fetal skull bones to adjust to the size and shape of the birth canal.

monitoring: Determining a client's status on a periodic or ongoing basis.

monocular: Pertaining to one eye.

monocyte: A circulating phagocytic leukocyte that can differentiate into a macrophage upon migration into tissue.

mood: Pervasive and sustained emotion that, when extreme, can color one's whole view of life; generally refers to either elation or depression.

morbidity: Illness or abnormal condition.

mores: Very strong norms; often laws.

morphogenesis: The morphological transformation, including growth, alterations of germinal layers, and differentiation of cells and tissues, during development.

mortality: Being subject to death.

motivation: Individual drives toward the mastery of certain goals and skills; may be intrinsic or involve inducements and incentives.

motivational theory: Theory in which motivation is described as an arousal to action, initiating molding and sustaining specific action patterns. Certain reinforcers may be used to increase or decrease motivation. Internal rewards appear to be better motivators than extrinsic ones.

motor control: The ability of the central nervous system to control or direct the neuromotor system in purposeful movement and postural adjustment by selective allocation of muscle tension across appropriate joint segments.

motor coordination: Functions that are traditionally defined as motoric. Includes gross motor, fine motor, and motor planning functions.

motor deficit: Lack or deficiency of normal motor function that may be the result of pathology or other disorder. Weakness, paralysis, abnormal movement patterns, abnormal timing, coordination, clumsiness, involuntary movements, or abnormal postures may be manifestations of impaired motor function (motor control and motor learning).

motor development: Growth and change in the ability to do physical activities, such as walking, running, or riding a bike.

motor dysfunction/deficit/disorder/disturbance: Generic terms for any type of disorder found in learning and pathology leading to problems in movement in disabled children that have a motor component.

motor function: The ability to learn or demonstrate the skillful and efficient assumption, maintenance, modification, and control of voluntary postures and movement patterns.

motor lag: A prolonged latent period between the reception of a stimulus and the initiation of the motor response.

motor learning: The acquisition of skilled movement based on previous experience. A set of processes associated with practice or experience leading to relatively permanent changes in the capability for producing skilled action.

motor neuron: A nerve cell that sends signals from the brain to the muscles throughout the body.

motor planning: The ability to organize and execute movement patterns to accomplish a purposeful activity.

motor skill: The ability to execute coordinated motor actions with proficiency.

motor strip: Precentral sulci in the brain that control movement of all muscles.

motor time (MT): In a reaction time (RT) test, the time from the onset of electromyographic activity to the initiation of the movement.

motor unit: One alpha motor neuron, its axon, and all muscle fibers attached to that axon.

mouse: A device that moves on a horizontal plane and controls the cursor on a computer monitor.

mouthstick: Assistive device; tool that has a mouthpiece with a pen, pencil, eraser, or paintbrush attached to it. It can also be used to push the buttons on a computer keyboard.

movement decomposition: Distortion of voluntary movement in which the movement occurs in a distinct sequence of isolated steps, rather than in a normal, smooth, flowing pattern.

movement speed: The time elapsed between the initiation of a movement and its completion.

mucous plug: An accumulation of mucous in lung diseases or a plug produced by the endocervical glands to seal the cervical canal and extruded from the vagina in early labor.

multicultural counseling: Process in which a therapist from one ethnic or racial background interacts with a person of a different background in order to assist in the psychological and interpersonal development and adjustment to the dominant culture.

multiculturalism: Awareness and knowledge about human diversity in ways that are translated into more respectful human interactions and effective interconnections.

multidimensional maps: Pictures of self and environment that are created within the central nervous system after receipt and analysis of multisensory input.

multidisciplinary team: Health care workers who are members of different disciplines, each one providing specific services to the patient/client.

multigenerational model: Model of family therapy that focuses on reciprocal role relationships over a period of time and thus takes a longitudinal approach.

multigravida: A woman who has completed two or more pregnancies to the stage of viability.

multi-infarct dementia: Form of organic brain disease characterized by the rapid deterioration of intellectual functioning and caused by vascular disease.

multilingual: Speaking many languages fluently.

multiparity: Refers to a condition of having two or more children.

multiparous: Refers to having given birth to two or more offspring in separate pregnancies.

multiple myeloma: Primary malignant tumor of the plasma cells usually arising in bone marrow.

multiple regression: Making predictions of one variable (using the multiple R) based on measures of two or more others.

multiple sleep latency test: Test that measures the degree of daytime sleepiness and rapid eye movement (REM) sleep of an individual.

multiskilled practitioner: Person from one profession who has established competence in specific skills usually associated with another profession.

murmur: A gentle blowing auscultatory sound caused by friction between parts, a prolapse of a valve, or an aneurysm.

muscle endurance: Sustained muscular contraction measured as repetitions of submaximal contraction (isotonic) or submaximal holding time (isometric).

muscle fiber types: Classification of muscle fibers based on anatomic, physiologic, and functional characteristics.

muscle performance: Execution or accomplishment of a movement resulting from muscle activity for effective, coordinated functioning.

muscle spindles: Sensory receptors in the tendons of muscles that monitor tension of muscles.

muscle strength: Nonspecific term relating to muscle contraction, often referring to the force generated by a single maximal isometric contraction.

muscle testing: Method of evaluating the contractile unit, including the muscle, tendons, and associated tissues, of a moving part of the body by neurologic or resistance testing.

muscle tone: The amount of tension or contractibility among the motor units of a muscle; often defined as the resistance of a muscle to stretch or elongation.

muscle weakness: Lack of the full tension-producing capability of a muscle needed to maintain posture and create movement.

muscular atrophies: Diseases of unknown etiology that are caused by the breakdown of cells in the anterior horn of the spinal cord.

muscular system: Framework of voluntarily controlled skeletal muscles in the body.

musculoskeletal: System in the human body that is associated with the muscles and the bones to which they attach.

mutability: The muscle fiber's ability to change in response to a new demand.

mutation: An error in gene replication that results in a change in the molecular structure of genetic material.

mutual support group: Type of group in which members organize to solve their own problems, usually led by the group members themselves who share a common goal and use their own strengths to gain control over their lives.

myalgia: Pain in a muscle or muscles.

myelin: A fat-like substance forming the principle component of the sheath of nerve fibers in the central nervous system.

myelination: The process of forming the "white" lipid covering of nerve cell axons; myelin increases the conduction velocity of the neuronal impulse and forms the "white matter" of the brain and spinal cord.

myelitis: Inflammation of the spinal cord with associated motor and sensory dysfunction.

myelography: Radiograph process used to view spinal lesions in the subarachnoid space after injection with dye or air.

myelopathy: A general term denoting functional disturbances and/or pathological changes in the brain.

myoclonus: Sudden, quick spasms of a muscle or group of muscles.

myoelectric prosthesis: Artificial limb that is operated electronically using the client's remaining muscle function.

myofascial release (MFR): Techniques used to release fascial tissue restrictions secondary to tonal dysfunction and decrease binding down of the fascia around a muscle.

myokymia: Continual irregular twitching of a muscle often seen around the eye in the facial region.

myoma: Benign tumor consisting of muscle tissue.

myometrium: Fixed, smooth muscle forming the middle layer of the uterine wall.

myopathy: Abnormal muscle function.

myorrhaphy: Suture of a muscle.

myosin: A protein in muscles.

myotasis: Stretching of muscle.

myringoplasty: Reconstruction of the eardrum.

myringotomy: Puncture of the eardrum with evacuation of fluids from the middle ear.

myxoma: A tumor composed of mucous tissue.

N **narcissism:** Egocentricity; dominant interest in one's self.

narcolepsy: Chronic sleep disorder manifested by excessive and overwhelming daytime sleepiness.

narrative: The interpretation of events through stories.

narrative documentation: System of documentation that uses summary paragraphs to describe evaluation data and treatment progress.

narrative reasoning: An aspect of clinical reasoning requiring an understanding of "life stories" of patients/clients.

national health insurance: Form of insurance sponsored by a national government intended to pay for health services used by its citizens.

natural environments: All integrated community settings.

naturalistic observation: Technical term that refers to a qualitative research technique of observing an individual in his or her natural environment.

natural killer cell (NK): A large granular lymphocyte capable of killing certain tumor and virally infected cells.

natural kinds: Method of grouping objects, usually animals, based on common external characteristics that are intrinsic to all members of that category.

nature/nurture controversy: Debate over the extent to which inborn, hereditary characteristics as compared to life experiences and environmental factors determine a person's identity and psychological makeup.

natriuresis: The excretion of sodium in the urine.

nebulizer: An atomizer; a device for throwing a spray or mist.

neck extension splint: Holds the neck extended and prevents the fusion of the chin to the chest.

neck righting reflex: Involuntary response in newborns in which turning the head to one side while the infant is supine causes rotation of the shoulders and trunk in the same direction. The reflex enables the child to roll over from supine to prone position.

necrosis: Death of tissue usually resulting in gangrene.

necrotic: Dead; avascular.

needs assessment: Systematic gathering of information about strengths, problems, resources, and barriers in a given population or community. Results of needs assessment are the basis of program planning.

negative reinforcement: Removing an aversive stimulus following an inappropriate response.

negligence: Commission of an act that a prudent person would not have done or the omission of a duty that a prudent person would have fulfilled, resulting in injury or harm to another person. It may be the basis for a malpractice suit.

neocerebellum: Those parts of the cerebellum that receive input via the corticopontocerebellar pathway.

neologism: A new, meaningless word, often spoken by fluent aphasic clients.

neonate: Represents the first 4 weeks of an infant's life.

nephrotoxicity: The quality of being toxic or destructive to kidney cells.

nerve conduction tests: Measurement of electrical conductivity of motor and sensory nerves by application of an external electrical stimulus to the nerve and evaluation of parameters such as nerve conduction time, velocity, amplitude, and shape of the resulting response as recorded from another site on the nerve or from a muscle supplied by the nerve.

nervous system: The network of neural tissues in the body comprised of the central and peripheral divisions, which are responsible for the processing of impulses.

network: Communication link between computers, a central computer, and users, or any group of computers that are connected in order to send messages to each other.

networking: Process that links people and information in order to accomplish objectives; often informal.

neuralgia: Attacks of pain along the entire course or branch of a peripheral sensory nerve.

neurapraxia: Interruption of nerve conduction without loss of continuity of the axon.

neuritic plaque: Normative age-related change in the brain involving the collection of amyloid protein on dying or dead neurons. A discrete structure found outside the neuron that is composed of degenerating small axons, some dendrites, astrocytes, and amyloid. Also known as *senile plaque*.

neuritis: Condition causing a dysfunction of a cranial or spinal nerve; in sensory nerves, paresthesia is present.

neuroanatomy: Structures within the central, peripheral, and autonomic nervous systems.

neurobehavioral approach: Analysis of tactile, kinesthetic, visual, auditory, and olfactory sensations and their required motor, visual, and verbal responses for each activity. Neurological integration of the input from the senses and muscular responses are included.

neuroblastoma: A malignant tumor of the nervous system composed chiefly of neuroblasts.

neurodevelopment: The progressive growth and development of the nervous system.

neurofibrillary tangle (NFT): A darkly stained, thick, and twisted band of material found in the cytoplasm of aging neurons. Associated with dementias of the Alzheimer's type.

neurofibromatosis: Growth of multiple tumors from the nerve sheath (ie, von Recklinghausen's disease).

neurogenic pain: Pain in the limbs caused by neurologic lesions.

neurography: The study of the action potentials of nerves.

neurohypophysis: The posterior lobe of the pituitary gland.

neuroleptic: Drug or agent that modifies psychotic behavior; antipsychotic.

neurologic impairment: Any disability caused by damage to the central nervous system (brain, spinal cord, ganglia, and nerves).

neurologist: Specialist who diagnoses and treats diseases of the nervous system.

neurolysis: Destruction of nerve tissue or loosening of adhesions surrounding a nerve.

neuroma: Tumor or growth along the course of a nerve or at the end of a lacerated nerve, which is often very painful.

neuromechanism: A neurologic system whose component parts work together to produce central nervous system function.

neuromuscular: Pertaining to the nerves and the muscles.

neuromuscular facilitation: Increasing the activity of the muscles through sensory stimuli.

neuromuscular inhibition: Decreasing the activity of the muscles through the specific application of sensory stimuli.

neuromuscular re-education: Specific treatment regimens provided by occupational and physical therapists to improve motor strength and coordination in persons with brain or spinal cord injuries.

neuron: Nerve cell.

neuronal sprouting: The process of regrowing a neuronal process (eg, an axon, in an injured neuron, attempting to re-establish innervation with a target structure).

neuropathy: Any disease or dysfunction of the nerves.

neuropharmacology: The study of the effects of drugs on the brain.

neuroplasty: Surgical repair of nerves.

neurosis: Mental disorder in which reality testing is not seriously disturbed, but the individual is fearful or overly anxious about various elements of his or her life.

neurosyphilis: Syphilis of the central nervous system.

neurotic: Analytic concept that reflects psychodynamic conflicts that cause difficulty for an individual to remain in contact with reality.

neurotmesis: Damage to the axon or complete transection of a nerve. Regeneration is less successful than in axonotmesis.

neurotransmitters: Chemical substances that are released from presynaptic cells and travel across the synapse to stimulate or inhibit postsynaptic cells, thereby facilitating or inhibiting neural transmission.

neurotrophic: Nutrition and maintenance of tissues as regulated by nervous influence.

neutrophil: A phagocytic leukocyte characterized by a multilobed nucleus and many intracellular granules.

nociceptor: A peripheral nerve ending that appreciates and transmits painful or injurious stimuli.

nominal (or categorical) data: Numbers are utilized to name mutually exclusive categories.

nominal scales: Measurement scales that contain information that is categorical and mutually exclusive (ie, it can only be contained in one category).

nonfenestrated trach: The inability to create an opening through the trachea.

nonhuman environment: Everything that is not human.

nonjudgmental acceptance: Therapist or group therapist lets the client know that his or her ideas and thoughts will be valued and not rejected.

nonmaleficence: Obligation to avoid doing harm to another individual or creating a circumstance in which harm could occur.

nonmaterial culture: Nontangible aspects of a society, such as language, knowledge, skills, beliefs, and values.

nonparametrics: Statistical tests that do not predict the population parameter, μ, or normality of the underlying population distribution.

nonrapid eye movement (NREM): Sleep state in which brain waves become slower and less regular.

norepinephrine: A hormone secreted by the adrenal medulla in response to splanchnic stimulation and stored in the chromaffin granules, being released predominantly in response to hypotension. Stimulates the sympathetic nervous system.

normal curve: When scores and frequency of occurrence are plotted on the x and y axes, respectively, this frequency distribution curve ensues.

normality: Range of behavior considered acceptable by a social group or culture.

normative ethics: Examination of daily debates between group members about what is right and what is wrong.

norm-referenced test: Any instrument that uses the typical scores of members of a comparison group as a standard for determining individual performance.

norms: Standards of comparison derived from measuring an attribute across many individuals to determine typical score ranges.

nosocomial: Diseases originating in hospitals.

noticing: Act of knowing; awareness of critical issues.

novitiate: Beginning stages or apprenticeship within a professional career.

noxious: Harmful to health; injurious (eg, noxious gas, noxious stimuli).

nuchal rigidity: Reflex spasm of the neck extensor muscles resulting in resistance to cervical flexion.

null hypothesis: In research, a hypothesis that predicts that no difference or relationship exists among the variables studied that could not have occurred by chance alone.

nyctalopia: The inability to see well in faint light or at night.

nystagmus: Rhythmic, constant, and rapid involuntary movement of the eyeball. A series of automatic, back-and-forth eye movements. Different conditions produce this reflex. A common way of producing nystagmus is by an abrupt stop following a series of rotations of the body. The duration and regularity of postrotary nystagmus are some of the indicators of vestibular system efficiency.

O **objective measure:** Method of assessment that is not influenced by the emotions or personal opinion of the assessor.

object relations: In psychoanalytic theory, the investment of psychic energy in objects and events in the world; sometimes seen exclusively as the bond(s) between two persons.

obligatory reflexive response: Reflex that is consciously present in a motor pattern; this reflex may dominate all other movement components.

observer bias: When the previous experiences of the individual influence his or her observations and interpretation of behaviors being assessed or evaluated.

obsession: Irresistible thought pattern, usually anxiety provoking, which intrudes on normal thought processes.

obsessive-compulsive disorder: Anxiety disorder characterized by recurrent uncontrollable thoughts, irresistible urges to engage repetitively in an act, or both, such that they cause significant anxiety or interfere with daily functioning.

obtrusive observation: When the individual is aware of being observed by the therapist for the purpose of evaluation of cognitive, physical, and/or psychosocial performance.

occipitofrontal: A line from the root of the nose to the most prominent portion of the occipital bone of the fetus at term.

occipitomental: Diameter from the chin of the fetus to the most prominent portion of the occipital bone; the correct angle for the application of forceps during delivery.

occiput anterior: Fetal occiput to the mother's symphysis pubis.

occupational capacity evaluation: Assessment of the match between the person's capabilities and the critical demands of a specific job.

occupational performance areas: Tasks related to self-care/self-maintenance, work/education, play/leisure, and rest/relaxation.

occupational performance component: Any subsystem that contributes to the performance of self-care/self-maintenance, work/education, play/leisure, and rest/relaxation.

occupational therapy (OT): Therapeutic use of self-care, work, and play activities to increase independent function, enhance development, and prevent disability. May include adaptation of a task or environment to achieve maximum independence and to enhance the quality of life. The American Occupational Therapy Association's definition can be found at www.aota.org. According to the AOTA's position paper, *Occupational Performance: Occupational Therapy's Definition of Function,* OT is a health profession that helps people address challenges or difficulties that threaten or impair their ability to perform activities and tasks that are basic to the fulfillment of their roles as worker, parent, spouse or partner, sibling, and friend to self or others.

occupational therapy aide: According to the American Occupational Therapy Association's position paper, *Use of Occupational Therapy Aides in OT Practice,* this is an individual assigned by an occupational therapy practitioner to perform delegated, selected, skilled tasks in specific situations under the direction and close supervision of an occupational therapy practitioner.

ocular dysmetria: The eyes are unable to fix on an object or follow a moving object with accuracy.

oculomotor: Pertains to movement of the eyeballs.

old age: Arbitrary or societally defined period of life; specifically, over 65 years of age in the United States.

older person: Term used to refer to individuals in the later years of the life span. Arbitrarily set between 65 and 70 years old in American society for the purpose of age-related entitlements.

oldest old: Persons over 85 years of age.

old old: Persons over 75 years of age.

olfactory: Pertaining to the sense of smell.

oligoclonal banding: A process by which cerebrospinal fluid IgG is distributed, following electrophoresis, in discrete bands. Approximately 90% of clients with multiple sclerosis show oligoclonal banding.

oligodendroglia: Myelin-producing cells in the central nervous system.

oligomenorrhea: Longer intervals between menstrual periods from 38 days to 3 months.

oliguria: Diminished amount of urine formation and excretion.

ombudsman: An official appointed to receive and investigate complaints made by individuals against public officials and institutions.

one-tail (directional) test: A test of the null hypothesis in which only one tail of the distribution is utilized.

on-line: Monitor linked to an off-site computer.

onlooker play: Level of social play in which a child watches other children at play. The child may verbally interact but does not participate in the activity.

on-screen keyboard: Virtual keyboard provided on the computer monitor by specific software. An individual can then touch the on-screen keyboard with an alternate access device, such as an optical scanner or head pointer.

on-the-job evaluation: Assesses the physical demands, psychosocial factors, cognitive factors, analysis of essential functions, tools and machines used, description of the work environment, and hazards and stress factors in a competitive employment situation, as well as the person's ability to perform under such circumstances.

ontogeny: Course of development during an individual's lifetime.

onychia: Inflammation of the nail bed.

onychogryphosis: Ingrown nail, either finger or toe.

onychosis: Any disease of the nails.

oocyte: A primitive cell in the ovary that becomes an ovum after meiosis.

open-chain movements: The distal end of a kinetic chain moves.

open-ended question: Question that may have multiple correct responses rather than a finite correct answer.

open enrollment period: Period of time in which new subscribers may elect to enroll in a health insurance plan.

open system: System of structures that functions as a whole and maintains itself by means of input from the environment and organismic change occurring as needed.

operant conditioning: A form of conditioning in which positive or negative reinforcement is contingent upon the occurrence of the desired response.

ophthalmoplegia: Paralysis of ocular muscles.

opioid: Terminology used to refer to synthetic drugs that have pharmacological properties similar to opium or morphine.

opisthotonos: Position of extreme hyperextension of the vertebral column caused by a tetanic spasm of the extensor musculature.

opposition: The movement in which the thumb is brought across to meet the little finger.

Optacon: Camera that allows blind people to read by converting print to an image of letters, which are then produced onto the finger using vibrations.

optical character recognition: Technology used in scanning to convert the images of typed text into a computer code (ie, translating the analog signal from the voltage of reflected light to a digital value readable by the computer).

optical pointers: Devices that sense light and feedback the stimulus to indicate in which direction the device is pointing.

optokinetic nystagmus: Nystagmus induced by watching stripes on a drum revolving around one's face.

oral defensiveness: Avoidance of certain textures of food and irritation with activities using the mouth.

oral-motor control: Coordinated ability of opening and closing the mouth and being able to manage chewing, swallowing, and speaking.

order: The desired state of affairs, which is an absence of disease in medicine and competence in the performance of work, play, or self-care. Disorder is defined as a disease in medicine and performance dysfunction.

ordinal data: Rank-ordered data.

ordinal scales: Measurement scales that contain information that can be rank ordered.

ordinate: In the coordinate system, the ordinate is the vertical axis. Synonym: y axis.

organismic view: Concept that an individual is active in determining and controlling his or her own behavior and can change that behavior if it is desirous to do so.

organization: Group of individuals organized for the attainment of a common goal.

organizational patterns: Hierarchic patterns of personnel ranking that indicate the underlying chain of command in an organization.

orgasm: The apex and culmination of sexual excitement.

orientation: The initial stage of group development, which includes a search for structure, goals, and dependency on the leader.

origin: Proximal attachment of a muscle that remains relatively fixed during normal muscular contraction.

orthokinetic cuff: Device made from an elastic bandage applied to a weak muscle to provide tactile stimulation to the muscle via movement of the cuff-skin interface during muscle contraction.

orthopedic: Branch of medical science that deals with the prevention or correction of disorders involving locomotor structures of the body.

orthopedic impairment: Any disability caused by disorders to the musculoskeletal system.

orthopnea: The inability to breathe except in an upright position.

orthosis/orthotic: Device added to a person's body to support, position, or immobilize a part; correct deformities; assist weak muscles and restore function; or modify tone.

orthostatic hypotension: A dramatic fall in the blood pressure when a patient assumes an upright position, usually caused by a disturbance of vasomotor control decreasing the blood supply returning to the heart.

orthotic: An external device utilized to apply forces to a body part to limit movement, increase the velocity or power of a movement, stop movement, or hold the body part in a particular position. Previously called a *brace*.

orthotics: External devices used to support and correct deformities or add stability to enhance control and function.

oscilloscope: Instrument that displays a visual representation of an electrical wave, such as a muscle contraction.

osmosis: The passage of pure solvent from the lesser to the greater concentration when two solutions are separated by a membrane, which selectively prevents the passage of solute molecules but is permeable to the solvent. An attempt to equalize concentrations on both sides of a membrane.

osteoblast: Any cell that develops into bone or secretes substances producing bony tissue.

osteochondrosis: A disease of one or more of the growth or ossification centers in children that begins as a degeneration or necrosis followed by regeneration or recalcification.

osteoclast: Any of the large multinucleate cells in bone that absorb or break down bony tissue.

osteokinematics: Gross angular motions of the shafts of bones in sagittal, frontal, and transverse planes.

osteoplasty: Plastic surgery of the bones; bone grafting.

osteotomy: Operation to cut across a bone.

otitis media: Inflammation of the inner ear, which usually causes dizziness.

otosclerosis: Hardening of the bony tissue of the ear, resulting in conductive hearing loss.

ougenics movement: Set of policies from the early 1900s that viewed people with disabilities as "defectives" and "deviates."

outcome: The way something turns out; result; consequence. Outcomes are the result of patient/client management. They relate to remediation of functional limitation and disability, primary or secondary prevention, and optimization of patient/client satisfaction.

outcome analysis: A systematic examination of patient/client outcomes in relation to selected patient/client variables (eg, age, sex, diagnosis, interventions performed); outcome analysis may be used in quality assessment, economic analysis of practice, and other processes.

outcome measure: Instrument designed to gather information on the efficacy of service programs; a means for determining if goals or objectives have been met.

out-of-pocket payment or costs: Costs borne solely by an individual without the benefit of insurance.

outpatient services: Ambulatory care provided in outpatient departments of health facilities.

outreach services: Services that seek out and identify hard-to-reach individuals and assist them in gaining access to needed services.

outrigger: Projecting support attached to a splint from which finger loops are suspended.

overflow: Clinical term for unwanted movement in a part of the body inappropriate to the action being performed.

overuse syndrome: Musculoskeletal disorder manifested from repetitive upper extremity movements occurring during activities. Symptoms include persistent pain in joints, muscles, tendons, or other soft tissues of the upper extremities. Synonyms: cumulative trauma disorder, repetitive strain disorder.

ovoid of motion: The curved path of motion through which a bone moves. It is always convex away from the joint at which motion occurs.

oximeter: A photoelectric device for determining the oxygen saturation of the blood.

oxygen consumption (VO$_2$): The amount of oxygen used by the tissues of the body, usually measured in oxygen uptake in the lung; normally about 250 mL/minute and it increases with increased metabolic rate. The difference between the oxygen inspired and the oxygen exhaled is the amount of oxygen used. Maximum oxygen consumption is the highest amount of oxygen used during exercise (VO$_{2MAX}$). The oxygen consumption will not increase even if the exercise intensity increases. This value is often used to measure maximal exercise capacity.

oxygen saturation: The degree to which oxygen is present in a particular cell, tissue, organ, or system.

oxytocin: A hormone stored in the pituitary that causes contraction of the uterus.

p

pacemaker: Electrical device implanted to control the beating of the heart.

pachymeningitis: Acute inflammation of the duramater.

pacing: Accommodating for time in a test or treatment session; the rate at which instruction is given or practice is provided.

pain: A sensation of hurting or strong discomfort in some part of the body caused by an injury, disease, or functional disorder and transmitted through the nervous system.

pain character measurements: Any of the tools used to define the character of a patient's/client's pain.

pain estimate: A pain intensity measurement in which a patient's/client's pain is rated on a scale of 0 to 100.

pain intensity measurements: Any of the scales used to quantify pain intensity.

pain management: Use of treatment to control chronic pain, including the use of behavioral modification, relaxation training, physical modalities and agents, medication, and surgery.

pain modulation: Variation in the intensity and appreciation of pain secondary to CNS and ANS affects on the nociceptors and along the pain pathways, as well as secondary to external factors such as distraction and suggestion.

pain pathway: The route along which nerve impulses arising from painful stimuli are transmitted from the nociceptor to the brain, including transmission within the brain itself.

pain quality: A description of the nature, type, or character of pain (eg, burning, dull, sharp, throbbing, etc).

paired *t* ratio: Statistical test between two sample means in which the sample selection is not independent.

pallesthesia: The ability to sense mechanical vibration.

palliative care: Care rendered to temporarily reduce or moderate the intensity of an otherwise chronic medical condition.

pallor: Paleness; absence of skin coloration.

palmar: Palm of the hand.

palpate: To examine by touching or feeling.

palpation: Examination using the hands (eg, palpation of muscle spasm, palpation of the thoracic cage, etc).

palpitation: Rapid, violent, or throbbing pulsation in a body part.

palsy: The loss of movement or ability to control movement.

pancreatitis: Inflammation of the pancreas, with pain and tenderness of the abdomen, tympanites (ie, gaseous pockets), and vomiting.

panic attack: State of extreme anxiety, usually including sweating, shortness of breath, chest pains, and fear. May come on unpredictably or as a result of a particular stimulus.

papilledema: Edema and hyperemia of the optic disc.

paracrine: The method of extracellular hormonal communication.

paracyesis: Pregnancy that develops outside the uterus in the abdominal cavity.

paradigm: Refers to the organization of knowledge, as well as the changes in scientific thought over time; an organizing framework.

paradox: A statement to the contrary of belief. A statement that is self-contradictory and, hence, false.

paraffin bath: A superficial thermal modality using paraffin wax and mineral oil.

parallel processing: Learning or solving a problem through a global approach integrating data into a whole experience.

parallel talk: A form of speech used during play therapy with children in which the clinician verbalizes actions, such as what is happening or what the child is doing without requiring "answers" from the child. For instance, "I'm building a tower. My tower is tall. You're building a tower, too. Your tower is tall, too." The clinician often repeats utterances of the child correctly and parallels the child's activities.

paralysis: Condition in which one loses voluntary motor control over a section of the body due to trauma or injury.

paranodal myelin intussusception: The ultra structural change that occurs at Ranvier's node because of acute focal compression of a nerve, resulting in a neuropraxic lesion.

paranoia: Thought pattern that reflects a belief that others are persecuting or attempting to harm one, in the absence of a realistic basis for such fears.

paraplegia (PARA): Paralysis of the spine affecting the lower portion of the trunk and legs. The impairment or loss of motor and/or sensory function in the thoracic, lumbar, or sacral (but not cervical) segments of the spinal cord secondary to damage of neural elements within the spinal canal.

parasomnia: Abnormal sleep behavior, including sleepwalking and bruxism (ie, grinding the teeth).

parasympathetic nervous system: Autonomic nervous system that serves to relax the body's responses and is the opposite of the sympathetic nervous system.

parasympatholytic: Producing the effects resembling those of interruption of the parasympathetic nerve supply to a part. An agent that opposes the effects of impulses conveyed by the parasympathetic nerves.

parasympathomimetic: Producing effects resembling those of stimulation of the parasympathetic nerve supply to a part. An agent that produces effects similar to those produced by stimulation of the parasympathetic nerves.

paraxial: Lying near the axis of the body.

parenchyma: Essential parts of an organ, which are concerned with its function rather than its framework.

parenteral: Administration by subcutaneous, intramuscular, or intravenous injection, thereby bypassing the gastrointestinal tract.

paresis: Weakness in voluntary muscle with slight paralysis.

paresthesia: Abnormal sensation, such as burning, pricking, tickling, or tingling.

parietoalveolar: Pertaining to the cavities of the alveoli in the lungs.

parity: A condition of having produced viable offspring. The state or condition of being the same in power, value, and rank. Equality.

paroxysm: Sudden, periodic attack, recurrence, or intensification of symptoms of a disease (eg, paroxysmal atrial tachycardia).

partial thickness: Loss of epidermis and possible partial loss of dermis.

participant-observer: Descriptor that can be applied when a therapist observes and evaluates an individual's performance while engaged in an activity with the person.

parturition: The act or process of giving birth.

passive-aggressive personality disorder: Disorder that is characterized by resistance to social and occupational performance demands through procrastination, dawdling, stubbornness, inefficiency, and forgetfulness that appears to border on the intentional.

passive range of motion (PROM): Amount of motion at a given joint when the joint is moved by the therapist.

passive stretch: Stretch applied with external force.

paternalism: Acting or making decisions on behalf of others without their consent.

pathogen: Any disease-producing agent or microorganism.

pathology: The study of the characteristics, causes, and effects of disease, as observed in the structure and function of the body.

pathophysiology: An interruption or interference of normal physiological and developmental processes or structures.

patient management interview: Interview used by multiple professionals to identify the type of intervention or treatment needed.

patient-related consultation: When the health professional shares information with other professionals regarding individuals who are not presently receiving services.

patient/client: A person receiving care or treatment. Individual who is the recipient of physical therapy and direct intervention.

patient's rights: The right of a patient to be informed about his or her conditions and prognoses and to make decisions concerning his or her treatment.

patterned responses: The programs, either preprogrammed or created by the motor system, to succeed at the presented task in the most efficient and integrated response possible at that moment in time.

Paxil: An orally administered antidepressant. Generic name: paroxetine hydrochloride.

Pearson's *r*: Statistical technique that shows the degree of relationship between variables (also called the *product-moment correlation*).

pectus carinatum: Undue prominence of the sternum, called also *chicken* or *pigeon chest/breast*.

pectus excavatum: Undue depression of the sternum, called also *funnel chest* or *breast*.

pedagogy: The art and science of teaching children.

peer culture: Stable set of activities or routines, artifacts, values, and concerns that a group of individuals produce or share.

peer review: Appraisal by professional coworkers of equal status of the way health practitioners conduct practice, education, or research.

pelvic contraction: A condition in which one or more diameters of the pelvis is narrower than normal, not allowing for normal progression of labor.

pelvic floor: A sling arrangement of ligaments and muscles that supports the reproductive organs.

pelvimetry: A method of obtaining pelvic measurements by x-ray.

pendular knee jerk: Upon elicitation of the deep tendon reflex of the knee, the lower leg oscillates briefly like a pendulum after the jerk, instead of returning immediately to resting position.

percent body fat: Percent of body weight that is fat, includes storage fat (expendable), essential fat, and sex-specific fat reserve.

perception: The ability to organize and interpret incoming sensory information.

perceptual-motor: The interaction of the various channels of perception with motor activity, including visual, auditory, tactual, and kinesthetic channels.

perceptual-motor match: The process of comparing and collating the input data received through the motor system and through perception.

perceptual-motor skill: The ability to integrate perceptual (sensory) input with motor output in order to accomplish purposeful activities.

perceptual processing: The ability to integrate and understand perceptual (sensory) input in order to respond appropriately with motor output. The ability to find meaning.

perceptual trace: Memory for past movement; the internal reference of correctness.

percussion (diagnostic): A procedure in which the clinician taps a body part manually or with an instrument to estimate its density.

percussion: A procedure utilized with pulmonary postural drainage to loosen secretions from the bronchial walls.

percutaneous: Administration of a drug by inhalation, sublingual, or topical processes.

per diem rate: Fixed all-inclusive price for 1 day of hospital or nursing facility care, including all supplies and services provided to the patient during that day, excluding the professional fees of nonstaff physicians.

performance areas: Life tasks, such as activities of daily living, work or productive activities, and play or leisure.

performance components: Sensorimotor, cognitive, integration, psychosocial, and psychological skills and abilities.

performance improvement: Planned, systematic, and organization-wide approach to designing, measuring, assessing, and improving organizational performance.

performance subsystem: Subsystem in the Model of Human Occupation that includes neuromuscular skills, process skills, and communication/interaction skills.

perfusion: The act of pouring over or through, especially the passage of a fluid through the vessels of a specific organ or body part.

perinatal: Time period immediately before and after birth.

perineometer: A pressure sensitive device inserted vaginally to measure the strength of pelvic floor muscles.

perineum: The area bounded by the pubis, coccyx, and the thighs, which is between the external genitalia and the anus.

period of concrete operations: Stage in the child's cognitive development in which he or she is bound by immediate physical reality.

peripheral nerve: Any nerve that supplies the peripheral parts and is a branch of the central nervous system (eg, the spinal cord).

peripheral nerve injuries: Loss of precision pinch and grip due to crushing, severance, or inflammation/degeneration of the peripheral nerve fibers.

peripheral nervous system (PNS): Consists of all of the nerve cells outside the central nervous system, including motor and sensory nerves.

peripheral neuropathy: Any functional or organic disorder of the peripheral nervous system; degeneration of peripheral nerves supplying the extremities, causing loss of sensation, muscle weakness, and atrophy.

peripheral pain: Pain arising from injury to a peripheral structure.

peristalsis: Movement by which a tube in the body (primarily the alimentary canal) sends contents within it to another part of the body. This is accomplished through alternative contractions and relaxations, which resemble a wave- or worm-like movement.

peritonitis: Inflammation of the peritoneum; a condition marked by exudations of serum, fibrin, cells, and pus in the peritoneum. It is attended by abdominal pain and tenderness, constipation, vomiting, and moderate fever.

perseveration: The inability to shift from thought to thought; persistence of an idea even when the subject changes.

personal care services: Services performed by health care workers that assist patients in meeting the requirements of daily living.

personal protective equipment (PPE): Accessories provided at the worksite to protect workers from possible injuries and accommodate the physical requirements of workers and the job (eg, gloves, eye wear, vibration and ear protection).

personality: Individual's unique, relatively consistent, and enduring methods of behaving in relation to others and the environment.

personality trait: Distinguishing feature that reflects one's characteristic way of thinking, feeling, and/or adapting.

person-environment fit: Degree to which individuals have adapted to their unique environments.

person-environment interaction: Model proposing that behavior is a function of the person and his or her perceptions of the environment.

persons with disabilities: Individuals who experience substantial limitations in one or more major life activities, including, but not limited to, such functions as performing manual tasks, walking, seeing, hearing, speaking, breathing, learning, and working.

pessary: A circular ring device used to hold a prolapsing uterus in place when surgical repair is contraindicated.

petit mal: Type of seizure characterized by a momentary lapse of consciousness that starts and ends abruptly.

phacoemulsification: Method of treating cataracts by using ultrasonic waves to disintegrate the cataract, which is then aspirated.

phagocytosis: A process by which a leukocyte (monocyte, neutrophil) engulfs, ingests, and degrades a foreign particle or organism.

phalanges: Bones of the fingers and toes.

phantom limb pain: Paresthesia or severe pain felt in the amputated part of a limb.

pharmacodynamics: The study of how drugs affect the body.

pharmacokinetics: The study of how the body handles drugs, including the way drugs are absorbed, distributed, and eliminated.

phenol block: An injection of phenol (ie, hydroxybenzene) into individual nerves. Used as a topical anesthetic and produces a selective block of these nerves. Sometimes used to control severe spasticity in specific muscle groups.

phenotype: Observable characteristics of an organism that result from the interaction of the genotype with the organism's environment.

phenytoin: Anticonvulsant drug used to control major (ie, grand mal) epileptic fits. Common side effects include dizziness, nausea, and skin rashes. Trade name: Dilantin.

phlebitis: Inflammation of a vein.

phlebotomy: Opening or piercing the vein.

phobia: Characterized by an extreme fear of a person, place, or thing when the situation is not hazardous.

phocomelia: The congenital absence or poor development of the proximal portion of the extremities. The hands and feet are thus attached to the trunk by an irregularly formed bone.

phonophoresis: The use of ultrasound waves to drive chemical molecules into the tissues for therapeutic purposes.

phototherapy: Intervention using the application of light.

physical: Pertaining to the body.

physical agent: A form of thermal, acoustic, or radiant energy that is applied to tissues in a systematic manner to achieve a therapeutic effect; a therapeutic modality used to treat physical impairments.

physical agent modalities (PAMS): Modalities, such as hot packs, paraffin, electrical stimulation, and ultrasound, used by qualified practitioners to prepare for or as an adjunct to purposeful activity.

physical demands: Physical requirements made on the worker by the specific job-worker situation. As defined in the *DOT*, there are 20 demands: lifting, standing, walking, sitting, carrying, pushing, pulling, climbing, balancing, stooping, kneeling, crouching, crawling, reaching, handling, fingering, feeling, talking, hearing, and seeing.

physical environment: Part of the environment that can be perceived directly through the senses. The physical environment includes observable space, objects and their arrangement, light, noise, and other ambient characteristics that can be objectively determined.

physical function: Fundamental component of health status describing the state of those sensory and motor skills necessary for mobility, work, and recreation.

physical therapist (PT): A person who is a graduate of an accredited physical therapist education program and is licensed to practice physical therapy whose primary purpose is the promotion of optimal human health and function through the application of scientific principles to prevent, identify, assess, correct, or alleviate acute or prolonged movement dysfunction.

physical therapist assistant: A person who is a graduate of an accredited physical therapist assistant education program and who assists the physical therapist in the provision of physical therapy. The physical therapist assistant may perform physical therapy procedures and related tasks that have been selected and delegated by the supervising physical therapist.

physical therapy: Treatment of injury and disease by mechanical means, such as heat, light, exercise, massage, and mobilization.

physical therapy aide: A nonlicensed worker, trained under the direction of a physical therapist, who performs designated routine physical therapy tasks.

physician assistant: Health professional licensed or, in the case of those employed by the federal government, credentialed to practice medicine with physician supervision.

Physicians' Desk Reference **(PDR):** Provides a listing of medications, including both the trade and generic names, the manufacturing company, the side effects and/or adverse reactions and appropriate interventions, and any incompatible medications.

physiologic flexion: The excessive amount of flexor tone that is normally present at birth because of the existing level of central nervous system maturation and fetal positioning in utero or in adulthood, damage to the central nervous system.

physiology: Area of study concerned with the functions of the structures of the body.

pica: Compulsive eating of nonnutritive substances, like dirt. A bizarre appetite.

pinch meter: Type of dynamometer used to measure the strength of a client's pinch. It can be used to measure tip, lateral, and palmar pinching.

piriformis syndrome: A condition characterized by over activity of the piriformis muscle, causing external rotation of the leg and buttock pain.

Pitocin: A synthetic oxytocic hormone administered through intravenous drip to induce or augment uterine contractions.

placenta: The organ that develops within the uterus from which the fetus derives its nourishment; also serves as a filtering system.

placenta previa: Condition in which the placenta is implanted in the lower segment of the uterus, extending over the cervical opening. This often causes heavy bleeding during labor.

planes of motion: Imaginary lines that divide the body into right and left portions, front and back portions, and top and bottom portions.

plan of care: Statements that specify the anticipated long-term and short-term goals and the desired outcomes, predicted level of optimal improvement, specific interventions to be used, duration, and frequency of the intervention required to reach the goals, outcomes, and criteria for discharge.

plaque: A lesion characterized by loss of myelin and hardening of tissue in diseases such as multiple sclerosis (peripherally) or Alzheimer's disease (in the brain).

plasma cell: Mature antibody-secreting cell derived from the B cell.

plasmapheresis: A process by which blood is removed from the patient/client; plasma is discarded and replaced by normal plasma or human albumin. Reconstituted blood is then returned to the patient/client. This process is believed to rid the blood of antibodies or substances that are damaging.

plasticity: Neuroscience: The ability of the central nervous system to adapt structurally or functionally in response to environmental demands. Anatomical and electrophysiological changes in the central nervous system. Biomechanics: Defined as continued elongation of a tissue without an increase in resistance from within the tissue.

platform crutches: Crutches designed to redirect stress during ambulation from joints in the wrist and hand to the forearm.

play: Choosing, performing, and engaging in an intrinsically motivated activity (attitude or process) that is experienced as pleasurable.

plethysmography: Use of a plethysmograph to measure the volume of a body part.

pleura: The serous membrane investing the lungs and lining the thoracic cavity, completely enclosing a potential space known as the *pleural cavity*. There are two pleurae, right and left, entirely distinct from each other.

pleurisy: Inflammation of the pleural membrane surrounding the lungs. Synonym: pleuritis.

pneumoencephalogram: Radiographic examination of ventricles and subarachnoid spaces of the brain following withdrawal of cerebrospinal fluid and injection of air or gas via lumbar puncture.

pneumonectomy: The excision of lung tissue.

pneumopathology: Any disease involving the respiratory system.

pneumothorax: An accumulation of air or gas in the pleural cavity, which may occur spontaneously or as a result of trauma or a pathological process. It prevents the lung from expanding.

podalic version: Manipulation of a breech fetus presentation internally or externally.

point stimulation: The stimulation of sensitive areas of skin using electricity, pressure, laser, or ice for the purpose of relieving pain.

policy: A principle, law, or decision that guides actions (eg, the sources and distribution of services and funds).

poliomyelitis: Viral infection of the motor cells in the spinal cord.

polycythemia: An excess number of red corpuscles in the blood.

polydrug abuse: Abuse of several psychoactive drugs (eg, alcohol and cocaine).

polyhydramnios: Excess volume of amniotic fluid greater than 2000 mL.

polymyositis: Systemic connective tissue disease characterized by inflammatory and degenerative changes in the muscles. It leads to symmetric weakness and some degree of muscle atrophy; its etiology is unknown.

polyneuritis: Inflammation of many nerves at once.

polyneuropathy: A disease involving several nerves such as that seen in diabetes mellitus.

polyp: Tumor with a stem (pedicle) that projects from a mucous membrane surface.

polypharmacy: The excessive and unnecessary use of medications.

polyradiculopathy: Inflammation of multiple nerve roots.

polysomnogram: Instrument that continuously records an individual's sleep brain waves and a number of nerve and muscle functions while sleeping.

polysomnography: The study of sleep.

population at-risk: Group of people who share a characteristic that causes each member to be vulnerable to a particular event (eg, nonimmunized children exposed to the polio virus).

position in space: A person's awareness of the place of his or her body in space.

position of deformity: Position of hand in which the wrist is flexed, the metacarpals are in hyperextension, the interphalangeal joints are in flexion, and the thumb is adducted. Dorsal edema of the hand fosters this type of hand positioning.

positive reinforcement: Providing a desired reinforcer following an appropriate response.

positron emission tomography (PET): Dynamic brain imaging technique that produces a very detailed image of the brain that can reflect changes in brain activity.

posterior: Toward the back of the body.

postpartum: The period following birth.

postpolio syndrome: Collection of impairments occurring in persons who have had poliomyelitis many years ago; related to chronic mechanical strain of weakened musculature and ligaments.

postrotary nystagmus: Reflexive movement of the eyes that occurs after quick rotational movements have ceased; used to indicate the level of processing of vestibular information.

post-traumatic amnesia: The time elapsed between a brain injury and the point at which the functions concerned with memory are determined to have been restored.

post-traumatic stress disorder (PTSD): Characterized by intense negative feelings or terror in re-experiencing a traumatic or disastrous event either in thoughts, nightmares, or dreams experienced over time. May also include physiological responses such as excessive alertness, the inability to concentrate or follow through on tasks, or difficulty sleeping.

postural alignment: The relationship of all the body parts around the center of gravity. Relationship of one body segment to another in standing, sitting, or any other position. Maintaining biomechanical integrity among body parts; *see also* posture.

postural background movements: The subtle, spontaneous body adjustments that make overt movements of the hands easier (eg, reaching for a distant object). These postural adjustments depend on good vestibular and proprioceptive integration.

postural control: The ability to effectively correct for perturbation of the center of gravity and regain postural alignment without falling. Using righting and equilibrium adjustments to maintain balance during functional movements.

postural drainage: Positioning a person so that gravity aides in the drainage of secretions from the respiratory system.

postural hypotension: *See* orthostatic hypotension.

postural insecurity: Fearfulness of movement or change in posture.

postural tremor: A pathological tremor of 3 to 5 Hz that appears in a limb or the trunk when either is working against the pull of gravity.

posture: The attitude of the body. The position maintained by the body in standing or in sitting. The alignment and positioning of the body in relation to gravity, center of mass, and base of support. In the strictest sense, the position of the body or body part in relation to space and/or other body parts. Functionally, the anticipation of and response to displacement of the body's center of mass.

power: The ability to impose one's will upon the behavior of other persons. The ability to perform work over time.

powered wheelchair: Motorized wheelchair that allows a person to control speed and direction by pushing a button or using a joystick. It enables those without the use of their arms to move their wheelchairs without assistance.

power of attorney: Document authorizing one person to take legal action on behalf of another, acting as an agent for the grantor.

practice settings: Various environments in which physical therapy is rendered, such as acute care, subacute care, rehabilitation settings, skilled nursing facilities, outpatient departments, assisted-living environments, home care, fitness centers, and other community settings.

pragmatics: The study of language as it is used in context.

pragmatism: Practical way of solving problems.

praxis: The ability to conceive and organize a new motor act.

precipitate delivery: An unexpected or sudden birth following a very short labor.

predictive validity: Positive correlation between test scores and future performance.

preeclampsia: Illness of late pregnancy characterized by high blood pressure, swelling, and protein in the mother's urine. Synonym: toxemia.

preferred provider organization (PPO): Acts as a broker between the purchaser of health care and the provider.

preferred practice patterns: Boundaries within which physical therapists may select any number of clinical pathways, based on consideration of a wide variety of factors, such as individual patient/client needs; the profession's code of ethics and standards of practice; and patient/client age, culture, gender roles, race, sex, sexual orientation, and socioeconomic status. Preferred practice patterns for physical therapy are outlined and defined in the *Guide for Physical Therapy Practice* by the American Physical Therapy Association.

prefix: Word element of one or more syllables placed in front of a combining form in order to change its meaning.

pregnancy: Condition of carrying a fertilized ovum (zygote) in the uterus.

prejudice: Unreasonable feelings, opinions, or attitudes directed against a race, religion, or national group.

preload: Conditions in the heart prior to beating (eg, blood pressure, filling volume, etc).

premature: Child born before the 37th week of gestation; birth or infant.

premature rupture of the membranes: Rupture of the amniotic sac before the fetus is at full-term.

premenstrual syndrome (PMS): A set of symptoms that occur monthly after ovulation and usually cease at menstruation or shortly thereafter.

premium: Amount paid to an insurer or third party for insurance coverage under an insurance policy.

premorbid personality: Psychosocial factor referring to personality characteristics that are present before the development of a disease and have either a positive or negative effect on the rehabilitative process.

premotor time (PMT): In a reaction time (RT) test, the time between the stimulus onset to the onset of electromyographic activity.

prenatal period: Time between conception and birth. The body does not change this much again during the entire lifespan as it does in these 38 weeks.

prepaid health plan: An insurance plan provided by health maintenance organizations (HMOs) and competitive medical plans. Preventive and wellness services are available in addition to care for illnesses.

prepared learning: Form of learning to which an individual is biologically predisposed.

presbyastasis: Age-related disequilibrium in the absence of known pathology.

presbycusis: Age-related hearing loss in the absence of pathology.

presbyopia: Age-related farsightedness with the loss in the ability to focus on objects that are near.

presenile: Pertaining to a condition in which a person manifests signs of aging in early or midlife.

presenting part: The part of the fetus that is first engaged in the pelvis.

pressure point: Point over an artery where the pulse may be felt.

pressure sore: An area of localized tissue damage caused by ischemia due to pressure.

prevalence: The total number of persons with a disease in a given population at a given point in time. Prevalence is usually expressed as the percentage of the population that has the disease.

prevention: The act of preventing. Decreasing the risk of disease or disability. Activities that are directed toward slowing or stopping the occurrence of both mental and physical illness and disease, minimizing the effects of a disease or impairment on disability, or reducing the severity or duration of an illness; **primary p.** prevention of the development of disease in a susceptible or potentially susceptible population through such specific measures as general health promotion efforts; **secondary p.** efforts to decrease the duration of illness, reduce severity of diseases, and limit sequelae through early diagnosis and prompt intervention; **tertiary p.** efforts to limit the degree of disability and promote rehabilitation and restoration of function in patients/clients with chronic and irreversible diseases.

preventive intervention: Occurs when therapists use their expertise to anticipate problems in the future and design interventions to keep negative outcomes from occurring.

preventive medicine: Care designed to deter disease and maintain optimal health.

primacy effect: Tendency of an individual to remember the initial items of a list more accurately than those in the middle of the list.

primary aging: Term used to describe the characteristics of physical change, as a result of aging, that are part of the biological process and are inevitable to all humans.

primary appraisal: Part of the appraisal process in coping in which the individual determines whether a stressful episode poses a situation of potential harm, threat, or challenge.

primary care: Ongoing monitoring of health status to prevent disease and sequelae of disease. First encounter in time or order of care giving. Preventive interventions, such as diet and exercise, to prevent hypertension. The provision of integrated, accessible health care services by clinicians who are accountable for addressing the majority of personal health care needs, developing a sustained partnership with patients/clients, and practicing in the context of family and community.

primary care provider: Clinician who assumes ongoing responsibility for a client's overall health care needs.

primary health care: Basic level of health care that includes programs directed at health promotion, early diagnosis, and prevention of disease.

primary intracerebral hemorrhage: Syndrome in which bleeding occurs spontaneously in the brain.

primary prevention: Efforts that support or protect the health and well-being of the general population.

primary somesthetic area: Portion of the parietal lobe of the cerebrum that receives information about the general senses from receptors in the skin, joints, muscles, and body organs.

prime mover: Muscle with the principal responsibility for a given action. For example, the biceps brachii is the prime mover for flexing the arm at the elbow.

primigravida: A woman who is in her first pregnancy.

primitive reflex (reaction): Any reflex normal in an infant or fetus. Its presence in an adult usually indicates serious neurologic disease (eg, grasp reflex, Moro's reflex, sucking reflex, etc).

principle: A general truth or rule that emerges from the testing of assumptions and hypotheses; generally proven or tested.

principle of object permanence: The ability to realize that objects not within sight do exist; usually accomplished by children of 8 months of age.

principle of overload: Concept that repeated imposition of a stress above that normally experienced will produce physiologic adaptation.

proactive interference (PI): The inability to recall recent experiences as a result of the memory of earlier experiences.

problem-based learning: Process of learning through solving everyday problems as they evolve in life.

problem-focused coping: Strategies that are directed at the source of stress itself, rather than at feelings or emotions associated with the stress.

problem-oriented medical record (POMR): A method of documentation originated by Weed that has four basic components: data base, problems, plan, and progress notes.

problem-oriented process model: A conceptual model in which emphasis is on the process surrounding the problem definition.

problem solving: Ability to manipulate knowledge and apply the information to new or unfamiliar situations.

procedural memory: Knowledge for the necessary procedures to perform some activity; the so-called "knowing how."

procedures: The sequence of steps to be followed in performing an action; criteria for the way in which things are done.

prodromal: Preliminary phase of an illness that warns of upcoming major/primary symptoms.

productivity: It is viewed as a controlling mechanism for top-level management. It is the ratio between the output and the resources expended to obtain the desired output.

product line: Services that are labeled to ensure that consumers understand what they are purchasing.

progesterone: A hormone produced by the ovary responsible for changes in preparing the wall of the uterus for implantation.

prognosis: Prediction of the probable outcome. The determination of the level of optimal improvement that might be attained by the patient/client and the amount of time needed to reach that level.

program evaluation: Measuring the effectiveness or goal attainment of programs.

programmed cell death: Physiological process in which cells die in the body; thought to be involved in the aging process.

programming: Creating a set of instructions that a computer is able to follow; also a term used to refer to the structuring of activity or influencing of behavior through environmental design, organization, or manipulation.

progressive: Compilation of stages that increase in complexity toward maturity (eg, course of a disease or condition in which signs and symptoms become more prominent and severe over time).

prolapsed: Any organ that descends and protrudes through an external cavity due to weakness of the supporting structures (eg, prolapsed uterus, prolapsed bladder, etc).

pronation: The act of assuming the prone position. Rotation of the forearm medially so the palm is facing down toward the floor. Applied to the foot, a combination of eversion and abduction movements taking place in the tarsal and metatarsal joints and resulting in lowering of the medial margin of the foot, hence of the longitudinal arch, so that the plantar surface of the foot turns outward.

prone: Lying with face down.

prophylactic: Preventive.

proprietary (commercial) facilities: Refers to private profit-making institutions or facilities (eg, nursing homes).

proprioception: Awareness of posture, movement, and changes in equilibrium and the knowledge of position, weight, and resistance of objects in relation to the body. The reception of stimuli from within the body (eg, from muscles and tendons); includes position sense (the awareness of the joints at rest) and kinesthesia (the awareness of movement).

proprioceptive: Receptors that respond to stimuli originating primarily from muscle spindles, Golgi tendon organs, and joints. Interpreting stimuli originating in muscles, joints, and other internal tissues that give information about the position of one body part in relation to another. The state of proprioception.

proprioceptive neuromuscular facilitation (PNF): A form of therapeutic exercise in which accommodating resistance is manually applied to various patterns of movement for the purpose of strengthening and restraining the muscles guiding joint motion using proprioceptive input.

propriospinal tract: Contralateral intersegmental tract functioning during reflexes and integration. Synonym: spinospinal tract.

prosopagnosia: The inability to identify a familiar face, either by looking at the person or picture.

prospective memory: Remembering to carry out some action in the future.

prostaglandin: A lipid soluble hormone-like acetic compound occurring in nearly all tissues, used for inducing labor.

prostaglandin-synthetase inhibitors: Substances that inhibit the synthesis of prostaglandins.

prosthesis: Artificial substitutes, often mechanical or electrical, used to replace missing body parts.

protective devices: External supports to protect weak or ineffective joints or muscles, including braces, protective taping, cushions, and helmets.

protective extension response: Reflexive act consisting of extending one's arms in front of the head to protect the face and head during forward falling.

proteinemia: Excess protein in the blood.

proteinuria: The presence of protein in the urine.

protopathic sensation: Gross sensory abilities in the extremities, allowing one to detect light moving touch, pain, and temperature but without the ability to make fine discrimination of extent. Pertaining to the somatic sensations of fast, localized pain; slow, poorly localized pain; and temperature.

provider: Person or organization who actually provides the health care.

proxemics: The study of humans' use of space and the effects on interpersonal behavior.

proximal: In terms of anatomical position, located nearer to the trunk; near the attachment of an extremity to the trunk.

prudence: The ability to govern and discipline one's self through the use of reason.

pruritus gravidarum: Generalized itching not relieved by medication.

pruritus vulvae: Disorders marked by severe itching of the external female genitalia.

pseudodementia: Affective disorders, particularly depression, that mimic the signs and symptoms of dementia. Term used to describe the misdiagnosis of depression as dementia in the elderly.

pseudoelastin: A protein found in aging elastin tissue. The essential constituent of yellow elastic connective tissue.

psychoanalysis: Branch of psychiatry founded by Sigmund Freud using the techniques of free association, interpretation, and dream analysis.

psychoanalytic theory: Approach to the treatment of neuroses that emphasizes unlocking long-repressed feelings and past experiences in order to allow the patient to better understand his or her behavior.

psychodynamic: Any therapy that examines the forces motivating behavior.

psychogenic: Having an emotional or psychological origin.

psychological age: Definition of age based on the functional level of psychological processes rather than on calendar time.

psychological constructs: Psychological concepts; terms (without universal definitions) commonly used to describe mental states.

psychometric instruments: Apparatus and paper-and-pencil techniques for measuring general intelligence, achievement, abilities, and related characteristics.

psychometric techniques (tests): Methods for measuring personality, interest, and attitude (frequently used in psychology).

psychoneuroimmunology: Field of study that links psychological, neural, and immunological processes.

psychosis: A major mental disorder of organic or emotional origin that can cause extreme personality disorganization, loss of reality orientation, and inability to function appropriately in society.

psychosocial: Pertaining to interpersonal and social interactions that influence behavior and development.

psychosocial development: Erik Erikson's theory of human development throughout the lifespan as a progression of stages named according to the possible outcome.

psychosocial disability: Disorder, impairment, or handicap relating to interpersonal relationships and social interactions that influence behavior and development.

psychosomatic: Psychological foundation for physiological symptoms.

psychotic: Psychological state characterized by hallucinations and delusions.

ptosis: Drooping of the upper eyelid.

ptyalism: Increased saliva production.

puberty: Period in life when the individual becomes functionally capable of sexual reproduction.

public good: General welfare or benefit to the majority or large contingent of citizens.

puerperium: Period of 6 weeks following childbirth and expulsion of the placenta in which the reproductive organs of the mother return to normal.

pulmonary embolism: An obstruction of the pulmonary artery or one of its branches usually caused by an embolus from a lower extremity thrombosis.

pulmonary postural drainage: Placing the body in a position that uses gravity to drain fluid from the lungs.

pulse rate: Number of beats per minute as measured on the radial, carotid, femoral, and pedal arteries.

punishment: Providing an aversive stimulus following an appropriate response.

pure synergism: When a muscle moves several joints simultaneously, its force is divided among them.

pure tone audiogram: Standard method used to determine degree of hearing loss using a decibel scale of loudness.

Purkinje cells: Large neurons found in the cerebral cortex that provide the only output from the cerebellar cortex after the cortex processes sensory and motor signals from the rest of the nervous system.

purpose: The desire to engage in behavior to accomplish a goal.

purposeful activity: Actions that are goal directed.

purposefulness: An individual's plan of action to achieve a goal.

purpura: Hemorrhagic disease that leaves red to purple spots on the skin.

purulent: Consisting of or containing pus.

pus: Thick fluid indicative of infection containing leukocytes, bacteria, and cellular debris.

pyogenic: Producing pus.

pyosalpinx: Pus in the fallopian tube.

pyrosis: Burning sensation in the epigastric and sternal region with raising of acid liquid from the stomach; heartburn.

Q

quadrigeminal: Fourfold, or in four parts, such as the heart.

quadrilateral: Having four sides.

quadriplegia (QUAD): Paralysis of all four extremities.

qualification: A qualifying or being qualified with the skill, knowledge, and experience that fits a person for a position, office, or profession.

qualitative: Subjective elements.

qualitative research: Methods for knowing that consider the unique properties of a natural setting without a reliance on quantitative data.

quality assurance (QA): Maintenance of quality by constant measuring and comparison to set standards. Quality maintenance problems may be identified and corrected through this procedure.

quality improvement (QI): Continuous improvement of performance; sometimes referred to as *continuous quality improvement*, or *CQI*.

quality of care: Providing the optimal care in any practice setting.

quality of life: The degree of satisfaction that an individual has regarding a particular style of life. Concept defined by an individual's perceptions of overall satisfaction with his or her living circumstances, including physical status and abilities, psychological well-being, social interactions, and economic conditions; the degree of satisfaction that an individual has regarding a particular style of life.

quality performance dimensions: Set of nine fundamental elements for change identified by the Joint Commission on Accreditation of Healthcare Organizations: efficacy, appropriateness, availability, timeliness, effectiveness, continuity, safety, efficiency, respect, and caring.

quantitative: Measurable.

quantum: As in the quantum theory, a fixed elemental unit, as of energy, angular momentum, and other physical properties of physics.

quickening: The sensation of fetal movement, usually initially occurring between the 4th and 5th months of pregnancy.

R   **rachitis:** Inflammation of the spinal column due to vitamin D deficiency.

radical mastectomy: Removal of the entire breast and lymph nodes.

radicular: Pertaining to a radical or root. Commonly associated with a nerve root.

radiographic anatomy: The study of the structures of the body using x-rays.

radiography: Commonly referred to as an *x-ray*.

rale: *See* crackle.

ramus: A branch; used in anatomical nomenclature as a general term to designate a smaller structure given off by a larger one, such as a blood vessel or a nerve.

randomization: Process of assigning participants or objects to a control or experimental group on a random basis.

random practice: Tasks practiced in a mixed order.

range of motion (ROM): The path of motion a joint can move in any one direction, measured in degrees. The space, distance, or angle through which movement occurs at a joint or a series of joints.

rapid eye movement (REM): Sleep state in which brain waves show an active pattern; dreaming is occurring. This state is thought to be important for adequate rest, repair, immunity, and health.

rapport: Harmonious relationship between people.

rating of perceived exertion (RPE): Psychophysical scale for subjective rating of exertion during work.

ratio scales: Measurement scales that contain values that are equally distant from each other and are characterized by the presence of an absolute zero value.

raw score: Unadjusted score derived from observations of performance; frequently, the arithmetic sum of a subject's responses.

reaction of degeneration: The condition in which a short duration (usually less than 1 msec) electrical stimulus applied to a motor nerve results in a sluggish or absent muscle response rather than the normally brisk contraction. This electrophysiologic reaction can be used as a screening assessment of peripheral nerve integrity.

reaction time (RT): The interval between the application of a stimulus and the detection of a response. The time required to initiate a movement following stimulus presentation.

reactive hyperemia: Extra blood in vessels in response to a period of blocked blood flow.

reactivity: Characteristic of assessment instruments whereby the act of administering the assessment changes the behavior of the person being evaluated, thus distorting the representatives of the findings.

reality orientation: Therapeutic technique often used with confused or disoriented clients. Includes both group techniques to remind the client of facts and patterned environment, which provides memory cues.

reappraisal: In coping, reconsideration of a harm, threat, or loss episode after an initial appraisal has taken place. It is thought that during coping, individuals constantly reassess the stressful episode and their resources and alternatives for dealing with it.

reasonable accommodations (RA): In order to allow equal opportunity to a worker with a disability, a company may modify the work environment by doing things such as job restructuring, providing adaptable equipment, or making other such adjustments for modification.

reasoning: The use of one's ability to think and draw conclusions, motives, causes, or justifications, which will form the basis of actions.

rebound phenomenon: The inability to stop a resisted muscle contraction, such that movement of the limb occurs when the resistance is unexpectedly withdrawn from the limb.

recency effect: Tendency of an individual to remember the last items of a list better than those in the middle.

receptive aphasia: The inability to comprehend normal speech.

receptive field: Receptor area served by one neuron.

receptor: Specific site at which a drug acts through forming a chemical bond.

reciprocal: Present or existing on both sides expressing mutual, corresponding, or complementary action.

reciprocal innervation: Excitatory innervation of synergists and inhibitory innervation of antagonists. The function is to permit the action of the group of synergists to reinforce one another while eliminating the action of the antagonistic muscles that would oppose the particular movement, either slowing the movement or preventing it.

reciprocal teaching: Instructional procedure used by Brown and Palincsar to develop cognitive monitoring. It requires students to take turns leading a study group in the use of strategies for comprehending and remembering text content.

reciprocity: Mutual exchange between entities. For instance, reciprocity between states for licensing of physical therapists whereby one state accepts the licensing qualifications of another state.

recognition: A recognizing or being recognized as an object, person, accomplishment, or place. Identification of a person, place, or object.

reconditioning: Restoration to good physical and mental condition.

reconstruction aides: Individuals who used physical and occupational therapy in World War I with the returning soldiers with disabilities. The use of reconstruction aides ultimately increased the visibility of rehabilitation therapies and resulted in strides in professional education and public policy.

rectocele: Herniation of the rectum with protrusion into the vaginal canal, or prolapse of the rectum into the perineum.

red nucleus: Large, vascular nucleus found in mesencephalon and involved in the transmission of cerebellar communications to the motor cortex and thalamus.

reduction: Realignment of a dislocated bone to its original position.

reductionistic: An approach to understanding in which the problem is broken into parts, and the parts are viewed and managed separately.

re-entry programs: Rehabilitation programs designed to maximize independence; usually the final rehabilitation program after hospitalization and rehabilitation programs are completed. Re-entry programs are often outpatient or community programs.

re-examination: The process by which patient/client status is updated following the initial examination (because of new clinical indications, failure to respond to interventions, or failure to establish progress from baseline data).

referral: A recommendation that a patient/client seek service from another health care provider or resource.

referred pain: Visceral pain felt in a somatic area away from the actual source of pain.

reflex: Subconscious, involuntary reaction to an external stimulus.

reflex incontinence: A form of incontinence caused by the inability to inhibit bladder stimulatory reflexes.

reflex integrity: The intactness of the neural path involved in a reflex.

reflux: Back flow of any substance (eg, urine from bladder to ureters or food returning to the esophagus from the stomach).

refractive error: Nearsightedness (ie, myopia), farsightedness (ie, hyperopia), astigmatism, or presbyopia. All conditions are improved with corrective lenses.

regression: A retreat or backward movement in conditions, signs, and symptoms (eg, returning to behavior patterns that were characteristic of a previous stage of development).

rehabilitation: Helping individuals regain skills and abilities that have been lost as a result of illness, injury or disease, disorder, or incarceration. The restoration of a disabled individual to maximum independence commensurate with his or her limitations.

rehabilitation frame of reference: Teaches clients to compensate for underlying deficits that cannot be remediated.

reimbursement: Compensation for services provided.

reinforcement: Desired outcome of behavior. In behavior therapy, reinforcement is provided to encourage specific activities; strengthened by fear of punishment or anticipation of reward.

relative endurance: Muscular endurance when force of contraction tested is based on percentage of measured strength.

relative value unit (RVU): An index of measure for Medicare resource-based relative value scale.

relaxation: Techniques that increase relaxation by reducing tension (eg, biofeedback, systematic relaxation exercises).

relaxation techniques: A cognitive treatment technique that addresses muscle tension accompanying pain.

relaxin: A polypeptide ovarian hormone secreted by the corpus luteum that possibly acts on the ligamentous structures of the body, slackening the ligaments to allow greater opening in the pelvic outlet.

release phenomenon: Ongoing action of one part of the central nervous system without modulation from a complementary functional component.

reliability: Predictability of an outcome regardless of observer. In diagnosis, refers to the probability that several therapists will apply the same label to a given individual.

reminiscence effect: Tendency for the recall of an item to improve for a short period of time after initial learning before being forgotten.

remission: Lessening in severity or abatement of symptoms of a disease.

renin: A proteolytic enzyme liberated by ischemia of the kidney or by diminished pulse pressure that changes hypertensinogen into hypertension.

repetition maximum (RM): Maximum weight that can be lifted in isotonic contraction. One RM = maximum weight that can be lifted one time, two RM = maximum weight that can be lifted twice, etc.

reprimand: Expression of disapproval of conduct.

reprivatize: Return responsibility to the private sector as opposed to public responsibility.

research: Systematic investigation, including development, testing, and evaluation design.

resistance: Amount of weight to be moved.

resistance exercise training: Exercise that applies sufficient force to muscle groups to improve muscle strength.

resonance: The prolongation and intensification of sound produced by the transmission of its vibrations to a cavity, especially a sound elicited by percussion. A decrease in resonance is called *dullness*; absence of resonance is called *flatness*.

resource-based relative value system (RBRVS): A system of reimbursement being developed by Medicare for outpatient service based on assessing the intensity and complexity of a service and assigning a numerical value and dollar amount related to that value.

respiration: The act or process of breathing; inhaling and exhaling air. The process by which a living organism or cell takes in oxygen from the air or water, distributes and utilizes it in oxidation, and gives off products of oxidation, especially carbon dioxide.

respiratory exchange ratio (VCO_2/VO_2): The ratio of the volume of carbon dioxide expired and the oxygen consumed.

respiratory failure: Failure of the pulmonary system in which inadequate exchange of carbon dioxide and oxygen occurs between an organism and its environment.

respite care: Short-term health services to the dependent adult, either at home or in an institutional setting.

response speed: The time elapsed between presentation of a stimulus and the patient's/client's initiation of movement.

responsivity: Level that the sensory input facilitates reaction or noticing.

restorative aide: A nursing assistant who works in a rehabilitation capacity and assists nursing home residents in carryover of learned functional mobility (ie, ambulation, transfers) and activity of daily living on the patient/client units.

restraints: Devices used to aid in immobilization of patients.

rest/relaxation: Performance during time not devoted to other activity and during time devoted to sleep.

retardation: A retarded person has had some degree of mental impairment throughout his or her entire life. A retarded person can also develop a delirium or dementia. A delirium or dementia differs from retardation in that there has been a change from what was normal for that person.

retention: Resistance to movement or displacement.

reticulospinal tract: Pathway that supports action of the flexors and extensors of the neck for postural control.

retirement planning: Preparing for retirement by preparing financially and considering aptitudes, developing interests and skill, and selecting appropriate leisure time pursuits, including planning residence and travel prior to retiring from a job or career.

retrograde amnesia: The inability to recall events that have occurred during the period immediately preceding a brain injury.

retrospective memory: Remembering information that occurred in the past.

retrospective recording: Waiting until the evaluation is completed to record observations of client function.

retroviruses: A group of ribonucleic acid (RNA) viruses causing a variety of diseases in humans. This group of viruses have RNA as their genetic code and are capable of copying RNA and deoxyribonucleic acid and incorporating them into an infected cell.

reverberating loops or circuits: A process by which closed chains of neurons, when excited by a single impulse, will continue to discharge impulses from collateral neurons back onto the original neuronal pool. The end result may produce a higher level of excitation than the original input itself.

Rh factor: Hereditary blood factor found in red blood cells determined by specialized blood tests; when present, a person is Rh positive; when absent, a person is Rh negative.

rhizotomy: A neurosurgical intervention at the level of the cauda equinus, or the lumbar level of the spine, to interrupt abnormal sensory feedback that appears to maintain hypertonus. The objective is to reduce hypertonus associated with central nervous system dysfunction to allow the expression of functional postural control.

rhonchus: A snoring sound; a rattling in the throat; also a dry, coarse rale in the bronchial tubes due to a partial obstruction.

ribonucleic acid (RNA): Basic genetic material in which nucleic acid is associated with the control of chemical activities within a cell.

righting reactions: Stimuli go through the labyrinths and to tactile receptors in the trunk, neck, and ears to keep the upper part of the body upright and to maintain the head and trunk in their proper relationship.

right-left discrimination: The ability to distinguish right from left. Differentiating one side from the other.

right to die: A person's right to die on his or her terms.

right-to-know law: Law that dictates that employers must inform their employees of any chemical hazards or health effects caused by toxic substances used in each workplace.

rigidity: Hypertonicity of agonist and antagonist that offers a constant, uniform resistance to passive movement. The affected muscles seem unable to relax and are in a state of contraction even at rest.

risk factors: Factors that cause a person or group of people to be particularly vulnerable to an unwanted, unpleasant, or unhealthy event.

risky shift: Type of group polarization of which the postdiscussion behaviors of individuals are less safe than before the group discussion.

robotics: Science of mechanical devices that work automatically or by remote control.

roentgenogram: An x-ray. A film produced by roentgenography.

role: Set of behaviors that has some socially agreed-upon functions and for which there is an accepted code of norms.

role competence: Achievement of the behaviors that have some socially agreed-upon function and for which there is an accepted code of behavioral norms or expectations.

role conflict: Occurs when a person encounters pressures within an important role that are in opposition to another valued role.

Rolfing: Technique of massage and deep muscular manipulation designed to realign the body with gravity; structured integration.

Romberg's sign: The inability to maintain body balance when the eyes open and then close with the feet close together; unsteadiness when eyes are closed indicates a loss of proprioceptive control.

rooting reflex: This normal reflex in infants up to 4 months of age consists of head turning in the direction of the stimulus when the cheek is stroked gently.

rotation: Movement around the long axis of a limb.

rotator cuff: The muscle complex of the shoulder that provides stability of the glenohumeral joint inclusive of the supraspinatus, infraspinatus, teres minor, and subscapularis muscles.

rote: Habit performance without meaning.

round ligament: A pair of ligaments that hold the uterus in place, extending laterally from the fundus between the folds of the broad ligaments to the lateral pelvic wall, terminating in the labia majora.

routines: Occupations with established sequences.

routine supervision: Direct contact at least every 2 weeks at the site of work, with interim supervision occurring by other methods, such as telephone or written communication.

rules-oriented style: Main assumption in this style is that people require reinforcement from the manager to function. This manager does things by the book; enforcing policies, rules, and procedures with employees ensures motivation and achievement.

rumination: Repetitive chewing of food; regurgitated after ingestion.

rupture: A bursting or the state of being broken apart.

S **SOAP (subjective, objective, assessment, plan):** The four parts of a written account of a health problem.

saccadic eye movement: Extremely fast voluntary movement of the eyes, allowing the eyes to accurately fix on a still object in the visual field as the person moves or the head turns.

saccadic fixation: A rapid change of fixation from one point in a visual field to another.

saccule: Organ in the inner ear that transmits information about linear movement in relation to gravity.

safety grab bars: Bars mounted on bath tub walls that provide a person with a secure fixture to hold and prevent falling.

safety procedures: Knowing and performing preventive and emergency procedures to maintain a safe environment and to prevent injuries.

sagittal plane: Runs from front to back, dividing the body into left and right segments.

salpingo-oophorectomy: Excision of an ovary and fallopian tube.

sample of behavior: Selected test items chosen because they constitute a subset of the behaviors that need to be assessed.

sandwich generation: Adults who have care-giving responsibilities for their dependent children and their aging parents.

sarcoidosis: A disorder that may affect any part of the body but most frequently involves the lymph nodes, liver, spleen, lungs, eyes, and small bones of the hands and feet; characterized by the presence in all affected organs or tissues of epithelioid cell tubercles, without caseation, and with little or no round-cell reaction, becoming converted, in the older lesions, into a rather hyaline featureless fibrous tissue.

sarcoma: Malignant tissue that originates in connective tissue and spreads through the bloodstream, often attacking bones.

scab: Dried exudate covering superficial wounds.

scaffolding: Teaching process that segments a task into separate subgoals in order to allow a child to perform tasks within his or her existing repertoire of skills, while the adult can model the skills and knowledge necessary to complete the entire task.

scanning: Technique for making selections on a device such as a communication aid, computer, or environmental control system. Scanning involves moving sequentially through a given set of choices and making a selection when the desired position is reached. Types of scanning include automatic, manual, row-and-column, and directed.

scanning speech: An abnormal pattern of speech characterized by regularly recurring pauses.

scapegoat: A symbolic person or thing blamed for other problems.

scapula: Flattened, triangular bone found on the posterior aspect of the body. It is part of the pectoral girdle, which joins the clavicle and humerus.

scar: Disposition of connective tissue as a result of the healing process.

schemata: Basic units of all knowledge. Each simple organization of experience and knowledge by the mind forms the original "schema" or framework that represents our everyday experiences. Each experience, thought, and idea is a structural element in an organizational matrix that integrates each person's experiences and history into a meaningful set of categories, each filled with data from one's memory of prior events.

schema theory: Notion that standard routine performances occur in given situations in a typical sequence and with typical kinds of participants; within the general framework or structure the details of a given performance may vary, but the basic structure remains consistent.

schemes: Structural elements of cognition; plans, designs, or programs to be followed.

schizophrenia (Sz): Pervasive psychosis that effects a variety of psychological processes involving cognition, affect, and behavior and is characterized by hallucinations, delusions, bizarre behavior, and illogical thinking.

school professionals: School principals, program directors, and directors of special education are committee members who interpret local administrative policies in special education.

sciatica: Nerve inflammation characterized by sharp pains along the sciatic nerve and its branches; area extends from the hip down the back of the thigh and surrounding parts.

scissors gait: Gait in which the legs cross the midline upon advancement.

scleroderma: Disease characterized by chronic hardening and shrinking of the connective tissue of any organ in the body.

scoliosis: Abnormal lateral curvature of the spine. This usually consists of two curves, the original abnormal curve and a compensatory curve in the opposite direction.

scooter board: Rectangular, flat board with wheels at each corner. It is used to evoke the pivot prone posture by being ridden.

scope of practice: Encompassing all of the skills, knowledge, and expertise required to practice a profession, such as physical therapy.

screening: The process of examining a population, usually a high risk population, for a given state or disease. A review of a client case to determine if services are necessary. Determining the need for further examination or consultation by a physical therapist or for referral to another health professional; **cognitive s.** brief assessment of the patient's/client's thinking process (eg, the ability to process commands).

screening instrument: Assessment device used for purposes of identifying potential problem areas for further in-depth evaluation.

script: General sequence of events about a common routine or scenario, usually with a common goal.

seasonal affective disorder (SAD): Mood disorder associated with shorter days and longer nights of autumn and winter. Symptoms include lethargy, depression, social withdrawal, and work difficulties.

seborrhea: Disease of the sebaceous glands marked by the increase in amount and quality of their secretions.

secondary aging: Changes in physical functioning, as a result of aging, that are not universal or inevitable but are commonly shared by humans as a result of environmental conditions or circumstances.

secondary care: Intervention provided once a disease state has been identified (eg, treating hypertension).

secondary conditions: Also called *secondary disabilities*. Pathology, impairment, or functional limitations derived from the primary condition.

secondary prevention: Efforts directed at populations who are considered "at risk" by early detection of potential health problems, followed by the interventions to halt, reverse, or at least slow the progression of that condition.

second stage of labor: Includes the time from 10 cm of dilation until the birth of the baby.

secretion: The process of elaborating a specific product as a result of the activity of a gland. This activity may range from separating a specific substance of the blood to the elaboration of a new chemical substance.

sedentary work: Exerting up to 10 pounds of force occasionally or a negligible amount of force frequently to lift, carry, push, pull, or otherwise move objects.

seizure disorders: Presence of abrupt irrepressible episodes of electrical hyperactivity in the brain.

selective abstraction: Focusing on one insignificant detail while ignoring the more important features of a situation.

self-actualization: Process of striving to achieve one's ultimate potential in life with accompanying feelings of accomplishment and personal growth.

self-care: The set of activities that comprise daily living, such as bed mobility, transfers, ambulation, dressing, grooming, bathing, eating, and toileting.

self-care activities: Personal activities an individual performs to prepare for and maintain a daily routine.

self-concept: View one has of one's self (eg, ideas, feelings, attitudes, identity, worth, capabilities, and limitations).

self-control: The ability to control one's behaviors. Modifying one's own behavior in response to environmental needs, demands, constraints, personal aspirations, and feedback from others.

self-deprecator: Type of person who seeks praise by devaluing him- or herself; successful "attention-getter" initially, but fails over the longer term when other group members become aware of circumstances.

self-efficacy: An individual's belief that he or she is capable of successfully performing a certain set of behaviors.

self-esteem: An individual's overall feeling of worth.

self-expression: An individual's ability to make his or her thoughts and feelings known. Using a variety of styles and skills to express thoughts, feelings, and needs.

self-fulfilling prophecy: A principle that a belief in or the expectation of a particular outcome is a factor that contributes to its fulfillment.

self-help: Various methods by which individuals attempt to remedy their difficulties without making use of formal care providers (eg, Alcoholics Anonymous).

self-identity skill: The ability to perceive one's self as holistic and autonomous and to have permanence and continuity over time.

self-image: Internalized view a person holds of him- or herself, which usually varies with changing social situations over one's lifespan.

self-monitoring: Process whereby the client records specific behaviors or thoughts as they occur.

self-report: Type of assessment approach in which the individual reports on his or her level of function or performance.

sellar articular surfaces: Synovial joint surfaces characterized by an egg-shaped articular surface that is concave in one plane and convex in the plane perpendicular to it.

semantic compaction: Technique for reducing the number of selections a user must make to generate a phrase on a voice-output communication aid. Symbols for semantic units are used rather than number or letter codes.

semantic memory: Memory for general knowledge.

semantics: The study of language with special attention to the meanings of words and other symbols.

semiautonomous: Individual is partially dependent upon another for the satisfaction of needs.

semicircular canals: Organ in the inner ear that transmits information about head position.

senescence: Aging; growing older. The process or condition of growing old.

senile dementia: An organic mental disorder resulting from generalized atrophy of the brain with no evidence of cerebrovascular disease.

senile plaque: *See* neuritic plaque.

sensation: Receiving conscious sensory impressions through direct stimulation of the body, such as hearing, seeing, touching, etc.

sense of control: Perception of being able to direct and regulate.

sense of security: Feeling of comfort in being able to trust and know that there is predictability in the environment.

sensitivity: Capacity to feel, transmit, and react to a stimulus; rating of how well changes will be measured on subsequent tests to show improvement.

sensitivity to stimuli: Due to low thresholds, persons who act in accordance with those thresholds tend to seem hyperactive or distractible. They have a hard time staying on tasks to complete them or to learn from their experiences, because their low neurological thresholds keep directing their attention from one stimulus to the next, whether it is part of the ongoing task or not.

sensitization: An acquired reaction; the process of a receptor becoming more susceptible to a given stimulus.

sensorimotor therapy: Therapy planned to enhance the integration of reflex phenomena and the emergence of voluntary motor behaviors concerned with posture and locomotion.

sensory: Having to do with sensations or the senses; including peripheral sensory processing (eg, sensitivity to touch) and cortical sensory processing (eg, two-point and sharp/dull discrimination).

sensory conflict: Situations in which sensory signals that are expected to match do not match, either between systems (vision, somatosensory, or vestibular) or within a system (left versus right sides).

sensory defensiveness: Constellation of symptoms that are the result of adversive or defensive reactions to non-noxious stimuli across one or more sensory modalities.

sensory deprivation: An involuntary loss of physical awareness caused by detachment from external sensory stimuli that can result in psychological disturbances. An enforced absence of the usual repertoire of sensory stimuli producing severe mental changes, including hallucinations, anxiety, depression, and insanity.

sensory environment: The conditions that exist in the real world around us and impact balance (ie, darkness, visual movement, complaint surfaces, etc).

sensory integration (SI): Ability of the central nervous system to process sensory information to make an adaptive response to the environment; also refers to a therapeutic intervention that uses strong kinesthetic and proprioceptive stimulation to attempt to better organize the central nervous system. The ability to integrate information from the environment to produce normal movement. The organization of sensory input for use, a perception of the body or environment, an adaptive response, a learning process, or the development of some neural function.

sensory integrative dysfunction: A disorder or irregularity in brain function that makes sensory integration difficult. Many, but not all, learning disorders stem from sensory integrative dysfunctions.

sensory integrative therapy: Therapy involving sensory stimulation and adaptive responses to it according to a patient's/client's neurological needs. Treatment usually involves full body movements that provide vestibular, proprioceptive, and tactile stimulation. The goal is to improve the brain's ability to process and organize sensations.

sensory memory: Memory store that holds sensory input in its uninterpreted sensory form for a very brief period of time.

sensory neuron: Nerve cell that sends signals to the spinal cord or brain.

sensory disregard: Condition characterized by lack of awareness of one side of the body. Synonym: body disregard.

sensory processing: The brain's ability to receive information and respond appropriately by interpreting sensory stimuli.

sensory registration: The brain's ability to receive input and select what will receive attention and what will be inhibited from consciousness.

sensory stimulation: Therapeutic intervention that makes use of patterned sensory input.

sensory testing: Evaluation of sensory system.

sensory training: General term for therapy aimed at enabling a person to regain contact with his or her environment; usually offered in groups, sensory training includes social introductions among the group, body-awareness exercises, and sensory activities utilizing objects.

sepsis: Poisoning that is caused by the products of a putrefactive process. Infection.

septicemia: Systemic disease associated with the presence and persistence of pathogenic microorganisms or toxins in the blood.

sequela: Morbid condition resulting from another condition or event.

sequencing: Putting things in order. The ability to accomplish a task in a logistical manner by placing information, concepts, and actions in order.

sequestrum: Fragment of necrosed bone that has become separated from the surrounding tissue.

serial casting: Process of applying casts of increasing degrees of joint position every few days to stretch a limb progressively away from a contracted spastic posture.

serial speech: Overlearned speech involving a series of words, such as counting and reciting the days of the week.

serology: The study of blood serum.

serous: Producing a serous secretion or containing serum.

service entrance: An entrance intended primarily for delivery of goods or services.

set: A belief or expectation one has about a person, place, or thing.

severe retardation: Within an IQ range of 20 to 34.

sex identification: Assigning of a masculine or feminine connotation to a given activity.

sexuality: The behaviors that relate psychological, cultural, emotional, and physical responses to the need to reproduce.

sexually transmitted disease (STD): A contagious disease usually acquired by sexual intercourse or genital contact.

shaken baby syndrome: A condition of whiplash-type injuries, ranging from bruises on the arms and trunk to retinal hemorrhages or convulsions, as observed in infants and children who have been violently shaken; a form of child abuse that often results in intracranial bleeding from tearing of cerebral blood vessels.

shear: Pressure exerted against the surface and layers of the skin as tissues slide in opposite but parallel planes. Trauma caused by tissue layers sliding against each other; results in disruption or angulation of blood vessels.

sheltered housing: Living arrangements that provide structure and supervision for individuals who do not require institutionalization but are not fully capable of independent living (eg, group homes).

shingles: Viral disease of the peripheral nerves with the eruption of skin vesicles along the path of the nerve.

shock therapy: Induced by delivering an electric current through the brain; a procedure used for treating depression.

short opponents: Splint that maintains the thumb in abduction and partial rotation under the second metacarpal.

short-term memory: Limited capacity memory store that holds information for a brief period of time; the so-called "working memory."

shoulder dystocia: Occurs when the presenting part in the pelvic inlet during delivery is the fetal shoulder, thereby arresting normal progression of labor.

shoulder separation: Separation of the acromioclavicular joint due to trauma, injury, or disease.

shoulder subluxation: Incomplete downward, usually partial, dislocation of the humerus out of the glenohumeral joint caused by weakness, stretch, or abnormal tone in the scapulohumeral and/or scapular muscles.

show: Refers to the blood and mucous plug that is extruded from the vagina in early labor.

shower seat: Chair placed in the shower, allowing a bather to sit.

shunt: Passage between two natural channels, especially blood vessels.

side effect: Other than the desired action (eg, effect produced by a drug).

sign: Clinically noted as the objective findings associated with an illness or dysfunction. Objective evidence of physical abnormality.

signage: Displayed verbal, symbolic, tactile, or pictorial information.

signal risk factors: Workers exposed to these factors are at greater risk for developing work-related musculoskeletal disorders. The factors are fixed or awkward work posture for more than 2 hours, performance of the same motion or motion pattern every few seconds for more than a total of 2 hours, use of vibrating or impact tools or equipment for more than a total of 1 hour, and unassisted frequent or forceful manual handling for more than 1 hour.

sign of behavior: Client responses that are viewed as "indirect manifestations" (or signs) of one's underlying personality.

simple fracture: Bone is broken internally but does not pierce the skin so that it can be seen.

simple reflex: Reflex with a motor nerve component that involves only one muscle.

single trait sample: Evaluation that focuses on the assessment of a single worker trait.

sinus tract: A course or pathway that can extend in any direction from the wound surface; results in dead space with the potential for abscess formation.

situational assessment: Assesses the person's performance under each circumstance of a realistic work situation by systematically altering variables such as production demands and stress factors.

situation-specific: In psychosocial assessment, those behaviors and tasks that must be mastered to function every day in a particular environment.

skeletal demineralization: The loss of bone mass due to loss of minerals from the bone as seen in conditions like osteoporosis.

skeletal system: Supporting framework for the body that is comprised of the axial and appendicular divisions.

skilled nursing facility (SNF): Institution or part of an institution that meets criteria for accreditation established by the sections of the Social Security Act that determine the basis for Medicaid and Medicare reimbursement. Provides care that must be rendered by or under the supervision of professional personnel such as a registered nurse. The care must be required daily and must be a continuation of the care begun in the hospital.

skin fold measurement: Method for estimating percent body fat by measuring subcutaneous fat with skin fold calipers.

sleep apnea: Disorder characterized by period of an absence of attempts to breathe; the person is momentarily unable to move respiratory muscles or maintain air flow through his or her nose and mouth.

sleep paralysis: Temporary inability to talk or move when falling asleep or waking up.

slough: Loose, stringy, necrotic tissue.

social: Having to do with human beings living together as a group in a situation in which their dealings with one another affect their common welfare. Availability and expectations of significant individuals, such as spouse, friends, and caregivers. Also includes larger social groups that are influential in establishing norms, role expectations, and social routines.

social age: Definition of age emphasizing the functional level of social interaction skills rather than calendar time.

social climate: Combined variables in the social environment that directly or indirectly influence individual behavior and are influenced by individual behavior.

social clock: Set of internalized beliefs that forms the standards that individuals use in assessing their conformity to age-appropriate expectations.

social conduct: Interacting by using manners, personal space, eye contact, gestures, active listening, and self-expression appropriate to one's environment. Behavior in a group.

social disadvantage or handicap: Results when an individual is not able to fulfill a role that he or she expects or is required to fill.

social environment: Those social systems or networks within which a given person operates; the collective human relationships of individuals, whether familial, community, or organizational in nature, constitute the social environment of that individual.

social identity theory: Social psychologist Henry Taifel's theory that when individuals are assigned to a group, they invariably think of that group as an in-group for them. This occurs because individuals want to have a positive image.

social indicators: An approach to needs assessment that examines data from public records: census, county health department, police records, and housing offices.

socialization: Development of the individual as a social being and a participant in society that results from a continuing, changing interaction between a person and those who attempt to influence him or her.

social learning theory: View of psychologists who emphasize behavior, environment, and cognition as the key factors for development.

social modeling theory: Maintains that learning is accomplished through observing others. A person may learn a behavior or its consequences by watching another person experience that behavior.

social phobia: Intense fear of social situations stemming from fear of negative judgment by others. Social phobics feel scrutinized and tend to be overly critical of themselves.

social referencing: Communicating behavior in which babies keep a watchful eye on their caregiver's expression to see how they should interpret unusual events.

social skills training: Cognitive/behavioral approach to teaching skills basic to social interaction.

social support: Social relatedness and interactions with others that are perceived by the individual as supplying emotional, physical, and social resources.

social systems: Organized interactions among individuals, as within marriages, families, communities, and organizations, both formal and informal.

societal limitations: When societal policy, attitudes, and actions (or lack of actions) create a physical, social, or financial barrier to access health care, housing, or vocational/avocational opportunities.

sociodramatic play: Imaginary or make-believe play involving two or more children enacting various social roles.

sociological aging: Age-specific roles a person adopts within his or her context of society and individual environment. It includes the changes of a person's roles and functions, and the reflected behavior of these changes within society throughout life.

socket: The part of a prosthesis into which a stump of the remaining limb fits.

soft neurological signs: Mild or slight neurological abnormalities that are difficult to detect.

soft tissue: All neuromusculoskeletal tissues except bone and articular cartilage.

soft tissue integrity: Health of the connective tissue of the body.

software: Programs that run on computers.

solitary play: Play in which a child is completely involved in the activity and blocks out the surroundings both physically and psychologically.

soma: Cell body of a nerve that contains the nucleus.

somatic nervous system: Portion of the nervous system composed of a motor division that excites skeletal muscles and a sensory division that receives and processes sensory input from the sense organs.

somatoform disorders: Group of mental disorders characterized by loss or alteration in physical functioning, for which there is no physiological explanation; evidence that psychological factors have caused the physical symptoms; lack of voluntary control over physical symptoms; and indifference from the patient to the physical loss.

somatosensory evoked potential (SEP): Peripheral nerve stimulation produces potentials that can be recorded from the scalp, over the spine, or the periphery.

somatotopic: Organization of cells in the somatosensory system that enables one to identify the exact skin surface touched.

spasm: An involuntary muscle contraction.

spastic diplegia: An increase in postural tonus that is distributed primarily in the lower extremities and the pelvic area.

spastic gait: Stiff movement, toes drag, legs are together, and hip and knee joints are slightly flexed.

spasticity: Increase in the muscle tone and stretch reflex of a muscle, resulting in increased resistance to passive stretch of the muscle and hyperresponsivity of the muscle to sensory stimulation.

spastic quadriplegia: An increase in postural tonus that is distributed throughout all four extremities. These findings are often coexistent, with relatively lower tone in the trunk and severe difficulty in controlling posture.

spatial awareness: The ability to orient one's self in space, visualize what an object looks like from all angles, know from where sounds are coming, and know where body parts are in space.

spatial relations: The ability to perceive the self in relation to other objects.

special interest groups: Collectives of individuals and organizations who are bound by beliefs about specific issues or populations and who seek to influence decisions about the allocation of resources.

specialized battery: Tests that measure a specific component (eg, cognitive functioning, such as attention or language).

specificity: An instrument's ability to accurately identify subjects possessing a specific trait.

speculum: An instrument used to hold open and dilate the vagina during inspection.

speech: The meaningful production and sequencing of sounds by the speech sensorimotor system (eg, lips, tongue, etc) for the transmission of spoken language.

speech-language pathology and audiology: Science that specializes in the investigation of the scientific bases of the normal processes of communication and its disorders.

sphygmomanometer: Instrument used to measure arterial blood pressure indirectly.

spin: An arthrokinematic movement in which one point on a surface will always be in contact with a new point on another surface, such as in rotating around a stationary mechanical axis and/or the longitudinal axis. An osteokinematic movement denoting rotation of a bone around a longitudinal axis.

spinal: An injection of anesthesia into the spinal fluid to produce numbness.

spinal fusion: Joining together spinal vertebrae to prevent damage to the bones or spinal cord from disease processes.

spinal motion segment: Term used to denote those structures and entities that compose the functional unit of the spine, including two adjacent vertebrae, the intervertebral disc, the apophyseal joints, all the interconnecting ligaments, the two intervertebral foramen, and the spinal canal.

spinal nerve: The nerve extending from the spinal cord.

spinocerebellar tracts: Dorsal tract consisting of the afferent ipsilateral ascending tract to cerebellum, serving most lower extremities for touch, pressure, and proprioception. The ventral tract consisting of the afferent contralateral ascending tract to cerebellum serving lower extremities for proprioception.

spinothalamic tract: Afferent contralateral and ipsilateral ascending tract to thalamus for sensation of pain, temperature, and light (erude) touch; also known as the *anterolateral system (ALS)*.

spiritual: Nonphysical and nonmaterial aspect of existence, which contributes insight into the nature and meaning of a person's life.

spiritual meaning: Meaning, usually symbolic, related to one's concerns with matters that transcend physical life.

spirometry: The measurement of air inspired and expired.

splint: Supportive device used to immobilize, fix, or prevent deformities or assist in motion. Support of a body segment through application of an external device; **static s.** customized and prefabricated splints, inhibitory casts, and spinal and other braces that are designed to maintain joints in a desired position; **dynamic s.** customized and prefabricated supports that allow for or control motion while providing support.

splinter skills: Skills learned by rote that are not intended to be generalized into other situations.

spondylitis: Inflammation of the vertebrae.

spondylolisthesis: Forward displacement of one vertebra over another, usually of the fifth lumbar vertebra over the body of the sacrum or the fourth lumbar over the fifth.

spontaneous remission: Unusual occurrence (eg, when cancer cells revert back to normal without aid or apparent cause).

Spork: Utensil that combines the bowl of a spoon and the tines of a fork and eliminates the need to change utensils.

sprain: Injury to a joint that causes pain and disability, with the severity depending on the degree of injury to ligaments or tendons.

spreadsheet: Type of computer software organized in section or table format and used in financial management and accounting systems.

sputum: Substance expelled by coughing or clearing the throat. Matter ejected from the lungs, bronchi, and trachea through the mouth.

stabilizer: Any muscle that acts to fix one attachment of a prime mover or hold a bone steady to provide a foundation for movement; equipment or device used to maintain a particular position.

staff development: Various educational resources for professionals that are used to attain new skills and knowledge.

staging: Classification of tumors by their spread through the body.

standard assessment: Tests and evaluation approaches with specific norms, standards, and protocol.

standard deviation: Mathematically determined value used to derive standard scores and compare raw scores to a unit normal distribution.

standard error: Possible range in the variability of a person's "true" score in a test; a number that recognizes the amount by which a score might vary on different days or in different situations.

standard error of the mean: Standard deviation of the entire distribution of random sample means successively selected from a single population.

standardization: Method by which test scores of a typical population are derived, thus allowing subsequent test scores to be analyzed in light of that broad population; standardization requires a rigorous process of data collection and comparison.

standardized battery: A battery of tests in which the testing and scoring procedures are well defined and fixed and the interpretation involves the use of standardized norms.

standard scores: Raw scores mathematically converted to a scale that facilitates comparison.

Standards of Practice for Physical Therapy: Guidelines assembled to assist physical therapy practitioners in the delivery of physical therapy services.

stasis: Stagnation of blood caused by venous congestion.

static equilibrium: The ability of an individual to adjust to displacements of his or her center of gravity while maintaining a constant base of support.

static flexibility: Range of motion in degrees that a joint will allow.

statics: The study of objects at rest.

static splint: Rigid orthosis used for the prevention of movement of a joint or for the fixation of a displaced part.

static strength: Holding the lengthened position without movement.

steatorrhea: Fatty stools, seen in pancreatic diseases; increased secretion of the sebaceous glands.

stenosis: A narrowing of any canal (ie, spinal stenosis denoting a state of decreased diameter of the spinal canal and the intervertebral foramen).

stent: Any material used to hold in place or to provide a support for a graft or anastomosis while healing takes place.

step test: Graded exercise test in which a person is required to rhythmically step up and down steps of gradually increasing heights.

stereognosis: The ability to identify common objects by touch with vision occluded.

stereopsis: Quality of visual fusion.

stereotypic behavior: Repeated, persistent postures or movements, including vocalizations.

stereotyping: Applying generalized and oversimplified labels of characteristics, actions, or attitudes to a specific socioeconomic, cultural, religious, or ethnic group. Often used to belittle or discount a particular group.

stertorous: Respiratory effort that is strenuous and struggling; sounds like snoring.

stethoscope: Instrument used to listen to heart and lung sounds.

stigma: An undesirable difference that becomes a basis for separating an individual bearing such traits from the rest of society.

stillbirth: Refers to the birth of a baby who has died in utero.

stimulation: Arousal of attention, interest, or tension.

stimulus-arousal properties: Alerting potential of various sensory stimuli, generally thought to be related to their intensity, pace, and novelty.

storage fat: Adipose tissue found primarily subcutaneously and surrounding the major organs.

strabismus: Oculomotor misalignment of one eye.

strain: Usually a muscular injury caused by the excessive physical effort that leads to a forcible stretch. Refers to the percent change in original length of a deformed tissue.

strain counterstrain techniques: Physical therapy techniques that assist with elongation of the muscle by using the force of the contracting muscle.

strategic planning: Goals that are essential, basic, or critical to the continuation of an institution or organization. It involves the use of resources to achieve long-range goals.

strategy: A plan of action.

strength: Nonspecific term relating to muscle contraction, often referring to the force generated by a single maximal isometric contraction. Force-generating capacity of a muscle.

strengthening: active s. a form of strength-building exercise in which the physical therapist applies resistance through the range of motion of active movement; **assistive s.** a form of strength-building exercise in which the physical therapist assists the patient/client through the available range of motion; **resistive s.** any form of active exercise in which a dynamic or static muscular contraction is resisted by an outside force. The external force may be applied manually or mechanically.

streptokinase: An enzyme produced by streptococci that catalyzes the conversion of plasminogen to plasmin.

stress: An individual's general reaction to external demands or stressors. Stress results in psychological as well as physiological reactions; **biomechanical s.** the force developed in a deformed tissue divided by the tissue's cross-sectional area.

stress incontinence: A type of urinary incontinence that occurs when the intravesicular pressure exceeds bladder resistance and sphincter activity is weak or absent.

stress management techniques: Methods of relieving or controlling chronic stress by interrupting reflexive neurologic stress reactions.

stressors: External events that place demands on an individual above the ordinary.

stretch: Temporary lengthening of tissues that is not maintained for a sufficient period of time to encourage collagen remodeling.

stretch weakness: A clinical term denoting the effect on muscles from prolonged immobilization in a lengthened position, in other words, beyond the neutral or physiologic rest position.

striae gravidarum: Stretch marks appearing on the distended skin caused by the rupture of elastic fibers due to excessive distention.

stridor: A harsh, high-pitched respiratory sound, such as the inspiratory sound often heard in laryngeal or bronchial obstruction. Sometimes heard through a tracheostomy tube.

strip: A term used in wound care that denotes the removal of epidermis by mechanical means. Synonym: denude.

stripping and ligation: Removal and tying off of a vein.

stroke: Syndrome characterized by a sudden onset in which blood vessels in the brain have become narrowed or blocked. Synonym: cerebrovascular accident.

stroke volume (SV): The amount of blood ejected from the left ventricle on one beat. Maximum stroke volume is the highest volume of blood expelled from the heart during a single beat. This value is usually reached when exercise is only about 40% to 50% of maximum exercise capacity.

structural theory: Dividing of the mind into three structures: the id, the ego, and the superego.

structured activities: Activities that have rules and can be broken down into manageable steps, which have been preplanned and preorganized.

sty, stye: Localized circumscribed inflammatory swelling of one of the sebaceous glands of the eyelid. Synonym: hordeolum.

subacute care: Short-term, comprehensive inpatient level of care.

subacute patient: Medically complex cases requiring a longer period of rehabilitation and recovery, usually 1 to 6 weeks.

sub-ASIS Bar: Orthotic bar included in seating and positioning systems placed snugly below the anterior superior iliac spine of the pelvis to maintain a forward tilt of the pelvis and better postural alignment.

subcortical: Region beneath the cerebral cortex.

subculture: Ethnic, regional, economic, or social group exhibiting characteristic patterns of behavior sufficient to distinguish it from others within an embracing culture or society. Does not usually include rejection of the larger culture. Most people are members of several subcultures.

subjective measure: Assessment designed to identify the client's own view of problems and performance.

sublingual: Under the tongue.

subluxation: Partial or incomplete dislocation (eg, shoulder of client with cerebrovascular accident).

sudomotor: Stimulating the sweat glands.

suffix: Word element of one or more syllables added to the end of a combining form in order to change its meaning.

sundowning: Condition in which persons tend to become more confused or disoriented at the end of the day.

superficial: Area of the body that is located closest to the surface.

superior: Toward the head or upper portion of a part or structure. Synonym: cephalad.

supervisor: Any person having authority in the interests of the employer to hire, transfer, lay off, recall, promote, assign, reward, or discipline other employees.

supination (sup): The act of assuming the supine position. Rotation of the forearm laterally so the palm is facing up toward the ceiling. Applied to the foot, it implies movement resulting in raising of the medial margin of the foot, hence of the longitudinal arch, so that the plantar surface of the foot is facing inward.

supine: Lying on the spine with the face up.

supported employment: Paid employment for people with disabilities without employment or for those whose employment has been interrupted as a result of a severe disability and need support services to perform job-related tasks.

supportive devices: External supports to protect weak or ineffective joints or muscles. Supportive devices include supportive taping, compression garments, corsets, slings, neck collars, serial casts, elastic wraps, and oxygen.

supportive services: Those that enable and empower an individual to function more independently within a community or facility.

suppression: The ability of the central nervous system to screen out certain stimuli so that others may be attended to more carefully.

surfactant: A surface agent.

surrogate: A person or thing that replaces another (eg, substitute parental figure).

swan neck deformity: Condition of the hand characterized by hyperextension of the proximal interphalangeal joint and flexion of the distal interphalangeal joint.

swing: Any osteokinematic motion other than a spin. A pure swing (cardinal swing) is when a bone swings without any accompanying spin. The arc of motion created is the shortest distance between two points. An impure swing (arcuate swing) is when a bone swings and simultaneously undergoes some spin. The arc of motion created is other than the shortest distance between two points.

symbolic associations: An object's broader, cultural connotations and its narrower, idiosyncratic associations for individuals or families.

symbolic deficit hypothesis: Lack of representational skills.

symbolic play: Imagining or assigning roles to objects or other people (eg, playing house).

symbols: Abstract representations of perceived reality.

symmetrical: Equal in size and shape; very similar in relative placement or arrangement about an axis.

sympathetic nervous system: Autonomic nervous system that mobilizes the body's resources during stressful situations.

sympatholytic: Opposing the effects of impulses conveyed by adrenergic postganglionic fibers of the sympathetic nervous system. An agent that opposes the effects of impulses conveyed by adrenergic postganglionic fibers of the sympathetic nervous system.

sympathomimetic: Mimicking the effects of impulses conveyed by adrenergic postganglionic fibers of the sympathetic nervous system. An agent (ie, drug) may be used to do this.

symptom (Sx): Subjective indication of a disease or a change in condition as perceived by the individual. Clinically noted as the subjective findings associated with an illness or dysfunction.

synapse: Minuscule space that exists between the end of the axon of one nerve cell and the cell body or dendrites of another.

synaptogenesis: The process of forming "synaptic connections" between nerve cells, or between nerve cells and muscle fibers; the basis of neuronal communication.

syncope: Fainting or brief lapse in consciousness caused by transient cerebral hypoxia.

syndactyly: Webbing of the fingers (or toes) involving only the skin or in complex cases the fusing of adjacent bones. Syndactyly is usually seen in children and can be surgically corrected.

syndrome: Combination of symptoms resulting from a single course or commonly occurring together that they constitute a distinct clinical picture.

synergism: Action of two or more substances, organs, or organisms to achieve an effect of which each is not individually capable.

synergist: Any muscle that functions to inhibit extraneous action from a muscle that would interfere with the action of a prime mover.

synergy: Fixed set of muscles contracting with a present sequence and time of contraction.

synovectomy: Excision of the synovial membrane (eg, as in the knee joint).

syringomyelia: Chronic progressive degenerative disorder of the spinal cord characterized by the development of an irregular cavity within the spinal cord.

systematic desensitization: Behavioral procedure that uses relaxation paired with an anxiety-provoking stimulus in an attempt to reduce the anxiety response.

systemic: Involving the whole system, such as in systemic rheumatoid arthritis.

systems interactions: The ways the various central nervous systems affect or interact with each other in order to provide a more integrative and functional nervous system.

systems model: A conceptual representation that incorporates a set of major functional divisions or systems within the central nervous system, which interlock and interrelate to create the functional whole. Although each division may be considered a whole in and of itself with multiple subsystems interlocking to form its entire division, each major component or division influences and is influenced by all others and thus the totality of the central nervous system is based on the summation of interactions, not individual function.

systems model/approach: A cyclical framework for understanding postural control that includes environmental stimuli; sensory reception, perception, and organization; and motor planning, execution, and modification.

systems theory: A theory describing movements emerging as a result of an interaction among many peripheral and central nervous system components with influence changing depending on the task.

systole: Contraction of the heart, especially of the ventricles, during which blood is forced into the aorta and pulmonary artery. Systolic blood pressure occurs during systole.

T cell: A heterogeneous population of lymphocytes comprising helper/inducer T cells and cytotoxic/suppressor T cells.

T score: Converted standard score in which the mean equals 50 and the standard deviation equals 10.

T-test: Parametric statistical test comparing differences of two data sets.

TENS (transcutaneous electrical nerve stimulation): Application of mild electric stimulation to skin electrodes placed over the region of pain to cause interference with the transmission of painful stimuli.

tachycardia: Rapid heartbeat.

tachypnea: Excessively rapid respiration marked by quick, shallow breathing.

tacit: Implied understanding that is not verbalized.

tactile defensiveness: Adverse reaction to being touched. A sensory integrative dysfunction characterized by tactile sensations that cause excessive emotional reactions, hyperactivity, or other behavioral problems.

tactile discrimination: The ability to discriminate among objects by the sense of touch.

tactile fremitus: A thrill or vibration that is perceptible on palpation. A thrill, as in the chest wall, that may be felt by a hand applied to the thorax while the patient is speaking.

talipes: Deformities of the foot, especially those congenital in origin. Synonym: clubfoot.

tamponade: Acute compression of the heart, which is due to effusion of fluid into the pericardium or collection of blood in the pericardium from rupture of the heart or a coronary vessel.

target site: Desired site for a drug's action within the body.

task: Work assigned to, selected by, or required of a person related to development of occupational performance skills; collection of activities related to accomplishment of a specific goal.

taxonomy: Laws and principles for classification of living things and organisms; also used for learning objectives.

technology transfer: In occupational therapy, the process by which knowledge is applied; occupational therapy knowledge is technology, which is transferred by administering evaluation and treatment.

telecommunication device for the deaf (TDD) or teletype-writer (TTY): Devices connected to a telephone by special adapters that allow telephone communication between a hearing person and a person with impaired hearing.

telemedicine: Provision of consultant services by off-site physicians to health care professionals on the scene using closed-circuit television.

telereceptive: The exteroceptors of hearing, sight, and smell that are sensitive to distant stimuli.

temporal environment: Manner in which social and cultural expectations influence behavior by organizing the time during which activities occur and the amount of time devoted to them.

tendon: Bands of strong, fibrous tissue that attach muscles to bones.

tendon injuries: Lacerations, avulsion-type injuries, and crash injuries to the flexor or extensor tendons of the hand; frequently work- or sports-related.

tenodesis: Surgical fixation of a tendon.

tenodesis splint: Orthosis fabricated to allow pinch and grasp movements through use of wrist extensors in substitution for finger flexors.

tenotomy: Surgical section of a tendon used, in some cases, to treat severe spasticity and contractures.

tensile force: Resistive force generated within a tissue in response to elongation or stretch.

tensiometer: Device used to measure force produced from an isometric contraction.

teratogen: Any agent that causes malformation in a developing embryo (eg, radiation, chemicals, drugs, alcohol, and pollutants).

teratogenic: Substances that harm the developing fetus, causing birth defects.

terbutaline: Drug given to mothers to stop premature labor.

tertiary care: Rehabilitation of disabilities resulting from disease/pathology to optimize and maximize an individual's functional status (eg, hypertension leading to stroke, tertiary care would prevent progression of disability).

tertiary circular reaction: Child's repetition of behavior with adaptations to make a new or different behavior.

tertiary prevention: Efforts that attempt to maximize function and minimize the detrimental effects of injury or illness.

test protocol: Specific procedures that must be followed when assessing a patient; formal testing procedures.

test-retest reliability: Extent to which repeated administrations of a test to the same people produce the same results.

tests and measures: Specific standardized methods and techniques used to gather data about the patient/client after the history and systems review have been performed.

test sensitivity: An instrument's ability to detect change within a measured variable.

tetany: A syndrome manifested by sharp flexion of joints, especially the wrist and ankle joints, muscle twitching, cramps, and convulsions, sometimes with attacks of difficult breathing.

tetraplegia: Impairment or loss of motor and/or sensory function in the cervical segments of the spinal cord due to damage of neural elements within the spinal cord.

text-to-speech synthesis: Translation of written communication into speech sounds and messages.

thalamic pain: Central nervous system pain caused by injury to the thalamus and characterized by contralateral and sometimes migratory pain brought on by peripheral stimulation.

theoretical rationale: Reason, based on theory or empirical evidence, for using a particular intervention for a specific person.

theory: Set of interrelated concepts used to describe, explain, or predict phenomena.

therapeutic activities: Activities within the limits of the patient's/client's physical, social, or cognitive capacity.

therapeutic community: Structured inpatient environment designed to provide a rehabilitative experience.

therapeutic environment: Organizing all aspects of the environment in a systematic way so that they enhance a patient's/client's abilities to perform desired tasks and activities (mental, emotional, functional).

therapeutic exercise: Exercise interventions directed toward maximizing functional capabilities. A broad range of activities intended to improve strength, range of motion (including muscle length), cardiovascular fitness, or flexibility or to otherwise increase a person's functional capacity.

therapeutic play programs: Hospital-based programs offering children play materials as a means of confronting fear, anxiety, and hostility.

therapeutic touch: The exchange of energy from one person to another for the purpose of healing.

there-and-then experience: Past experience used as a means to understand present conflicts.

thermistor: An electrical resistor that uses a semiconductor whose resistance varies sharply in a known manner with the ambient temperature; used in determining temperature.

thermotherapy: The use of heat or cold for therapeutic purposes.

third-party payment: Payment for services by someone other than the person receiving them.

third stage of labor: Birth of the placenta.

thoracic: Pertaining to the chest.

thoracocentesis: Surgical puncture of the chest wall with drainage of fluid.

thought disorder: Disturbance in thinking, including distorted content (eg, ideas, beliefs, sensory interpretation) and distorted written and spoken language (eg, word salad, loose associations, echolalia).

threat minimization: Psychological coping strategy in which emotions are managed through "playing down" the importance or significance of a stressor.

three-point pressure splints: Type of splint in which the middle force is directed opposite to the two distal or end forces. These splints operate through a series of reciprocal forces. Most splints incorporate the three-point pressure design.

threshold: Level at which a stimulus is recognized by sensory receptors.

thrombin: The enzyme derived from prothrombin that converts fibrinogen to fibrin.

thrombocytopenia: A condition in which the blood platelets are destroyed, causing severe bleeding if injury occurs.

thrombolytic: Dissolving or splitting up a thrombus.

thrombophlebitis: Inflammation of a vein associated with thrombus formation.

thromboplastin: Enzyme that assists in the process of blood clotting.

thrombosis: Coagulation of the blood in the heart or a blood vessel forming a clot.

thrust technique: A high velocity, short amplitude joint motion performed at the end of the available range of motion, but within the anatomical range of motion.

thyrotropin-releasing hormone: A hormone of the anterior pituitary gland having an affinity for and specifically stimulating the thyroid gland.

tibial torsion: Rotation occurring inherently in the shaft of the tibia from proximal to distal ends.

tic: Spasmodic muscular contraction usually involving the face, head, and neck.

time-related measures: Assessment in which the client records the thoughts, feelings, and/or behaviors that occur during a specific time period; time sampling and duration are included.

tinnitus: Subjective ringing or tinkling sound in the ear.

tissue approximation: Motion is prevented by compression of soft tissue when one body part is engaged against the other.

titer: The required quantity of a substance needed to produce a reaction to a given amount of another substance. Titer is synonymous with level.

titration: Volumetric determinations by means of standard solutions of known strength.

tolerance: Physiological and psychological accommodation or adaptation to a chemical agent over time.

tone: State of muscle contraction at rest; may be determined by resistance to stretch.

tongue-thrust swallow: An immature form of swallowing in which the tongue is projected forward instead of retracted during swallowing.

tonic-clonic: Muscle stiffening and falling into unconsciousness followed by rhythmic jerking, breathing problems, drooling, loss of bladder control, and finally confusion and sleepiness.

tonic labyrinthine reflex: A normal postural reflex in animals, abnormally accentuated in decerebrate humans, characterized by extension of all four limbs when the head is positioned in space at an angle above the horizontal in quadrupeds or in the neutral, erect position in humans. Synonym: decerebrate rigidity.

tonic neck reflex: A normal response in newborns to extend the arm and the leg on the side of the body to which the head is quickly turned while the infant is supine and to flex the limbs of the opposite side. Integrated at 3 to 4 months of age. Absence of persistence of the reflex may indicate central nervous system damage. Synonym: asymmetric tonic neck reflex.

tonotopic: Organization of cells within the auditory system that enables one to identify the exact sound heard.

top-down processing: When processing starts with higher-order stored knowledge and depends upon contextual information or is "conceptually driven."

topographic: Organization of cells in the visual system that enables one to identify the exact location and features of the stimulus.

torque: Rotating tendency of force; equals the product of force and the perpendicular distance from the axis of a lever to the point of application of the same force.

torsion dystonia: A condition in which twisting occurs in the alignment of body parts due to a lack of normal muscle tone secondary to infection or disease of the nervous system.

torticollis: Irresistible turning of the head that becomes more persistent, so that eventually the head is held continually to one side. The spasm of the muscles is often painful, and this condition may be caused by a birth injury to the sternocleidomastoid muscle. Synonym: wryneck.

total hip arthroplasty: Type of hip surgery involving the removal of the head and neck of the femur and replacement with a prosthetic appliance.

total lymphoid irradiation (TLI): Radiation therapy targeted to the body's lymph nodes; the goal is to suppress immune system functioning (reduce the number of lymphocytes in the blood).

total quality management (TQM): Paradigm for management developed by Deming; emphasized three themes: continuous quality improvement, empowerment of workers at all levels, and having a standard to do things right the first time.

toxicology: Branch of pharmacology that examines harmful chemicals and their effects on the body.

tracheotomy: Incision of the trachea through the skin and muscles of the neck for establishment of an airway, exploration, removal of a foreign body, obtainment of a biopsy specimen, or removal of a local lesion.

trachoma: Chronic infectious eye disease of the conjunctiva and cornea.

trackball: Control device used to move and operate the cursor on the computer screen.

traction: The therapeutic use of manual or mechanical tension created by a pulling force to produce a combination of distraction and gliding to relieve pain and increase tissue flexibility.

training effect: As a result of exercise, heart rate and blood pressure become less than previously required for the same amount of work.

tranquilizer: Drug that produces a calming effect, relieving tension and anxiety.

transcutaneous electrical nerve stimulation (TENS): The use of electrical energy to stimulate cutaneous and peripheral nerves via electrodes on the skin's surface. A procedure in which electrodes are placed on the surface of the skin over specific nerves and electrical stimulation is done in a manner that is thought to improve central nervous system function, reduce spasticity, and control pain.

transfer: The process of relocating a body from one object or surface to another (eg, getting into or out of bed, moving from a wheelchair to a chair).

transfer appropriate processing: The concept that the cognitive processes used while learning determine the type of criteria task on which one will best perform when evaluated for what has been learned.

transfer of learning: Practice and learning of one task can influence the learning of another task.

transient ischemic attack (TIA): Episode of temporary cerebral dysfunction caused by impaired blood flow to the brain. TIAs have many symptoms, such as dizziness, weakness, numbness, or paralysis of a limb or half of the body. TIA may last only a few minutes or up to 24 hours but does not have any persistent neurologic deficits.

transudate: A fluid substance that has passed through a membrane or been extruded from a tissue, sometimes as a result of inflammation. A transudate, in contrast to an exudate, is characterized by high fluidity and a low content of protein, cells, or of solid materials derived from cells.

traumatic brain injury (TBI): Injury caused by impact to the head. An insult to the brain caused by an external physical force that may produce a diminished or altered state of consciousness, which results in impairment of cognitive abilities or physical functioning.

treatment: The sum of all interventions provided by the physical therapist to a patient/client during an episode of care. Application of or involvement in activities/stimulation to effect improvement in abilities for self-directed activities, self-care, or maintenance of the home.

tremor: Involuntary shaking or trembling.

Trendelenburg's position: A position with the patient on his or her back on a plane inclined 30 to 40 degrees and the legs and feet hanging over the end of the table.

trephination: Process of making a circular hole in the skull.

treppe: Type of muscle contraction in which the first few contractions increase in strength when a rested muscle receives repeated stimuli.

TriAlliance of Health and Rehabilitation Professions: Created in September 1991 between the American Physical Therapy Association, American Occupational Therapy Association, and the American Speech-Language-Hearing Association as a forum to represent and address the concerns of health and rehabilitation professions.

trigeminal neuralgia: A neurologic condition of the trigeminal facial nerve characterized by a brief but frequent flashing, stab-like pain radiating usually throughout mandibular and maxillary regions. Caused by degeneration of the nerve or pressure on it; also known as *tic douloureux*.

trigeminy: The condition of occurring in threes, especially the occurrence of three pulse beats in rapid succession.

trigger point: Highly sensitive point within the muscle or myofascial tissue.

triglyceride: Any of a group of esters derived from glycerol and three fatty acid radicals; the chief component of fats and oils.

trigonal: Relating to a triangular shape.

trophic: Changes that occur as a result of inadequate circulation, such as loss of hair, thinning of skin, and ridging of nail.

trophotropic: Combination of parasympathetic nervous system activity, somatic muscle relaxation, and cortical beta rhythm synchronization. Resting or sleep state.

truncal ataxia: Uncoordinated movement of the trunk.

tuberosity: Medium-sized protrusion on a bone.

tunnel vision: The visual field is limited to one side; the peripheral fields are lost, usually due to damage to the optic chiasm.

two-tail (nondirectional) test: A statistical test of the null hypothesis in which both tails of the distribution are utilized.

tympany: A tympanic, or bell-like, percussion note. A modified tympanic note heard on percussion of the chest in some cases of pneumothorax.

type A behavior: A cluster of personality traits that include high achievement motivation, drive, and a fast-paced lifestyle. Associated with stress-related diseases, such as heart disease.

type B behavior: A cluster of personality traits that include low achievement motivation, laziness, and a laid-back lifestyle. Associated with inactivity, lack of exercise, and sedentary-related diseases, such as heart disease.

U **ulcer:** An open sore on the skin or some mucous membrane characterized by the disintegration of tissue and, often, the discharge of serous drainage.

ultrasound: A diagnostic or therapeutic technique using high-frequency sound waves to produce heat; **pulsed u.** the application of therapeutic ultrasound using predetermined interrupted frequencies.

ultraviolet: A form of radiant energy using light rays with wavelengths beyond the violet end of the visible spectrum.

unconditional positive regard: Unconditional love and acceptance.

undermine: Tissue destruction underlying intact skin along wound margins.

universal: Pertaining to any group, need, or environment.

universal access design: Concept of designing the built environment to permit access regardless of physical or sensory capability.

universal assessments: Used to evaluate the environmental needs of any group using all sizes and types of settings.

universal cuff: Device used on the dominant hand to hold tools, such as a pencil or brush.

universal goniometer: Instrument used to measure joint motion. It consists of a protractor, an axis, and two arms.

universal hemiplegic sling: Sling that is used to support a nonfunctional shoulder and prevent shoulder subluxation by restricting active motion and keeping the humerus in adduction and internal rotation.

universal precautions: An approach to infection control designed to prevent transmission of blood-borne diseases such as AIDS and hepatitis B; includes specific recommendations for the use of gloves, protective eye wear, and masks.

unobtrusive observation: Observation for assessment that minimizes reactivity.

upper motor neuron (UMN): Neurons of the cerebral cortex that conduct stimuli from the motor cortex of the brain to motor nuclei of cerebral nerves of the ventral gray columns of the spinal cord.

urbanization: Fundamental belief and societal attitude that men were to provide financial support and women were to care for their families. This is a 19th-century concept.

uremia: Toxic condition associated with renal insufficiency in which urine is present in the blood.

urethrocele: Prolapse of the urethra with bulging into the vaginal opening.

urgency: Need to excrete urine immediately.

urogenital diaphragm: The perineal membrane; the deep muscle layer of the deep fascial layer that supports the pelvic organs.

urokinase: A substance found in the urine of mammals, including humans, that activates the fibrinolytic system, acting enzymatically by splitting plasminogen.

uterine dysfunction: The inability of the uterus to contract and relax in a coordinated fashion.

uterus: The pear-shaped organ in which the fetus grows; also called *the womb*.

uterine inversion: When the uterus loses its shape and comes out toward its opening.

utilization review: Assessment of the appropriateness and economy of an admission to a health care facility or a continued hospitalization.

V **VO₂ max:** Maximum oxygen consumption, usually expressed as a volume of oxygen consumed per minute. It is used as an indicator of maximal exercise power and to standardize exercise rate between individuals (eg, exercising at 60% of one's VO_2 max).

vagina: A 5- to 6-inch long elastic canal from the vulva to the uterus.

vaginismus: Painful spasms of the vagina from contraction of the muscles surrounding the vagina.

valgus: An angulation that does not conform to an imaginary circle in which the patient is placed. A limb deformity in which the extremity is moved away (ie, laterally) from the midline.

validity: Degree to which a test measures what it is intended to measure.

Valsalva's maneuver: A process in which the intra-abdominal pressure is increased by holding the breath and pushing down during exertion or excretion.

values: Operational beliefs that one accepts as one's own and that determine behavior.

valvuloplasty: Replacement of a cardiac valve with a prosthetic valve.

valvulotomy: Incision of a valve, such as valve of the heart.

variance: Measure that demonstrates how scores in a distribution deviate from the mean.

varicocele: Enlargement of the veins in the spermatic cord.

varicose veins: Refers to the enlargement of veins when the valves in the veins become swollen and have retrograde flow within them.

varus: An angulation that conforms to an imaginary circle in which the patient is placed. Directed toward the center.

vasomotor center: A regulatory center in the lower pons and medulla oblongata that regulates the diameter of blood vessels, especially the arterioles.

vasopneumatic compression device: A device to decrease edema by using compressive forces that are applied to the body part.

vasopressor: Stimulating contraction of the muscular tissue of the capillaries and arteries. An agent that stimulates the contraction of the muscular tissue of the capillaries and arteries.

vector: Arrow that indicates direction and magnitude of a force.

ventilation: The circulation of air; to aerate (blood); oxygenate. Mechanical ventilation is the use of equipment to circulate oxygen to the respiratory system.

ventilatory equivalent (V_E/VO_2): The ratio of minute ventilation to oxygen consumption. The normal ratio is 25:1, meaning that for 25 L of air breathed, 1 L of oxygen has been consumed.

ventilatory pump: Thoracic skeleton and skeletal muscles and their innervation responsible for ventilation. The muscles include the diaphragm; the intercostal, scalene, and sternocleidomastoid muscles; accessory muscles of ventilation; and the abdominal, triangular, and quadratus lumborum muscles.

ventilatory pump dysfunction: Abnormalities of the thoracic skeleton, respiratory muscles, airways, or lungs that interrupt or interfere with the work of breathing or ventilation.

ventral: In terms of anatomical position, located toward the front or the belly.

veracity: Obligation of the client and the therapist to tell the truth at all times.

verbal communication: Process of interpreting another's words and expressing one's own thoughts and emotions through words.

verbal rating scale: A pain intensity measurement in which patients/clients rate pain on a continuum that is subdivided from left to right into gradually increasing pain intensities.

verbal therapies: Any therapy in which talk and discussion are the primary modes of intervention.

vergence: Movement of the two eyes in the opposite direction.

vermis: Forms the unpaired medial region of the cerebellum.

versions: Movement of the two eyes in the same direction.

vertigo: One's sensation of revolving in space or of having objects move around him or her.

vestibular: Pertaining to a vestibule, a cavity, or space at the entrance of a canal, such as the inner ear. Describing the sense of balance located in the inner ear. Interpreting stimuli regarding head position and movement based on the shift of fluid and inner ear receptors.

vestibular-bilateral disorder: A sensory integrative dysfunction characterized by shortened duration nystagmus, poor integration of the two sides of the body and brain, and difficulty in learning to read or compute. The disorder is caused by underreactive vestibular responses.

vestibular function: Pertaining to the sense of balance.

vestibulocochlear nerve: Combined portions of the eighth cranial nerve.

vestibulo-ocular reflex: A normal reflex in which eye position compensates for movement of the head, induced by excitation of vestibular apparatus.

vicarious reinforcement: Idea that one person's observation of another person's experiencing a positive consequence as a result of a particular behavior increases the probability that the observer will exhibit that behavior.

videofluoroscopy: Radiological study that allows visualization of the pharyngeal and esophageal phases of swallow.

vigorometer: Alternative measurement of hand strength that requires the person to squeeze a rubber bulb.

virtual reality: Term describing any optical or sensory simulation of something real, to the point of confounding the senses into accepting that simulation.

viscosity: Describes the extent to which a tissue's resistance to deformation is dependent on the rate of the deforming force.

visual: Connected with or used in seeing. Interpreting stimuli through the eyes, including peripheral vision and acuity.

visual acuity: Measure of visual discrimination of fine details of high contrast.

visual agnosia: The inability to name objects as viewed.

visual analog scale: A tool used in a pain examination that allows the patient/client to indicate his or her degree of pain by pointing to a visual representation of pain intensity.

visual evoked response (VER): Presentation of a particular visual stimulus evokes consistent electrocortical activity that can be recorded from electrodes placed on the scalp.

visualization: An effective means of deepening relaxation and desensitizing a real-life situation that is generally met with stress and tension.

visual motor coordination: The ability to coordinate vision with the movements of the body or parts of the body.

visual motor function: The ability to draw or copy forms or to perform constructive tasks.

visual motor integration: The ability to integrate vision with movements of the body or parts of the body by coordinating the interaction of information from the eyes with body movement during activity.

visual neglect: Inattention to visual stimuli occurring in the space on the involved side of the body.

visual orientation: Awareness and location of objects in the environment and their relationship to each other and to one's self.

visual perception: The brain's ability to understand sensory input to determine size, shape, distance, and form of objects.

visual perceptual dysfunction: May include deficits in any of the areas of visual perception: figure-ground, form constancy, or size discrimination. Distinct from deficits in functional visual skills and tested separately.

vision screening: Can include distance and near visual acuities, oculomotilities, eye alignment or posture, depth perception, and visual fields.

vital capacity (VC): Measurement of the amount of air that can be expelled at the normal rate of exhalation after a maximum inspiration, representing the greatest possible breathing capacity.

vital signs: Measurements of pulse rate, respiration rate, and body temperature.

vocational activities: Participating in tasks associated with performance of work-related activities and skills.

vocational maturity: Scale along which people are placed during their working lives. Maturity is reached when occupational activities are aligned with what is expected of the corresponding age group.

volar: Palm of the hand or the sole of the foot.

volar splint: Splint that runs from the lower third of the forearm to the individual's fingertips, with the thumb extended and abducted. The phalangeal joint should be slightly flexed, thus enabling this type of splint construction to prevent stiffening of the phalangeal joints in extension. This splint is often used as a night splint for inpatients.

volitional postural movements: Movement patterns under volitional control that relate specifically to controlling the center-of-gravity, as in skating, ballet, gymnastics, etc.

Volkmann's contracture: Permanent contracture of a muscle due to replacement of destroyed muscle cells with fibrous tissue that lacks the ability to stretch. Destruction of muscle cells may occur from interference with circulation caused by a tight bandage, splint, or cast.

volume measurement: The amount of fluid that has been displaced from a container (of any size) following the introduction of part or all of the body.

voluntary muscle: Type of muscle tissue that can be controlled by the brain to produce movement.

volvulus: Twisting of the bowel upon itself.

vulva: External female genitalia.
vulvadynia: Painful intercourse.
vulva vestibulitis: Irritation of the vestibule of the external genitalia.

waddling gait: Gait pattern in which the feet are wide apart, resembling that of a duck.

wallerian degeneration: The physical and biochemical changes that occur in a nerve because of the loss of axonal continuity following trauma.

wandering cells: Connective cells usually involved with short-term activities, such as protection and repair.

warm-up: Exercise that prepares the person for the experience to follow.

waxy rigidity: Symptom of catatonia in which an individual will assume any position in which he or she is placed and remain there until moved again.

wear-and tear theory: Theory that describes the biological effects of aging as the body deteriorates.

wearing schedule: Amount of time the splint is to be worn and when it should be off.

weight: Measure of matter that incorporates the effect of gravity on an object; a kinematic measurement.

weight shift: Bearing the body's weight from one leg to another; shifting the center of gravity.

wellness: Dynamic state of health in which an individual progresses toward a higher level of functioning, achieving an optimum balance between internal and external environments. Concepts that embrace positive health behaviors (eg, exercise, nutrition, stress reduction).

Wharton's jelly: Connective tissue with a jelly-like quality within the umbilical cord that supports the umbilical vessels.

wheelchair pushing cuffs: Soft gloves worn to protect the hands and to provide traction when pushing a wheelchair.

wheeze: A whistling sound made in breathing resulting from constriction and/or partial obstruction of the airways. Heard on auscultation; however, in severe cases of asthma and chronic obstructive pulmonary disease, it can often be audible without the use of a stethoscope.

whiplash injury: Injury caused by sudden hyperextension and flexion of the neck, traumatizing cervical ligaments; common in rear-end car accidents or falls.

white matter: Area of the central nervous system that contains the axons of the cells.

within normal limits (WNL): The normal range of motion at a given joint.

Wolff's law: States that bone is formed in areas of stress and reabsorbed in areas of nonstress.

work behaviors: Behaviors that are necessary for successful participation in a job or independent living (eg, cooperative behavior). Synonyms: prevocational readiness or personal skills.

work capacity evaluation: Comprehensive process that systematically uses work, real or simulated, to access and measure an individual's physical abilities to work.

work conditioning: An intensive, work-related, goal-oriented, conditioning program designed specifically to restore systemic neuromuscular functions (eg, strength, endurance, movement, flexibility, motor control) and cardiopulmonary functions. The objective of a work conditioning program is to restore physical capacity and function to enable the patient/client to return to work.

work/education: Skill and performance in purposeful and productive activities in the home, employment, school, and community.

work hardening: Type of treatment program that is graded work simulation to increase an individual's productivity to an acceptable level to be able to function in a work environment. Highly structured, goal-oriented, individualized treatment program designed to return the client to work. Work hardening programs, which are interdisciplinary in nature, use real or simulated work activities designed to restore physical, behavioral, and vocational functions. Work hardening addresses issues of productivity, safety, physical tolerances, and worker behaviors.

work practice controls: Techniques to improve worker safety, such as education and training in safe and proper work techniques.

work samples: Well-defined work activity involving tasks, materials, and tools that are identical or similar to those in an actual job or cluster of jobs. It is used to access an individual's vocational aptitude, worker characteristics, and vocational interests.

work setting: Any environment in which an individual performs productive activity.

work site analysis: Formal assessment of the relationship between worker habits, specific work tasks, and the work environment.

work space: Physical area in which one performs work.

work tolerance: Refers to how a person deals with his or her work environment. This includes being able to handle the stress and pressures that are part of the job and maintain one's productivity, quality, and effort time after time.

work-up: The process of performing a complete evaluation of an individual, including history, physical examination, laboratory test, and x-ray or other diagnostic procedures, to acquire an accurate database on which a diagnosis and treatment plan may be established.

wound: An area of disrupted or discontinuous skin or tissue.

wound base: Uppermost viable tissue layer of a wound; may be covered with slough or eschar.

wound care: Procedures used to achieve a clean wound bed, promote a moist environment, facilitate autolytic debridement, or absorb excessive exudation from a wound complex.

wound management: Comprehensive physical therapy intervention to reduce pressure points and manage the interdisciplinary efforts to facilitate wound care and healing.

wound margin: Rim or border of a wound.

wound repair: Healing process. Partial thickness involves epithelialization; full thickness involves contraction granulation and epithelialization.

wrist system: Computerized glove that measures range of motion.

xenophobia: Fear and/or hatred of any person or thing that is strange or foreign.

xeroderma: Condition of rough and dry skin.

X-linked recessive: Trait transmitted by a gene located on the X chromosome. These traits are passed on by a carrier mother to an affected son.

yarn cone: Object used to measure thumb abduction and extension and can also be adapted to measure the first web space of burned hands. There are no norms for this measurement. It is used to measure a patient's progress over time.

young old: Persons between 60 and 75 years of age.

Z

z score (standard score): Numerical value from the transformation of a raw score into units of standard deviation.

zero-to-three infant stimulation groups: Groups that provide therapeutic services for children from birth to 3 years of age, because this age-group is not yet eligible for public school placement.

zip disk: Disk that stores 100 megabytes of data.

zone of proximal development: Difference between what a child can do alone and what he or she can do with the assistance of a more skilled helper.

zygote: Single cell formed at conception by the union of the 23 chromosomes of the sperm and the 23 chromosomes of the ovum.

BIBLIOGRAPHY

Accreditation Manual for Hospitals. Oakbrook Terrace, Ill: Joint Commission on Accreditation of Healthcare Organizations; 1998.

American Heritage Dictionaries. *Compact American Medical Dictionary: A Concise and Up-to-Date Guide to Medical Terms.* Philadelphia, Pa: Chapters Publishing; 1998.

American Physical Therapy Association. Guide to physical therapy practice. *J Am Phys Assoc.* 1997;77(11).

Bailey D. *Research for the Health Professional: A Practical Guide.* Philadelphia, Pa: FA Davis; 1991.

Bottomley JM, Lewis CB. *Geriatric Rehabilitation: A Clinical Approach.* 2nd ed. Upper Saddle River, NJ: Prentice Hall Publishers; 2003.

Commonwealth of Massachusetts. *Architectural Access Board Rules and Regulations 521 CMR.* Boston, Mass: Architectural Access Board; 1996.

Dilberti W, Eccles M. *Thesaurus of Aging Terminology, Ageline.* 5th ed. Washington, DC: American Association of Retired Persons; 1994.

Guccione AA, ed. *Geriatric Physical Therapy.* St. Louis, Mo: Mosby-Year Book; 1993.

Jablonski S. *Dictionary of Medical Acronyms and Abbreviations.* Philadelphia, Pa: Hanley & Belfus Publishers; 1997.

Jacobs K. *Quick Reference Dictionary for Occupational Therapy.* 2nd ed. Thorofare, NJ: SLACK Incorporated; 1999.

Merriam-Webster's Medical Desk Dictionary. Springfield, Mass: G&C Merriam Co Publishers; 1998.

Miller-Keane Encyclopedia & Dictionary of Medicine, Nursing, & Allied Health. 5th ed. Philadelphia, Pa: WB Saunders; 1992.

Mosby's Medical, Nursing & Allied Health Dictionary. 4th ed. St. Louis, Mo: Mosby-Year Book; 1994.

Physicians' Desk Reference. 49th ed. Montvale, NJ: Medical Economics; 1995.

Spencer JW, Jacobs JJ. *Complementary Alternative Medicine: An Evidence-Based Approach.* St. Louis, Mo: Mosby-Year Book; 1999.

Stedman's Medical Dictionary. 26th ed. Baltimore, Md: Williams & Wilkins; 1995.

Thomas CL. *Taber's Cyclopedic Medical Dictionary.* 18th ed. Philadelphia, Pa: FA Davis; 1997.

Umphred DA, ed. *Neurological Rehabilitation.* 4th ed. St. Louis, Mo: Mosby-Year Book; 2001.

World Health Organization. *International Classification of Impairments, Disabilities, and Handicaps: A Manual of Classification Relating to the Consequences of Disease.* Albany, NY: Author; 1980.

List of Appendices

Suggested Reading

American Physical Therapy Association. Guide to physical therapy practice. 2nd ed. *J Am Phys Assoc.* 2001;81(1).

Angelo J, Jane SJ, eds. *Assistive Technology for Rehabilitation Therapists.* Philadelphia, Pa: FA Davis; 1997.

Anson DK. *Alternative Computer Access: A Guide to Selection.* Philadelphia, Pa: FA Davis; 1997.

Bailey D. *Research for the Health Professional: A Practical Guide.* Philadelphia, Pa: FA Davis; 1991.

Bolton B. *Handbook of Measurement and Evaluation in Rehabilitation.* Baltimore, Md: Paul H. Brookes; 1987.

Bottomley JM, Lewis CB. *Geriatric Rehabilitation: A Clinical Approach.* 2nd ed. Upper Saddle River, NJ: Prentice Hall Publishers; 2003.

Bruckner J. *The Gait Workbook: A Practical Guide to Clinical Gait Analysis.* Thorofare, NJ: SLACK Incorporated; 1998.

Cech D, Martin S. *Functional Movement Development Across the Life Span.* 2nd ed. Philadelphia, Pa: WB Saunders; 2002.

Commonwealth of Massachusetts. *Architectural Access Board Rules and Regulations 521 CMR.* Boston, Mass: Architectural Access Board; 2002.

Curtis KA. *The Physical Therapist's Guide to Health Care.* Thorofare, NJ: SLACK Incorporated; 1999.

Davis CM. *Patient Practitioner Interaction: An Experiential Manual for Developing the Art of Health Care.* 3rd ed. Thorofare, NJ: SLACK Incorporated; 1998.

Davis CM. *Complementary Therapies in Rehabilitation: Evidence for Efficacy in Therapy, Prevention, and Wellness.* 2nd ed. Thorofare, NJ: SLACK Incorporated. In press.

DeLisa J, Gans B, eds. *Rehabilitation Medicine: Principles and Practice.* 2nd ed. Philadelphia, Pa: JB Lippincott; 1993.

Dutton R. *Clinical Reasoning in Physical Disabilities.* Baltimore, Md: Lippincott, Williams & Wilkins; 1995.

Fisher SV, Helm PA, eds. *Comprehensive Rehabilitation of Burns.* Baltimore, Md: Lippincott, Williams & Wilkins; 1984.

Fuhrer MJ, ed. *Rehabilitation Outcomes: Analysis and Measurement.* Baltimore, Md: Paul H. Brookes; 1987.

Goldstein TS. *Geriatric Orthopaedics: Rehabilitative Management of Common Problems.* 2nd ed. Gaithersburg, Md: Aspen Publication; 1999.

Goodman CC, Boissonnault WG. *Pathology: Implications for the Physical Therapist.* Philadelphia, Pa: WB Saunders Company; 1998.

Guccione AA, ed. *Geriatric Physical Therapy*. 2nd ed. St. Louis, Mo: Mosby-Year Book; 2000.

Hopp JW, Rogers EA. *AIDS and the Allied Health Professions*. Philadelphia, Pa: FA Davis; 1989.

International Classification of Diseases: Clinical Modification. 10th revision. New York, NY: World Health Organization; 2000.

Kane RL, Ouslander JG, Abrass IB. *Essentials of Clinical Geriatrics*. 4th ed. New York, NY: McGraw-Hill; 1999.

Kauffman TL. *Geriatric Rehabilitation Manual*. Philadelphia, Pa: Churchill Livingstone; 1999.

Kendall FP, McCreary EK, Provance PG. *Muscles: Testing and Function*. 4th ed. Baltimore, Md: Lippincott, Williams & Wilkins; 1993.

Konin JG, Wiksten DL, Isear JA Jr, Brader H. *Special Tests for Orthopedic Examination*. 2nd ed. Thorofare, NJ: SLACK Incorporated; 2002.

Malone TR, ed. *Physical and Occupational Therapy: Drug Implications for Practice*. Philadelphia, Pa: JB Lippincott; 1989.

Norkin C, Levangie P. *Joint Structure and Function: A Comprehensive Analysis*. Philadelphia, Pa: FA Davis; 1992.

O'Connor LJ, Gourley RJ. *Obstetric and Gynecologic Care in Physical Therapy*. Thorofare, NJ: SLACK Incorporated; 1990.

O'Sullivan SB, Schmitz TJ. *Physical Rehabilitation: Assessment and Treatment*. 2nd ed. Philadelphia, PA: FA Davis Company; 1988.

Outcomes Effectiveness in Physical Therapy: An Annotated Bibliography. Alexandria, VA: American Physical Therapy Association; 1995.

Palmer ML, Toms JE. *Manual for Functional Training*. 3rd ed. Philadelphia, Pa: FA Davis; 1993.

Perry J. *Gait Analysis: Normal and Pathological Function*. Thorofare, NJ: SLACK Incorporated; 1992.

Pomeroy B. *BeginnerNet in Rehabilitation: A Beginner's Guide to the Internet and the World Wide Web*. Thorofare, NJ: SLACK Incorporated; 1996.

Roberge RA, Roberts SO. *Exercise Physiology: Exercise, Performance, and Clinical Applications*. St. Louis, Mo: Mosby-Year Book; 1997.

Roggow PA, Berg DK, Lewis MD. *The Home Rehabilitation Program Guide*. Thorofare, NJ: SLACK Incorporated; 1994.

Spencer JW, Jacobs JJ. *Complementary Alternative Medicine: An Evidence-Based Approach*. St. Louis, Mo: Mosby-Year Book; 1999.

Tan JC. *Physical Medicine and Rehabilitation: Diagnostics, Therapeutics, and Basic Problems*. St. Louis, Mo: Mosby-Year Book; 1998.

Trott M, Laurel M, Windeck S. *Sense Abilities: Understanding Sensory Integration*. Tucson, Ariz: Therapy Skill Builders; 1993.

Umphred DA, ed. *Neurological Rehabilitation*. 4th ed. St. Louis, Mo: Mosby-Year Book; 2001.

Van Deusen J, Brunt D. *Assessment in Occupational and Physical Therapy.* Philadelphia, Pa: WB Saunders; 1997.

Zoltan B. *Vision, Perception, and Cognition: A Manual for the Evaluation and Treatment of the Neurologically Impaired Adult.* 3rd ed. Thorofare, NJ: SLACK Incorporated; 1996.

General Acronyms and Abbreviations

(A): assisted, assistance
A: accommodation
a.: artery
AAE: active assistive exercise
AAROM: active assistive range of motion
abd: abduction
ABG: arterial blood gas
ABI: ankle brachial index
ABNORM: abnormal
ABR: absolute bed rest
A/C: acromioclavicular
AC: alternating current
ACA: anterior cerebral artery
ACCE: Academic Coordinator of Clinical Education
ACDV: acute cardiovascular disease
ACLF: adult congregate living facility
ACLS: advanced cardiac life support
ACHF: acute congestive heart failure
ACT: adaptive control of thoughts
ACTH: adrenocorticotropic hormone
ACVD: arterial cardiovascular disease
AD: Alzheimer's disease; autogeneic drainage; admitting diagnosis
ADA: Americans with Disabilities Act
add: adduction
ADD: attention deficit disorder
ADH: antidiuretic hormone
ADHD: attention deficit hyperactivity disorder
ADL: activities of daily living
ad lib: as desired
ADM: administration
ADP: adenosine diphosphate
ADS: alternative delivery system
A/E: above elbow
AED: automated external defibrillation
AF: atrial fibrillation
AFB: acid-fast bacillus
AFDC: Aid to Families with Dependent Children

AFO: ankle foot orthosis

AI: aortic insufficiency

AICD: automatic implantable cardioverter-defibrillator

AID: acute inflammatory disease

AIDS: acquired immunodeficiency syndrome

AJ: ankle jerk

AJPT: *American Journal of Physical Therapy*

A/K: above knee

Alb: albumin

ALOS: average length of stay

ALS: amyotrophic lateral sclerosis

A-M: Austin-Moore prosthesis

AMA: against medical advice

Am't: amount

ANCOVA: analysis of covariance

ANOVA: analysis of variance

ANS: autonomic nervous system

Ant: anterior

AOB: alcohol on breath

AP: anterior-posterior

APE: anterior pituitary extract

APG: Ambulatory Patient (Payment) Group

Approx: approximately

Aq: water

ARD: acute respiratory distress

ARF: acute rheumatic fever

AROM: active range of motion

ART: active resistive training

AS: aortic stenosis

ASA: aspirin (acetyl salicylic acid)

ASAP: as soon as possible

ASCII: American Standard Code for Information Interchange

ASD: atrial septal defect

ASHD: arterial sclerotic heart disease

ASIS: anterior superior iliac spine

ASO: arteriosclerosis obliterans

ASROM: assistive range of motion

AT: assistive technology

ATNR: asymmetrical tonic neck reflex

ATP: adenosine triphosphate

(B): both, bilateral

BADL: basic activities of daily living

Ba Enema: barium enema

BBA: Balanced Budget Act
BBS: bulletin board system
B/E: below elbow; base equivalent
BFP: biologic false positive
BG: blood glucose
b.i.d.: twice a day
Bilat: bilateral
B/K: below knee
BKA: below knee amputee
Bl: blood
BLS: basic life support
BM: bowel movement
bm: body mechanics
BMD: bone mineral density
BMI: body mass index
BMR: basal metabolic rate
BOS: base of support
BP: blood pressure
BPH: benign prostatic hypertrophy
BPM: beats per minute
BR: bedrest
BRB: bright red blood
BRP: bathroom privileges
BS: blood sugar; breath sounds
BSA: body surface area
BSF: benign senescent forgetfulness
BT: brain tumor
BUN: blood urea nitrogen
Bx: biopsy
C: centigrade; Celsius; cervical
Ca: cancer, carcinoma
Ca++: calcium
CABG: coronary artery bypass graft
CAD: coronary artery disease
cal: calorie
CAMP: cyclic adenosine monophosphate
CAO: chronic airway obstruction
cap: capsules
CAPD: continuous ambulatory peritoneal dialysis
CART: classification and regression trees
CAT: computer-assisted tomography
CAVH: continuous arteriovenous hemofiltration
CBC: complete blood count

CBI: closed brain injury
CBR: complete bedrest
CBS: chronic brain syndrome
CC: chief complaint
cc: cubic centimeter(s)
CCCE: clinical coordinator of clinical education
CCS: cardiopulmonary certified specialist
CCU: coronary care unit
CD: cardiovascular disease; compact disk
CDC: Centers for Disease Control and Prevention
CDH: congenital dislocated hip; congenital hip dysplasia
CDM: Charge Description Master (HCFA)
CE: continuing education
CEO: chief executive officer
CEU: continuing education unit
CF: cystic fibrosis
CFR: code of federal regulations
CHAMPUS: Civilian Health and Medical Program of the Uniformed Services
CHD: coronary heart disease
CHF: congestive heart failure
CHI: closed head injury
CHT: certified hand therapist
CK: creatine kinase
CKC: closed kinetic chain
Cl: chloride; chlorine; cardiac index; clinical instructor
CICU: coronary intermediate care unit
cm: centimeter(s)
CMP: competitive medical plan
CMS: Centers for Medicare & Medicaid Services (formerly HCFA)
CNS: central nervous system
CO: carbon monoxide
CO_2: carbon dioxide
c/o: complains of
COB: coordination of benefits
COG: center of gravity
COJ: *Classification of Jobs According to Worker Trait Factors*
COLA: cost of living adjustment
COLD: chronic obstructive lung disease
COM: center of mass or center of motion
CONTRA: contraindication
COPD: chronic pulmonary obstructive disease
CORF: comprehensive outpatient rehabilitation facility

COTA: certified occupational therapy assistant
CP: chest pain; cold pack
CPAP: continuous positive airway pressure
CPE: certified professional ergonomist; continuing professional education
CPEF: Clinical Performance Evaluation Form (developed by the New England Consortium of Academic Coordinators of Clinical Education)
CPI: consumer price index
CPK: creatine phosphokinase
CPM: continuous passive motion
CPR: cardiopulmonary resuscitation
CPT: *Current Procedural Terminology*
CPU: central processing unit
CQI: continuous quality improvement
CRF: chronic renal failure
CRI: chronic renal insufficiency
C-section: cesarean section
CSF: cerebrospinal fluid
CSHN: children with special health needs
CSM: Combined Sections Meeting—APTA
C&S: culture and sensitivity
CST: convulsive shock treatment
CT: computed tomography
CTD: connective tissue disease
CTS: carpal tunnel syndrome
CTX: cervical traction
cu: cubic
CV: cardiovascular
CVA: cerebrovascular accident
cva: costovertebral angle
cva T: costovertebral angle tendon
CVD: cardiovascular disease; *see also* CD
CVI: cardiovascular insufficiency
CVP: central venous pressure
CXR: chest x-ray
D: distal
d/c: discharge
D&C: dilation and curettage
DD: developmental disabilities; differential diagnosis
D&E: dilation and evacuation
Dep: dependent
Derm: dermatology

DFF: directions for the future
dia: diameter
DIP: distal interphalangeal
DJD: degenerative joint disease
DKA: diabetic ketoacidosis
dL: deciliter (= 100 mL)
DM: diabetes mellitus
DME: durable medical equipment
DMEPOS: durable medical equipment prostheses, orthotics, and supplies
DMERC: DME regional carrier (HCFA)
DMG: dimethylglycerine
DNA: deoxyribonucleic acid
DNR: "do not resuscitate" orders
DPT: Doctor of Physical Therapy
DOA: dead on arrival
DOB: date of birth
DOE: dyspnea on exertion
doff: take off clothing
DOMS: delayed onset muscle soreness
don: put on clothing
DOT: *Dictionary of Occupational Titles*
DRG: diagnosis-related groups
DRS: disability rating scale
DSD: dry sterile dressing
DSR: dynamic spatial reconstructor
DT: delirium tremens; distance test
D-T-P: diphtheria-tetanus-pertussis (vaccine)
DTP: distal tingling on percussion
DTR: deep tendon reflex
DTs: delirium tremors
DVT: deep vein thrombosis
DVR: Department of Vocational Rehabilitation
Dx: diagnosis
DZ: disease
EAP: employee-assistance program
ECF: extended care facility
E.C.F.: extracellular fluid
ECG: electrocardiogram
ECHO: echo-encephalogram
ECT: electroconvulsive therapy
ECU: environmental control unit
ED: effective dose

EDM: extensor digitorum minimi
EEG: electroencephalogram
EENT: eye, ear, nose, and throat
EKG: electrocardiogram
EMA: external moment arm
EMC: encephalomyocarditis
EMF: erythrocyte maturation factor
EMG: electromyelogram
EMI: educable mentally impaired
EMS: electrical muscle stimulation; emergency medical service
ENT: ear, nose, and throat
EOB: end of bed
e.o.d.: every other day
EOM: edge-of-mat
E.O.M.: extraocular movement
EPL: extensor pollicis longus
EPR: electrophrenic respiration
EPSDT: Early and Periodic Screening, Diagnostic, and Treatment
ER: external rotation; emergency room
ERG: electroretinogram
ERPF: effective renal plasma flow
ERV: expiratory reserve volume
ESF: erythropoietic stimulation factor
ESR: erythrocyte sedimentation rate
ESRD: end-stage renal disease
EST: electric shock treatment
ESTR: electrical stimulation for tissue repair
ETIOL: etiology
EVAL: evaluation, evaluate
EX: exercise
Ex: example
EXC: excision
Exp: exploratory
Ext: extension
Ext. rot.: external rotation
F-: fair (40%) minus muscle strength grade
F: fair (50%) muscle strength grade, full ROM against gravity, no resistance
F+: fair (60%) plus muscle strength grade
F: Fahrenheit; female
FAPTA: Fellow of the American Physical Therapy Association
FAS: fetal alcohol syndrome
FBS: fasting blood sugar

FCU: flexor carpi ulnaris
FEF: forced expiratory flow
FEMS: functional electrical muscle stimulation
FES: functional electrical stimulation
FET: forced expiratory technique
FEV$_1$: forced expiratory volume
FFA: free fatty acid
FFC: fixed flexion contracture
FH: family history
FIM: functional independence measure
FiO$_2$: fraction of inspired oxygen
FLEX: flexion
FNA: femoral neck anteversion
FOR: frame of reference
F.P.: freezing point
FR: flocculation reaction
FRC: functional residual capacity
FRG: functional related groups
FS: frozen section
FSH: follicle-stimulating hormone
ft: foot, feet
FUNC: function
FUO: fever of undetermined origin
FWB: full weight bearing
FWW: front-wheeled walker
Fx: fracture
FY: fiscal year
G-: good (70%) minus muscle strength grade
G: good (80%) muscle strength grade, full ROM against gravity
with moderate resistance
G+: good (90%) plus muscle strength grade
GABA: gamma-aminobutyric acid
Galv.: galvanic
GAS: general adaptation syndrome
GAU: geriatric assessment unit
GBS: Gillian-Barré syndrome
GCE: general conditioning exercises
GCRC: general clinical research center
GCS: geriatric certified specialist
GEC: geriatric education center
GED: general educational development
GER: gerontology
GFR: glomerular filtration rate

GG: gamma globulin
GI: gastrointestinal
Gluc.: glucose
gm: gram(s)
GME: graduate medical education
GNP: gross national product
GOE: *Guide for Occupational Exploration*
GOK: God only knows
G.P.: general paralysis
GPT: glutamic-pyruvic transaminase
Gr: grain
GSR: galvanic skin response
GSW: gun shot wound
GTT: glucose tolerance test
GU: genitourinary
GYN: gynecology
H/A: headache
H$_2$: histamine
Hb: hemoglobin
HBP: high blood pressure
HCFA: Health Care Finance Administration
HCO$_3$: bicarbonate
HCPCS: Health Care Financing Administration Common Procedure Coding System
HCS: Health Communication Services
HCVD: hypertensive cardiovascular disease
Hct: hematocrit
HD: hearing distance
HDL: high density lipoprotein
HDN: hemolytic disease of newborn
HEA: Higher Education Act
Hemi: hemiplegia
HEP: home exercise program
HF: heart failure
Hg: mercury
Hgb: hemoglobin
HHA: home health agency
HHE: home health equipment
HI: head injury; hearing impaired; hospital insurance
HIV: human immunodeficiency virus
HL: human leukocyte
HMO: health maintenance organization
HNP: herniated nucleus propolsus

H&P: history and physical
HP: hot pack
HPI: history of present illness
H/O: history of
HOP: high oxygen pressure
HR: heart rate
Hr: hour
HS: hours of sleep
h.s.: at bedtime
HSA: health systems agency
HSN: hospital satellite network
HTN: hypertension
HU: hyperemia unit
HVPS: high-voltage pulsed stimulation
Hx: history
Hyper: beyond or excessive
Hypo: under or lacking
HYPO: hypodermic
Hz: hertz (cycles/second)
I: independent
IABP: intra-aortic balloon pump
IADL: instrumental activities of daily living
IAT: interagency transfer
IB: inclusion body
IC: integrated circuit; inspiratory capacity
ICD: *International Classification of Diseases*
ICD-9: *International Classification of Diseases*, 9th revision
ICF: intermediary care facility
I.C.F.: intracellular fluid
ICIDH: *International Classification of Impairments, Disabilities, and Handicaps*
ICIDH-2: *International Classification of Impairments, Disabilities, and Handicaps-2*
ICSH: interstitial cell-stimulating hormone
I.C.T.: inflammation of connective tissue
ICT: insulin coma therapy
ICU: intensive care unit
I&D: incision and drainage
I.D.: infective dose
IDDM: insulin-dependent diabetes mellitus
IDEA: Individuals with Disabilities Education Act
IDT: interdepartmental transfer
I:E: inspiratory to expiratory ratio

IEP: individualized education plan
IFSP: individual family service plan
IgA etc: immunoglobulin A, etc
IH: infective hepatitis
IHSS: idiopathic hypertrophic subaortic stenosis
ILC: independent living center
IM: intramuscular
IME: indirect medical education
IMP: impression (tentative diagnosis)
I.M.Rod: intramedullary rod
IMV: intermittent mandatory ventilation
in: inch(es)
IND: indications
Indep: independent
inf: inferior
infra: occurring beneath
Inhal: inhalation
Inj: injection
in situ: in the normal place
int. rot.: internal rotation
in vitro: in a test tube
in vivo: in a living body
IOP: intraocular pressure
IP: interphalangeal; intraperitoneal
IPA: independent practice association
IPF: idiopathic pulmonary fibrosis
IPPB: inspiratory positive pressure breathing
I.Q.: intelligence quotient
IR: internal rotation
I.R.: internal resistance
IRV: inspiratory reserve volume
IS: intercostal space
ITC: information technology and communications
ITP: individual transition plan
IU: international unit(s); immunizing unit(s)
IUD: intrauterine device
IV: intravenous
IVDU: intravenous drug user
IVP: intravenous pyelogram; intravenous pressure
IVT: intravenous transfusion
JOGPT: *Journal of Geriatric Physical Therapy*
JOSPT: *Journal of Sports Physical Therapy*
JRA: juvenile rheumatoid arthritis

JROM: joint range of motion
Jt: joint
K: potassium
Ka: cathode
KAFO: knee-ankle-foot orthosis
KB: kilobyte
Kc: kilocycle
kcal: kilocalorie (food calorie)
KCC: cathodal closing
KCT: cathodal closing tetanus
KDT: cathodal dration tetanus
kerato: corneal or horny growth
kg: kilogram(s)
kino: relating to movement
KJ: knee jerk
k.k.: knee kick (knee jerk)
kL: kiloliter
KO: knee orthosis
KOC: cathodal opening contraction
K.P.: keratitis precipitate
KUB: kidney, ureter, bladder
kv: kilovolt
kw: kilowatt
(L): left
L: liter(s); lumbar
L&A: light and accommodation
LAD: language acquisition device
lat: lateral
lat. dol.: to the painful side
lb: pound(s)
LBP: low back pain
LC: locus ceruleus
LCPD: Legg-Calvé-Perthes disease
LCR: lifetime clinical record
LD: learning disabilities; lethal dose
LDH: lactic dehydrogenase
LDL: low-density lipoprotein
LDLR: labor and delivery, recovery, postpartum
LE: lower extremity
L.E.: lupus erythematosus
L.E.D.: lupus erythematosus disseminate
les: local excitatory state
LFA: low friction arthroplasty

L.F.D.: least fatal dose
LH: luteinizing hormone
L.I.F.: left iliac fossa
LLB: long leg brace
LLD: leg length discrepancy
LLE: left lower extremity
LLQ: left lower quadrant (of abdomen)
LMD: local medical doctor
LMN: lower motor neuron
LMP: last menstrual period
LOA: leave of absence
LOC: loss of consciousness
loc. dol.: to the painful spot
LOS: length of stay
LP: lumbar puncture
LPF: leukocytosis-promoting factor
LS: lumbosacral
L-S: low salt
LTC: long-term care
LTG: long-term goals
LTH: luteotropic hormone
LUE: left upper extremity
LUL: left upper lobe
LUQ: left upper quadrant
LVH: left ventricular hypertrophy
L&W: living and well
M: male; micrococcus; mix
m: meter(s)
m.: muscle
MA: mechanical advantage
ma: milliampere(s)
MAC: maximal allowable concentration
mam: milliamps/minute
MAO: monoamine oxidase
MAS: mobile arm support
Max: maximum
MBD: minimal brain damage
MC: metacarpal
mc: millicurie
Mc: megacycle
MCA: middle cerebral artery
MCC: medical center computing
MCE: medical care evaluation

mcg: microgram(s)
MCH: mean corpuscular hemoglobin; maternal and child health
MCHC: mean corpuscular hemoglobin concentration
MCO: managed care organizations
MCP: metacarpophalangeal
Mcps: megacycles per second
MCV: mean corpuscular volume
MD: muscular dystrophy
M.D.: Doctor of Medicine
M.D.A.: motor discrimination acuity
Mdn: median
MDS: minimum data set
M.E.D.: minimum effective dose
MED: minimal erythema dose
med: medium, medial, median
MEPS: motor evoked potentials
mEq: milliequivalent(s)
MFR: myofascial release
MFT: muscle function test
MG: myasthenia gravis
mg: milligram(s)
Mg: magnesium
MH: mental health
MHB: maximum hospital benefit
MHC: myosin heavy chain
M.H.D.: minimum hemolytic dose
MI: myocardial infarction; mitral insufficiency
M.I.D.: minimal infective dose
MIN: minimal
min: minute
M.I.O.: minimal identifiable odor
MIS: medical information system
M.K.S.: meter-kilogram-second
ml: milliliter(s)
M.L.D.: minimal lethal dose
mm: millimeter(s)
M.M.: mucous membrane
mm: muscles
MMSE: mini-mental status exam
MMT: manual muscle testing
MNE: motor neuron excitability
mo: month

Mod: moderate
MOHO: model of human occupation
mol. wt.: molecular weight
MOM: milk of magnesia
MP: metacarpophalangeal joint
mp: melting point
M.P.D.: maximal permissible dose
mph: miles per hour
MPSMS: materials, products, subject matter, or services
mr: milliroentgen
M.R.D.: minimum reactive dose
MRI: magnetic resonance imaging
MRSA: methicillin-resistant *Staphylococcus aureus*
MS: mitral stenosis; multiple sclerosis
msec: millisecond
MSH: melanocyte-stimulating hormone
M.S.L.: midsternal line
MSP: Medicare secondary payer
MSQ: mental status questionnaire
MTEWA: machines, tools, equipment, and work aids used
mU: milliunit
μm: micron
MUGA: multigated acquisition
MUP: motor unit potential
mv: millivolt
MVA: motor vehicle accident
MVC: maximum voluntary contraction
MVE: maximum voluntary effort
Mx: multiple
My: myopia
N: normal; nitrogen; normal muscle strength through complete range of motion against gravity with maximal resistance
n.: nerve
Na: sodium
N/A: not applicable or not available
NaC: normal saline
N.A.D.: no appreciable disease
NAD: no acute distress
NCS: neurology certified specialist
NCV: nerve conduction velocity
ND: new drugs
NDT: neurodevelopmental treatment
Neg: negative

n.g.: nanogram
NG-tube: nasogastric tube
NICU: neonatal intensive care unit
NIDDM: noninsulin-dependent diabetes mellitus
NKA: no known allergy
NKDA: no known drug allergy
nn: nerves
non rep: do not repeat
NP: neuropsychiatry; nursing procedure
NPH: neutral protein hagedorn (insulin)
NPN: nonprotein nitrogen
NPO: nothing by mouth
NPTE: National Physical Therapy Examination
NREM: nonrapid eye movement
NSAIDS: nonsteroidal anti-inflammatory drugs
NSG: nursing
NSR: normal sinus rhythm
n.t.p.: normal temperature and pressure
n.v.: normal vision
NWB: nonweightbearing
n.y.d.: not yet diagnosed
O_2: oxygen
OA: osteoarthritis
OB: obstetrics
OBRA '87: Omnibus Budget Reconciliation Act of 1987
OBS: observation
OCS: orthopedic certified specialist
OD: right eye (ocular dextra)
o.d.: once a day
O.D.: overdose
OKC: open kinetic chain
OLPR: online patient record
om: every morning
OOB: out of bed
OPD: outpatient department
OR: operating room
Orth: orthopedic
OS: left eye (ocular sinister)
OT: occupational therapy/occupational therapist
OTC: over the counter
OTD: organ tolerance dose
OTR: occupational therapist, registered
OTS: occupational therapy student

OU: both eyes

oz: ounce

P-: poor (10%) minus muscle strength grade

P: poor (20%) muscle strength with complete range in gravity eliminated position

P+: poor (30%) plus muscle strength grade

P: phosphorus; pressure

PA: posterior anterior

P&A: percussion and auscultation

PCO$_2$: carbon dioxide pressure (or tension)

PO$_2$: oxygen pressure (or tension)

Pa CO$_2$: arterial carbon dioxide pressure

PaO$_2$: arterial oxygen pressure; alveolar oxygen pressure

PAMS: physical agent modalities

PARA: paraplegia

PAS: para-aminosalicylic acid

PAT: paroxysmal atrial tachycardia

PATH: pathology

PATRA: professional and technical role analysis

PBI: protein-bound iodine

p.c.: after meals

PCA: personal care attendant; posterior cerebral artery

pcpt: perception

PCS: pediatric certified specialist

Pcs: preconscious

PCT: periarticular connective tissue

PCV: packed cell volume

p.d.: pupillary distance

PD: physical disabilities; postural drainage

PDD: pervasive developmental disorder

PDR: *Physicians' Desk Reference*

PE: physical examination; pulmonary embolism

Ped: pediatric

PEEP: positive end expiratory pressure

PEF: peak expiratory flow

P.E.G.: pneumoencephalogram

PEP: positive expiratory pressure

PERLA: pupils equal and react to light and accommodation

PES: professional examination service

PET: positron emission tomography

PFS: patient financial services

PFT: pulmonary function test

Phy Dys: physical disabilities
PHYS: physical; physiology
PI: present illness
P.I.: proactive interface; protein insulin
PICC: percutaneous inserted central catheter; peripherally inserted central catheter
PICU: pediatric intensive care unit
PID: pelvic inflammatory disease
PIP: proximal interphalangeal
PITR: plasma iron turnover rate
PKU: phenylketonuria
P.L.: light perception
P.M.B.: polymorphic basophil leukocyte
PMH: past medical history
PMR: physical medicine and rehabilitation
PMT: premotor time
P.N.: percussion note
PNF: proprioceptive neuromuscular facilitation
PNI: peripheral nerve injury
PNS: peripheral nervous system
p.o.: by mouth
PO: postoperative
POMR: problem-oriented medical record
Post: posterior
Postop: postoperative
PP&A: palpation, percussion, and auscultation
P.P.D.: purified protein derivative
PPE: personal protective equipment
ppm: parts per million
PPO: preferred provider organization
PPS: prospective payment system (Medicare)
P.Q.: permeability quotient
PRE: progressive resistive exercise
Pre-op: preoperative
PRN: whenever necessary
PRO: peer review organization
PROG: prognosis
PROM: passive range of motion
PROSTUD: Prospective Student Program Data Base
p.s.: per second
p.s.i.: pounds per square inch
PT: physical therapy/physical therapist; prothrombin time
Pt: patient

pt: pint(s)
PTA: physical therapist assistant; prior to admission
PTB: patella tendon bearing
PTCA: percutaneous transluminal coronary angioplasty
PTSD: post-traumatic stress disorder
PTT: partial thromboplastin time
PTX: pelvic traction
PUO: pyrexia of unknown origin
PVD: peripheral vascular disease
PVE: prevocational evaluation
PWA: person with AIDS
PWB: partial weightbearing
Px: physical examination
px: pneumothorax
PZI: protamine zinc insulin
Q: electric quantity
q: every
q2h: every 2 hours
QA: quality assurance
q.d.: every day
q.h.: every hour
QI: quality improvement
q.i.d.: four times daily
q.l.: as much as desired
q.m.: every morning
q.n.: every night
q.o.d.: every other day
q.p.: at will
q.r.s.: sufficient quantity
q.suff.: as much as suffices
qt: quart
q.v.: as much as you please
R, r: roentgen(s)
(R): right
RA: rheumatoid arthritis
RAM: random access memory
RAP: resident assessment protocol
RAS: reticular activating system
RBC: red blood count
RBE: relative biological effectiveness
RBRVS: resource-based relative value scale (Medicare)
RC: rehabilitation counselor
R.C.D.: relative cardiac dullness

RCR: right costal region
RD: retinal detachment
R.D.: reaction of degeneration
Re: regarding, about, concerning
R.E.: right eye
R.E.G.: radioencephalogram
Rehab: rehabilitation
REM: rapid eye movement
rep: repeat, repetition
RES: reticuloendothelial system
RET: rational emotive therapy
RF: renal failure; rheumatoid factor; rheumatic fever
RHC: Rural Health Clinic
RHD: rheumatic heart disease
R.H.D.: relative hepatic dullness
R.I.F.: right iliac fossa
RKY: roentgen kymography
RLE: right lower extremity
RLF: retrolental fibroplasia
R.L.L.: right lower lobe
RLQ: right lower quadrant
RM: repetition maximum; respiratory movement
R.M.L.: right middle lobe
RNA: ribonucleic acid
R/O: rule out
ROH: roster of honor
ROM: range of motion
ROS: review of systems
RPCH: rural primary care hospital
RPE: rating of perceived exertion
RPF: renal plasma flow
r.p.m.: revolutions per minute
R.P.S.: renal pressor substance
R.Q.: respiratory quotient
RROM: resistive range of motion
RSR: regular sinus rhythm
RT: radiation therapy
RTI: routine task inventory
RUE: right upper extremity
RUG: resource utilization grouping
R.U.L.: right upper lobe
RUQ: right upper quadrant
RV: residual volume

R.V.H.: right ventricular hypertension
RVU: relative value unit
Rx: prescription, treatment
S: social history; sacral
SaO$_2$: arterial oxygen saturation
SAD: seasonal affective disorder
sat: saturated
SAQ: short arc quad
SBA: stand by assistance
SBE: subacute bacterial endocarditis
SBF: skin blood cell flux
s.c.: subcutaneous(ly)
SCI: spinal cord injury
SCS: sports certified specialist; splint classification system
SD: streptodornase
S.D.: skin dose; standard deviation
S.D.A.: specific dynamic action
SE: side effects
S.E.: standard error
sec: second(s)
SED: Seriously emotionally disturbed
S.E.D.: skin erythema dose
SEP: somatosensory evoked potential
SGOT: serum glutamic-oxaloacetic transaminase
SGPT: serum glutamic-pyruvic transaminase
SH: social history; serum hepatitis
SHUR: system for hospital uniform reporting
SI: sensory integration
S.I.: soluble insulin
SICU: surgical intensive care unit
SIDS: sudden infant death syndrome
SK: streptokinase
SLB: short leg brace
SLE: systemic lupus erythematosus
SLH: state and local hospitalization
SLR: straight leg raise
SMI: supplemental medical insurance
SMS: shared medical systems
S.N.: according to nature
SNF: skilled nursing facility
SOAP: subjective, objective, assessment, plan
SOB: shortness of breath
SOL: space occupying lesion

sol: solution
SOP: standard operating procedure
SOS: if necessary
SOTT: synthetic medium old tuberculin trichloroacetic acid
s/p: status post
SP: speech
SPCA: serum thrombin conversion acceleratory
SPF: specific-pathogen free
sp. gr.: specific gravity
SPEM: smooth pursuit eye movement
SPI: serum precipitable iodine
SpO$_2$: pulse oxygen saturation
SPSS: *Statistical Package for Social Sciences*
SPT: student physical therapist
sq: square
SQ: subcutaneous
SR: systematic review
S.R.: sedimentation rate
SS: half
s.s.e.: soap suds enema
SSI: supplemental security income
SSS: specific soluble substance
SSV: under a poison label
St: let it stand
STA: serum thrombotic accelerator
stat: at once
STD: sexually transmitted disease; skin test dose
STG: short-term goals
STH: somatotropic (growth) hormone
STNR: symmetrical tonic neck reflex
S.T.S.: serology test for syphilis
S.T.U.: skin test unit
sub q: subcutaneous
SUDS: single use diagnostic system
Sup: supination
sup: superior
SV: simian virus
SVP: specific vocational preparation
Sx: symptom
SXI: severely multiply impaired
SYM: symptom
Sz: schizophrenia; seizure
T: trace (5%) muscle strength grade; temperature; thorasis

t: temporal
t$_{1/2}$: half-life
TA: alkaline tuberculin
T&A: tonsils and adenoids
T.A.: toxic-antitoxin
TAB: temporarily-abled body
T.A.F.: toxoid-antitoxin floccules
TAH: transabdominal hysterectomy
TAL: tendon-achilles lengthening
T.A.M.: toxoid-antitoxin mixture
TAP: turning and positioning program
T.A.T.: toxin-antitoxin
TB: tuberculosis
T.b.: tubercle bacillus
TBG: thyroxine-binding globulin
TBI: traumatic brain injury
TDD: telecommunication device for the deaf
t.d.s.: to be taken three times per day
TDWB: touch down weightbearing
Te: tetanus
TEFRA: Tax Equity and Fiscal Responsibility Act
Temp: temperature
TENS: transcutaneous electrical nerve stimulation; transepidermal necrotizing syndrome
T.F.: tuberculin filtrate
TGV: transplantation of great vessels
Th: thoracic
THR: total hip replacement
TI: tricuspid insufficiency
TIA: transient ischemic attack
t.i.d.: three times daily
TKA: trochanter-knee-ankle
TKE: terminal knee extension
TKR: total knee replacement
TLC: tender loving care; total lung capacity
TLR: tonic labyrinthine reflex
TO: original tuberculin
TOP: termination of pregnancy
TOWER: testing, orientation, and work evaluation in rehabilitation
T.P.: tuberculin precipitation
t-PA: tissue plasminogen activator
TPR: temperature, pulse, respiration
TQM: total quality management

tr: tincture
T.S.: test solution
TSH: thyroid-stimulating hormone
TTWB: toe touch weightbearing
TTY: teletypewriter
T.U.R.P.: transurethral resection procedure
TV: tidal volume
Tx: treatment
Ty: type
u: unit(s)
UA: urine analysis
UAP: university-affiliated programs
UBI: ultraviolet blood irradiation
UE: upper extremity
UFA: unestrified fatty acids
UGI: upper gastrointestinal
UMN: upper motor neuron
Un: unable
UR: utilization review
URI: upper respiratory infection
US: ultrasound
USA: unstable angina
UTI: urinary tract infection
UV: ultraviolet
V: vision
v.: vein; volt
Va: visual acuity
VC: vital capacity
V.C.: acuity of color vision
V.D.: venereal disease
V.D.A.: visual discriminatory acuity
V.D.H.: valvular disease of the heart
VDM: vasodepressor material
VEM: vasoexciter material
VER: visual evoked response
V.F.: vocal fremitus
v.f.: visual field
VI: volume index
VIA: virus inactivating agent
V.M.: voltmeter
VO: verbal order
VO$_2$ Max: maximum oxygen consumption
V.P.: venous pressure

V.R.: vocal resonance

VS: vestibular stimulation

V.S.: vibratory sense; volumetric solution

v.s.: vital signs

vs: venisection

VSD: ventricular septal defect

V.T.: vacuum tuberculin

V&T: volume and tension (of pulse)

V.W.: vessel wall

w.: watt

WBAT: weight bearing as tolerated

WBC: white blood cell count

WBQC: wide base quad cane

W/C or WC: wheelchair

WD: well-developed

WD/WN: well-developed/well-nourished

WFL: within functional limits

WIC: special supplemental nutrition program for women, infants, and children

Wk: week

WN: well-nourished

WNL: within normal limits

WORK: *Work: A Journal of Prevention, Assessment & Rehabilitation*

WP: whirlpool

wt: weight

x: times

y/n: yes/no

y/o: years old

yrs: years

Medical Roots: Etymology
(Greek and Latin Deriviations)

a-	negative prefix (n is added before words beginning with a vowel) (eg, ametria)
ab-	away from (eg, abducent)
abdomin-	abdomen (eg, abdominis, abdominoscopy)
ac-	*see* ad- (eg, accretion)
acet-	acid (eg, acetum vinegar, acetometer)
acid-	acid (eg, acidus sour, aciduric)
acou-	hear (eg, acouesthesia) (also spelled acu-)
acr-	extremity, peak (eg, acromegaly)
act-	drive, act (eg, reaction)
actin-	ray, radius (eg, actinogenesis)
acu-	hear (eg, osteoacusis)
ad-	toward (d changes to c, f, g, p, s, or t before words beginning with those consonants) (eg, adrenal)
aden-	gland (eg, adenoma)
adip-	fat (eg, adipocellular, adipose)
-aemia	blood (eg, polycythemia)
aer-	air (eg, anaerobiosis)
aesthe-	sensation (eg, aesthesioneurosis)
af-	*see* ad- (eg, afferent)
ag-	*see* ad- (eg, agglutinant)
-agogue	leading, inducing (eg, galactogogue)
-agra	catching, seizure (eg, podagra)
alb-	white (eg, albocinereous)
alg-	pain (eg, neuralgia, algesia)
all-	other, different (eg, allergy)
alve-	channel, cavity (eg, alveolar, alveus trough)
amb-	both, on both sides (eg, ambulate)
amph-	*see* amphi-; around, on both sides (eg, ampheclexis)
amphi- with	both, doubly (i is dropped before words beginning with a vowel) (eg, amphicelous)
amyl-	starch (eg, amylosynthesis)
an-	*see* ana- (eg, anagogic)
ana-	up, positive (final a is dropped before words beginning with a vowel) (eg, anaphoresis)
andr-	man (eg, gynandroid)
angi-	vessel (eg, angiemphraxis)

ankyl-	crooked, looped (eg, ankylodactylia); also spelled ancyl-
ant-	*see* anti- (eg, antophthalmic)
ante-	before (eg, anteflexion)
anti-	against, counter (i is dropped before words beginning with a vowel, or the word is hyphenated) (eg, antipyogenic, anti-inflammatory); *see also* contra-
antr-	cavern (eg, antrodynia)
ap-	*see* ad- (eg, append)
-aph-	touch (eg, dysaphia); *see also* hapt-
apo-	away from, detached, opposed (o is dropped before words beginning with a vowel) (eg, apophysis)
arachn-	spider (eg, arachnodactyly)
arch-	beginning, origin (eg, archenteron)
arter(i)-	elevator, artery (eg, arteriosclerosis, periarteritis)
arthr-	joint (eg, synarthrosis); *see also* articul-
articul-	articulus joint (eg, disarticulation); *see also* arthr-
as-	*see* ad- (eg, assimilation)
-ase	enzyme (eg, steatolase, proteolase)
at-	*see* ad- (eg, attrition)
aur-	ear (eg, aurinasal); *see also* ot-
aut-	self (eg, autechoscope)
auto-	self (eg, autoimmune)
aux-	increase (eg, enterauxe)
ax-	axis (eg, axofugal)
axon-	axis (eg, axonometer)
ba-	go, walk, stand (eg, hypnobatia)
bacill-	small staff, rod (eg, actinobacillosis); *see also* bacter-
bacter-	small staff, rod (eg, bacteriophage); *see also* bacill-
ball-	throw (eg, ballistics); *see also* bol-
bar-	weight (eg, pedobarometer)
bi-[1]	life (eg, aerobic)
bi-[2]	two, twice, double (eg, bipedal)
bil-	bile (eg, biliary)
blast-	bud, child, a growing thing in its early stages (eg, blastoma, zygotoblast)
blep-	look, see (eg, hemiablepsia)
blephar-	eyelid (eg, blepharoncus)
bol-	ball (eg, embolism)
brachi-	arm (eg, brachiocephalic)
brachy-	short (eg, brachycephalic)
brady-	slow (eg, bradycardia)
brom-	stench (eg, podobromidrosis)
bronch-	windpipe (eg, bronchoscopy)

bry-	be full of life (eg, embryonic)
bucc-	cheek (eg, distobuccal)
cac-	bad, evil, abnormal (eg, cacodontia, arthrocace); *see also* mal-, dys-
calc-¹	stone, limestone, lime (eg, calcipexy)
calc-²	heel (eg, calcaneotibial)
calor-	heat (eg, calorimeter); *see also* therm-
cancr-	cancer, crab (eg, camcrology); *see also* carcin-
capit-	head (eg, decapitate); *see also* cephal-
caps-	container (eg, encapsulation)
carbo-	coal, charcoal (eg, carbohydrate, carbonuria)
carcin-	crab, cancer (eg, carcinoma); *see also* cancr-
cardi-	heart (eg, lipocardiac)
cat-	*see* cata- (eg, cathode)
cata-	down, negative (final a is dropped before words beginning with a vowel) (eg, catabatic)
caud-	tail (eg, caudate)
cav-	hollow (eg, concave)
cec-	blind (eg, cecopexy)
-cele	tumor, hernia, cyst (eg, gastrocele)
cell-	room (eg, celliferous)
cen-	common (eg, cenesthesia)
cent-	one hundred (eg, centimeter, centipede)
cente-	puncture (eg, enterocentesis, amniocentesis)
centr-	central point, center (eg, neurocentral)
cephal-	relating to the head (eg, encephalitis)
cept-	take, receive (eg, receptor)
cer-	wax (eg, ceroplasty, ceromel)
cerebr-	relating to the cerebrum (eg, cerebrospinal)
cervic-	neck (eg, cervicitis, cervical)
chancr-	crab, cancer (eg, chancriform)
chir-	hand (eg, chiromegaly)
chlor-	green (eg, achloropsia)
chol-	bile (eg, hepatocholangeitis)
chondr-	cartilage (eg, chondromalacia)
chord-	string, cord (eg, perichordal)
chori-	protective fetal membrane (eg, endochorion)
chrom-	color (eg, polychromatic)
chron-	time (eg, synchronous)
chy-	pour (eg, ecchymosis)
-cid(e)	causing death, cut, kill (eg, infanticide, germicidal)
cili-	eyelid (eg, superciliary); *see also* blephar-
cine-	move (eg, autocinesis)

-cipient	take, receive (eg, incipient)
circum-	around (eg, circumferential); *see also* peri-
-cis-	cut, kill (eg, excision)
clas-	break (eg, osteoclast, cranioclast)
clin-	bend, incline, make lie down (eg, clinometer)
clus-	shut (eg, malocclusion)
co-	*see* con-, (eg, cohesion)
cocc-	seed, pill, (eg, gonococcus)
coel-	hollow, (eg, coelenteron); also spelled cel-
col-1	pertaining to the lower intestine (eg, colic)
col-2	*see* con- (eg, collapse)
colon-	lower intestine (eg, colonic)
colp-	hollow, vagina (eg, endocolpitis)
com-	*see* con- (eg, commasculation)
con-	with, together (becomes co- before vowels or h; col- before l; com- before b, m, or p; cor- before r) (eg, contraction)
contra-	against, counter (eg, contraindication); *see also* anti-
copr-	dung (eg, coproma); *see also* sterco-
cor-1	doll, little image, pupil (eg, isocoria)
cor-2	*see* con- (eg, corrugator)
corpor-	body (eg, intracorporal) (*see also* somat-)
cortic-	bark, rind (eg, corticosterone)
cost-	rib (eg, intercostal); *see also* pleur-
crani-	skull, cranium (eg, pericranium)
creat-	meat, flesh (eg, creatorrhea)
-crescent	grow (eg, excrescent)
cret-1	grow (eg, accretion)
cret-2	distinguish, separate off (eg, discrete)
crin-	distinguish, separate off (eg, endocrinology)
crur-	shin, leg (eg, brachiocrural)
cry-	cold (eg, cryesthesia)
crypt-	hide, conceal (eg, cryptorchism)
cult-	tend, cultivate (eg, culture)
cune-	wedge (eg, sphencuneiform)
cut-	skin (eg, subcutaneous); *see also* derm(at)-
cyan-	blue (eg, anthocyanin)
cycl-	circle, cycle (eg, cyclophoria)
cyst-	bag, bladder (eg, nephrocystitis); *see also* vesic-
cyt-	cell (eg, plasmocytoma); *see also* cell-
dacry-	tear (eg, dacryocyst)
dactyl-	finger, toe, digit (eg, hexadactylism)
de-	down from (eg, decomposition)

dec-[1]	ten, indicates multiple in metric system (eg, decagram)
dec-[2]	ten, indicates fraction in metric system (eg, decimeter)
deci-	tenth (eg, decibel)
demi-	half (eg, demipenniform)
dendr-	tree (eg, neurodendrite)
dent-	tooth (eg, interdental); *see also* odont-
derm-	skin (eg, endoderm, dermatitis); *see also* cut-
desm-	band, ligament (eg, syndesmopexy)
dextr-	handedness (eg, ambidextrous)
di-[1]	two (eg, dimorphic); *see also* bi-[2]
di-[2]	*see* dia- (eg, diuresis)
di-[3]	*see* dis- (eg, divergent)
dia-	through, apart, between, asunder (a is dropped before words beginning with a vowel) (eg, diagnosis)
didym-	twin, gemini (eg, epididymal)
digit-	finger, toe (eg, digital); *see also* dactyl-
diplo-	double (eg, diplomyelia)
dis-	apart, away from, negative, absence of (s may be dropped before a word beginning with a consonant) (eg, dislocation)
disc-	disk (eg, discoplacenta)
dors-	back (eg, ventrodorsal)
drom-	course (eg, hemodromometer)
-ducent	lead, conduct (eg, adducent)
duct-	lead, conduct (eg, oviduct)
dur-	hard, sclera (eg, induration)
dynam(i)-	power (eg, dynamoneure, neurodynamic)
-dynia	pain (eg, coxodynia)
dys-	bad, improper, malfunction, difficult (eg, dystrophic)
e-	out from (eg, emission)
ec-	out of, on the outside (eg, eccentric)
-ech-	have, hold, be (eg, synechotomy)
ect-	outside (eg, ectoplasm); *see also* extra-
-ectomy	a cutting out (eg, mastectomy)
ede-	swell (eg, edematous)
ef-	out of (eg, efflorescent)
-elc-	sore, ulcer (eg, enterelcosis); *see also* helc-
electr-	amber (eg, electrotherapy)
em-	in, on (eg, embolism, empathy, emphlysis); *see also* en-
-em-	blood (eg, anemia); *see also* hem(at)-
-emesis	vomiting (eg, nemesis)
-emia	blood (eg, bacteremia)
en-	in, on, into (n changes to m before b, p, or ph) (eg, encelitis)

end-	inside (eg, endangium); *see also* intra-
endo-	within (eg, endocardium)
enter-	intestine (eg, dysentery)
epi-	upon, after, in addition (i is dropped before words beginning with a vowel) (eg, epiglottis, epaxial)
erg-	work, deed (eg, energy)
erythr-	red, rubor (eg, erythrochromia)
eso-	inside (eg, esophylactic); *see also* intra-, endo-
esthe-	perceive, feel, sensation (eg, anesthesia)
eu-	good, normal, well (eg, eupepsia, eugeric)
ex-	out of (eg, excretion)
exo-	outside (eg, exopathic); *see also* extra-
extra-	outside of, beyond (eg, extracellular)
faci-	face (eg, brachiofaciolingual)
-facient	make (eg, calefacient)
-fact-	make (eg, artifact)
fasci-	band (eg, fascia)
febr-	fever (eg, febrile, febricide)
-fect-	make (eg, defective)
-ferent	bear, carry (eg, efferent, afferent)
ferr-	iron (eg, ferroprotein)
fibr-	fibre (eg, chondrofibroma)
fil-	thread (eg, filament, filiform)
fiss-	split (eg, fissure)
flagell-	whip (eg, flagellation)
flav-	yellow (eg, riboflavin)
-flect-	bend, divert (eg, deflection)
-flex-	bend, divert (eg, reflexometer, flexion)
flu-	flow (eg, fluid)
flux-	flow (eg, affluxion)
for-	door, opening (eg, foramen, perforated)
fore-	before, in front of (eg, forefront)
-form	shape, form (eg, ossiform, cuniform)
fract-	break (eg, fracture, refractive)
front-	forehead, front (eg, nasofrontal)
-fug(e)	to drive away, flee, avoid (eg, vermifuge, centrifugal)
funct-	perform, serve, function (eg, functional, malfunction)
fund-	pour (eg, infundibulum)
fus-	pour (eg, diffusible)
galact-	milk (eg, dysgalactia)
gam-	marriage, reproductive union (eg, agamont)
gangli-	swelling, plexus (eg, neurogangliitis)
gastro-	stomach, belly (eg, gastrostomy)

gelat-	freeze, congeal (eg, gelatin)
gemin-	twin, double (eg, quadrigeminal)
gen-	become, be produced, originate, formation (eg, genesis, cytogenic, gene)
germ-	bud, a growing thing in its early stages (eg, germinal, ovigerm)
gest-	bear, carry (eg, congestion)
gland-	acorn (eg, intraglandular)
-glia	glue (eg, neuroglia)
gloss-	relating to the tongue (eg, lingutrichoglossia)
glott-	tongue, language (eg, glottic)
gluc-	sweet (eg, glucose)
glutin-	glue (eg, agglutination)
glyc(y)-	sweet (eg, glycemia, glycyrrhiza)
gnath-	jaw (eg, orthognathous)
gno-	know, discern (eg, diagnosis)
gon-	produce, formulate (eg, gonad, amphigony)
grad-	walk, take steps (eg, retrograde)
-gram	scratch, write, record (eg, cardiogram)
gran-	grain, particle (eg, lipogranuloma, granulation)
graph-	scratch, write, record (eg, histography)
grav-	heavy (eg, multigravida)
gyn(ec)-	woman, wife (eg, androgyny, gynecologic)
gyr-	ring, circle (eg, gyrospasm)
haem(at)-	pertaining to blood (eg, haemorrhagia, Haematoxylon)
hapt-	touch (eg, haptometer)
hect-	one hundred, indicates multiple in metric system (eg, hectometer)
helc-	sore, ulcer (eg, helcosis)
hem(at)-	blood (eg, hematocyturia, hemangioma)
hemi-	half (eg, hemiageusia); *see also* semi-
hen-	one (eg, henogenesis)
hepat-	liver (eg, gastrohepatic)
hept(a)-	seven (eg, heptatomic, heptavalent)
hered-	heir (eg, heredity)
hetero-	other, indicating dissimilarity (eg, heterogeneous)
hex-[1]	six, sex-, hexly- (eg, hexagram)
hex-[2]	have, hold, be (eg, cachexy)
hexa-	six, sex-, hexly- (eg, hexachromic)
hidr-	sweat (eg, hyperhidrosis)
hist-	web, tissue (eg, histodialysis)
hod-	road, path (eg, hodoneuromere)
holo-	all (eg, hologenesis)

homo-	common, same (eg, homomorphic)
horm-	impetus, impulse (eg, hormone)
hydat-	water (eg, hydatism)
hydr-	pertaining to water (eg, achlorhydria)
hyp-	under (eg, hypaxial, hypodermic)
hyper-	over, above, beyond, extreme (eg, hypertrophy)
hypn-	sleep (eg, hypnotic)
hypo-	under, below (o is dropped before words beginning with a vowel) (eg, hypometabolism)
hyster-	womb (eg, hysterectomy)
-iasis	condition, pathological state (eg, hemiathriasis; *see also* -osis
iatr-	specialty in medicine (eg, pediatrics)
idio-	peculiar, separate, distinct (eg, idiosyncrasy)
il-	negative prefix (eg, illegible); in, on (eg, illinition)
ile-	pertaining to the ileum (ile- is commonly used to refer to the portion of the intestines known as the ileum) (eg, ileostomy)
ili-	lower abdomen, intestines (ili- is commonly used to refer to the flaring part of the hip bone known as the ilium) (eg, iliosacral)
im-	in, on (eg, immersion); negative prefix (eg, imperfection)
in-1	fiber (eg, inosteatoma)
in-2	in, on (n changes to l, m, or r before words beginning with those consonants) (eg, insertion)
in-3	negative prefix (eg, invalid)
infra-	beneath (eg, infraorbital)
insul-	island (eg, insulin)
inter-	among, between (eg, intercarpal)
intra-	inside (eg, intravenous)
ir-	in, on (eg, irradiation); negative prefix (eg, irreducible)
irid-	rainbow, colored circle (eg, keratoiridocyclitis)
is-	equal (eg, isotope)
ischi-	hip, haunch (eg, ischiopubic)
-ism	condition, theory (eg, hemiballism, agism)
iso-	equal (eg, isotonic)
-itis	inflammation (eg, neuritis)
-ize	to treat by special method (eg, specialize)
jact-	throw (eg, jactitation)
ject-	throw (eg, injection)
jejun-	hungry, not partaking of food (eg, gastrojejunostomy)
jug-	yoke (eg, conjugation)
junct-	yoke, join (eg, conjunctiva)

juxta-	near (eg, juxtaposed)
kary-	nut, kernel, nucleus (eg, megakaryocyte)
kerat-	horn (eg, keratolysis, keratin)
kil-	one thousand, indicates multiple in metric system (eg, kilogram)
kine-	move (eg, kinematics)
-kinesis	movement (eg, orthokinesis)
labi-	lip (eg, gingivolabial)
lact-	milk (eg, glucolactone, lactose)
lal-	talk, babble (eg, glossolalia)
lapar-	flank, loin, abdomen (eg, laparotomy)
laryng-	windpipe (eg, laryngendoscope)
lat-	bear, carry (eg, translation)
later-	side (eg, bentrolateral)
lent-	lentil (eg, lenticonus)
lep-	take, seize (eg, cataleptic, epileptic)
lepto-	small, soft (eg, leptotene)
leuk-	white (eg, leukocyte); also spelled leuc-
lien-	spleen (eg, lienocele)
lig-	tie, bind (eg, ligate)
lingu-	tongue (eg, sublingual)
lip-	fat (eg, glycolipid)
lith-	stone (eg, nephrolithotomy)
loc-	place (eg, locomotion)
log-	speak, give an account (eg, logorrhea, embryology)
lumb-	loin (eg, dorsolumbar)
lute-	yellow (eg, xanthluteoma)
ly-	loose, dissolve (eg, keratolysis)
-lysis	setting free, disintegration (eg, glycolysis)
lymph-	water (eg, hydrolymphadenosis)
macro-	long, large (eg, macromyoblast)
mal-	bad, abnormal (eg, malfunction)
malac-	soft (eg, osteomalacia)
mamm-	breast (eg, mammogram, mammary)
man-	hand (eg, maniphalanx, manipulation)
mani-	mental aberration (eg, kleptomania)
mast-	breast (eg, mastectomy, hypermastia)
medi-	middle (eg, medial, medifrontal)
mega-	great, large, indicates multiple (1,000,000) in metric system (eg, megacolon, megadyne)
megal-	great, large (eg, cardiomegaly, acromegaly)
mel-	limb, member (eg, symmelia)
melan-	black (eg, melanoma, melanin)

men-	month (eg, menopause, dysmenorrhea)
mening-	membrane (eg, encephalomeningitis)
ment-	mind (eg, dementia)
mer-	part (eg, polymeric)
mes-	middle (eg, mesoderm)
met-	after, beyond, accompanying (eg, metallurgy)
meta-	after, beyond, accompanying (a is dropped before words beginning with a vowel) (eg, metacarpal, metatarsal)
metr-[1]	measure (eg, stereometry)
metr-[2]	womb (eg, endometritis)
micr-	small (eg, photomicrograph)
mill-	one thousand, indicates fraction in metric system (eg, milligram, millipede)
mio-	smaller, less (eg, mionectic)
miss-	send (eg, intromission)
-mittent	send (eg, intermittent)
mne-	remember (eg, pseudoamnesia)
mon-	only, sole, single (eg, monoplegia)
morph-	form, shape (eg, morphonuclear)
mot-	move (eg, vasomotor, locomotion)
multi-	many (eg, multiple)
my-	muscle (eg, myopathy)
-myces	fungus (eg, myelomyces)
myc(et)-	fungus (eg, Ascomycetes, streptomycin)
myel-	marrow (eg, poliomyelitis)
myx-	mucus (eg, myxedema)
narc-	numbness (eg, toponarcosis, narcolepsy)
nas-	nose (eg, nasal)
ne-	new, young (eg, neocyte, neonate)
necr-	corpse, dead (eg, necrocytosis, necrosis)
nephr-	kidney (eg, nephron, nephric)
neur-	nerve (eg, neurology, esthesioneure)
nod-	knot (eg, nodosity)
nom-	deal out, distribute, law, custom (eg, nominal, taxonomy)
non-	nine, no (eg, nonacosane)
nos-	disease (eg, nosology)
nucle-	nut, kernel (eg, nucleus, nucleide)
nutri-	nourish (eg, malnutrition)
ob-	against, toward (b changes to c before words beginning with that consonant) (eg, obtuse)
oc-	*see* ob-, occlude

ocul-	eye (eg, oculomotor)
-od-	road, path (eg, periodic)
-ode¹	road, path (eg, cathode)
-ode²	form (eg, nematode)
odont-	tooth (eg, orthodontia)
-odyn-	pain, distress (eg, gastrodynia)
-oid	form (eg, hyoid)
-ol	oil (eg, cholesterol)
-old	form, shape, resemblance (eg, scaffold)
ole-	oil (eg, oleoresin)
olig-	few, small (eg, oligospermia)
-oma	tumor (eg, blastoma)
omo-	shoulder (eg, omosternum)
omphal-	navel (eg, periomphalic)
onc-	bulk, mass (eg, oncology, hematoncometry)
onych-	claw, nail (eg, anonychia)
oo-	egg, ovum (eg, perioothecitis)
oophor-	pertaining to the ovary (eg, oophorectomy)
ophthalm-	eye (eg, ophthalmic)
or-	mouth (eg, intraoral)
orb-	circle (eg, suborbital)
orchi-	testicle (eg, orchiopathy)
organ-	implement, instrument (eg, organoleptic)
orth-	straight, right, normal (eg, orthopedics)
-osis	condition, disease (eg, osteoporosis)
oss-	bone (eg, osseous, ossiphone)
ost(e)-	bone (eg, enostosis, osteonecrosis)
ot-	ear (eg, parotid); *see also* aur-
-otomy	cutting (eg, osteotomy)
ov-	egg (eg, synovia)
oxy-	sharp, acid (eg, oxycephalic)
pachy(n)-	thicken (eg, pachyderma, myopachynsis)
pag-	fix, make fast (eg, thoracopagus)
pan-	entire, all (eg, pancytosis, pandemic)
par-¹	bear, give birth to (eg, primiparous)
par-²	*see* para- (eg, parepigastric)
para-	beside, beyond, along side of (final a is dropped before words beginning with a vowel) (eg, paramastoid)
part-	bear, give birth to (eg, parturition)
path-	that which one undergoes, sickness, disease (eg, pathology, psychopathic)
pec-	fix, make fast (eg, sympectothiene); *see also* pex-
ped-	child (eg, pediatric, orthopedic)

pell-	skin, hide (eg, pellagra)
-pellent	drive (eg, repellent)
pen-	need, lack (eg, erythrocytopenia)
pend-	hang down (eg, appendix)
pent(a)-	five (eg, pentose, pentaploid)
peps-	digest (eg, bradypepsia)
pept-	digest (eg, dyspeptic)
per-	through, excessive (eg, pernasal)
peri-	around (eg, periphery)
pet-	seek, tend toward (eg, centripetal)
pex-	fix, make fast (eg, hepatopexy)
pha-	say, speak (eg, dysphasia)
phac-	lentil, lens (eg, phacosclerosis); also spelled phak-
phag-	eat (eg, lipphagic)
phak-	lentil, lens (eg, phakitis)
phan-	show, be seen (eg, diaphanoscopy)
pharmac-	drug (eg, pharmacology)
pharyng-	throat (eg, glossopharyngeal)
phen-	show, be seen (eg, phosphene)
pher-	bear, support (eg, periphery)
phil-	like, have affinity for (eg, eosinophilia, philosophy)
phleb-	vein (eg, periphlebitis, phlebotomy)
phleg-	burn, inflame (eg, adenophlegmon)
phlog-	burn, inflame (eg, antiphlogistic)
phob-	fear, dread (eg, claustrophobia)
phon-	sound (eg, echophony)
phor-	bear, support (eg, exophoria)
phos-	light (eg, phosphorus)
phot-	light (eg, photerythrous)
phrag-	fence, wall off, stop up (eg, diaphragm)
phrax-	fence, wall off, stop up (eg, emphraxis)
phren-	mind, midriff (eg, metaphrenia, metaphrenon)
phthi-	decay, waste away (eg, ophthalmophthisis)
phy-	beget, bring forth, produce, be by nature (eg, nosophyte, physical)
phyl-	tribe, kind (eg, phylogeny)
phylac-	guard (eg, prophylactic)
-phylaxis	protection (eg, prophylaxis)
-phyll	leaf (eg, xanthophyll)
phys(a)-	blow, inflate (eg, physocele, physalis)
physe-	blow, inflate (eg, emphysema)
pil-	hair (eg, epilation)
pituit-	phlegm (eg, pituitous)

placent-	cake (eg, extraplacental)
plas-	mold, shape (eg, cineplasty, plastazode)
platy-	broad, flat (eg, platyrrhine)
pleg-	strike (eg, diplegia, paraplegia)
plet-	fill (eg, depletion)
pleur-	rib, side (eg, peripleural)
plex-	strike (eg, apoplexy)
plic-	fold (eg, complication)
plur-	more (eg, plural)
pne-	breathing (eg, traumatopnea)
pneum(at)-	breath, air (eg, pneumodynamics, pneumatothorax)
pneumo(n)-	lung (eg, pneumocentesis, pneumonotomy)
pod-	foot (eg, podiatry)
poie-	make, produce (eg, sarcopoietic)
pol-	axis of a sphere (eg, peripolar)
poly-	much, many (eg, polyspermia)
pont-	bridge (eg, pontocerebellar)
por-[1]	passage, (eg, myelopore)
por-[2]	callus (eg, porocele)
posit-	put, place (eg, deposit, repositor)
post-	after, behind in time or place (eg, postnatal, postural)
pre-	before in time or place (eg, prenatal, prevesical)
press-	press (eg, pressure, pressoreceptive)
pro-	before in time or place (eg, progamous, prolapse)
proct-	anus (eg, ecteroproctia)
prosop-	face (eg, prosopus)
proto-	first (eg, prototype)
pseud-	false (eg, pseudoparaplegia)
psych-	soul, mind (eg, psychosomatic)
pto-	fall (eg, nephroptosis)
pub-	adult (eg, puberty, ischiopubic)
puber-	adult (eg, puberty)
pulmo(n)-	lung (eg, cardiopulmonary, pulmolith)
puls-	drive (eg, propulsion)
punct-	prick, pierce (eg, puncture, punctiform)
pur-	pus (eg, puration)
py-	pus (eg, nephropyosis)
pyel-	trough, basin, pelvis (eg, nephropyelitis)
pyl-	door, orifice (eg, pylephlebitis)
pyr-	fire (eg, galactopyra)
quadr-	four (eg, quadriplegic, quadrigeminal)
quinque-	five (eg, quinquecuspid)
rachi-	spine (eg, alorachidian)

radi-	ray (eg, irradiation)
re-	back, again (eg, retraction)
ren-	kidneys (eg, adrenal)
ret-	net (eg, retothelium)
retro-	backwards (eg, retrodeviation, retrograde)
rhag-	break, burst (eg, hemorrhagic)
rhaph-	suture, stitching (eg, gastrorrhaphy)
rhe-	flow, discharge (eg, diarrheal)
rhex-	break, burst (eg, metrorrhexis)
rhin-	nose (eg, basirhinal)
rot-	wheel (eg, rotator)
rub(r)-	red (eg, bilirubin, rubrospinal)
racchar-	sugar (eg, saccharin)
sacro-	pertaining to the sacrum (eg, sacroiliac)
salping-	tube, trumpet (eg, salpingitis)
sanguin-	blood (eg, sanguineous)
sarc-	flesh (eg, sarcoma)
schis-	split (eg, schistorachis, rachischisis)
scler-	hard (eg, sclerosis, scleroderma)
scop-	look at, observe (eg, endoscope)
sect-	cut (eg, sectile, resection)
semi-	half (eg, semiflexion)
sens-	perceive, feel (eg, sensory)
sep-	rot, decay (eg, sepsis)
sept-[1]	fence, wall off, stop up (eg, septal)
sept-[2]	seven (eg, septan)
ser-	whey, watery substance (eg, serum, serosynovitis)
sex-	six (eg, sexdigitate)
sial-	saliva (eg, polysialia)
sin-	hollow, fold (eg, sinobronchitis)
sit-	food (eg, parasitic)
solut-	loose, dissolve, set free (eg, dissolution)
-solvent	loose, dissolve (eg, dissolvent)
somat-	body (eg, somatic, psychosomatic)
-some	body (eg, dictyosome)
spas-	draw, pull (eg, spasm, spastic)
spectr-	appearance, what is seen (eg, spectrum, microspectro-scope)
sperm(at)-	seed (eg, spermacrasia, spermatozoon)
spers-	scatter (eg, dispersion)
sphen-	wedge (eg, sphenoid)
spher-	ball (eg, hemisphere)
sphygm-	pulsation (eg, sphygmomanometer)

spin-	spine (eg, cerebrospinal)
spirat-	breathe (eg, inspiratory)
splanchn-	entrails, viscera (eg, neurosplanchnic)
splen-	spleen (eg, splenomegaly)
spor-	seed (eg, sporophyte, sygospore)
squam-	scale (eg, squamous, desquamation)
sta-	make stand, stop (eg, genesistasis)
stal-	send (eg, peristalsis); *see also* stol-
staphyl-	bunch of grapes, uvula (eg, staphylococcus, staphylectomy)
stear-	fat (eg, stearodermia)
steat-	fat (eg, steatopygous)
sten-	narrow, compressed (eg, stenocardia)
ster-	solid (eg, cholesterol)
sterc-	dung (eg, stercoporphyrin)
sthen-	strength (eg, asthenia)
stol-	send (eg, diastole)
stom(at)-	mouth, orifice (eg, anastomosis, stomatogastric)
strep(h)-	twist (eg, strephosymbolia, streptomycin); *see also* stroph-
strict-	draw tight, compress, cause pain (eg, constriction)
-stringent	draw tight, compress, cause pain (eg, astringent)
stroph-	twist (eg, astrophic); *see also* strep(h)-
struct-	pile up (against) (eg, obstruction)
sub-	under, below (b changes to f or p before words beginning with those consonants) (eg, sublumbar)
suf-	*see* sub- (eg, suffusion)
sup-	*see* sub- (eg, suppository)
super-	above, beyond, extreme (eg, supermobility)
sy-	*see* syn- (eg, systole)
syl-	*see* syn- (eg, syllepsiology)
sym-	*see* syn- (eg, symbiosis, symmetry, sympathetic, symphysis)
syn-	with, together (n disappears before s, changes to l before l, and changes to m before b, m, p, and ph) (eg, myosynizesis)
ta-	stretch, put under pressure (eg, ectasis)
tac-	order, arrange (eg, atactic)
tact-	touch (eg, contact)
tax-	order, arrange (eg, ataxia, taxonomy)
tect-	cover (eg, protective)
teg-	cover (eg, integument)
tel-	end (eg, telosynapsis)

tele-	at a distance (eg, teleceptor, telescope)
tempor-	time, timely or fatal spot, temple (eg, temporomalar)
ten(ont)-	tight stretched band (eg, tenodynia, tenonitis, tenontagra)
tens-	stretch (eg, extensor)
test-	pertaining to the testicle (eg, testitis)
tetra-	four (eg, tetragenous)
the-	put, place (eg, synthesis)
thec-	repository, case (eg, thecostegnosis)
thel-	teat, nipple (eg, thelerethism)
therap-	treatment (eg, hydrotherapy)
therm-	heat (eg, diathermy)
thi-	sulfur (eg, thiogenic)
thorac-	chest (eg, thoracoplasty)
thromb-	lump, clot (eg, thrombophlebitis, thrombopenia)
thym-	spirit (eg, dysthymia)
thyr-	shield, shaped like a door (eg, thyroid)
tme-	cut (eg, axonotmesis)
toc-	childbirth (eg, dystocia)
tom-	cut (eg, appendectomy)
ton-	stretch, put under pressure (eg, tonus, peritoneum)
top-	place (eg, topesthesia)
tors-	twist (eg, extorsion)
tox-	arrow poison, poison (eg, toxemia)
trache-	windpipe (eg, tracheotomy)
trachel-	neck (eg, trachelopexy)
tract-	draw, drag (eg, protraction)
trans-	across (eg, transport)
traumat-	wound (eg, traumatic)
tri-	three (eg, trigonad)
trich-	hair (eg, trichoid)
trip-	rub (eg, entripsis)
trop-	turn, react (eg, sitotropism)
troph-	nurture, relating to nourishment (eg, atrophy)
tuber-	swelling, node (eg, tubercle, tuberculosis)
typ-	type (eg, atypical)
typh-	for, stupor (eg, adenotyphus)
typhl-	blind (eg, typhlectasis)
uni-	one (eg, unioval)
ur-	urine (eg, polyuria)
vacc-	cow (eg, vaccine)
vagin-	sheath (eg, invaginated)
vas-	vessel (eg, vascular)

ventro-	abdomen, in front of (eg, ventrolateral, ventrose)
vers-	turn (eg, inversion)
vert-	turn (eg, diverticulum)
vesic-	bladder (eg, vesicovaginal)
vit-	life (eg, devitalize)
vuls-	pull, twitch (eg, convulsion)
xanth-	yellow, blond (eg, xanthophyll)
-yl-	substance (eg, cacodyl)
zo-	life, animal (eg, microzoaria)
zyg-	yoke, union (eg, zygote, zygodactyly)
zym-	ferment (eg, enzyme)

Evaluation Acronyms

ABC: Activity-Specific Balance Confidence Scale
ABI: Ankle-Brachial Index
ABS: Adaptive Behavior Scale
ACIF: Acute Care Index of Function
ACL: Allen Cognitive Level Test
ADAPT: Additive Activities Profile Test
AIMS: Alberta Infant Motor Scale
ALSAR: Assessment of Living Skills and Resources
AMAS: Activity Marching Ability System
AMPS: Assessment of Motor and Process Skills
AOL: Ankle Osteoarthritis Scale
APIB: Assessment of Premature Infant Behavior
ARCET: Astrand Rhyming Cycle Ergometer Test
BADLS: Bristol Activities of Daily Living Scale
BaFPE: Bay Area Functional Performance Evaluation
BCT: Boston Cancellation Test
BDI: Beck Depression Inventory; Battelle Developmental Inventory
BGMA: Basic Gross Motor Assessment
BIT: Behavioral Inattention Test
BNBA: Brazelton Neonatal Behavioral Assessment
BOMC: Blessed Orientation-Memory-Test
BOTMP: Bruininks-Oseretsky Test of Motor Proficiency
BP: Blood Pressure
BSID-II: Bayley Scales of Infant Development–Second Version
BTE: Baltimore Therapeutic Equipment (Work Simulator)
BVRT: Benton Visual Retention Test
CAM: Cognitive Assessment of Minnesota
CARS: Childhood Autism Rating Scale
CBDI: Cognitive Behavioral Driver's Index
CBRS: Cognitive Behavior Rating Scales
CCS: Children's Coma Scale
CEBLS: Comprehensive Evaluation of Basic Living Skills
CES-D: Center for Epidemiological Studies Depression Scale
CFA: Comprehensive Functional Assessment
CHART: Craig Handicap Assessment and Reporting Technique
CIQ: Community Integration Questionnaire
CLM: Comprehensive Lifting Model

CMAP: Compound Muscle Action Potential
CMT: Contextual Memory Test
CO: Cardiac Output
COPM: Canadian Occupational Performance Measure
CPT: Cognitive Performance Test
CRS: Coma Recovery Scale
CTONI: Comprehensive Test of Nonverbal Intelligence
CTSIB: Clinical Test for Sensory Integration in Balance
CUE: Capabilities of the Upper Extremity
CVMT: Continuous Visual Memory Test
CVP: Central Venous Pressure
DDS: Descriptor Differential Scale (pain scale)
DDST-R: Denver Developmental Screening Test-Revised
DPQ: Dallas Pain Questionnaire
DPT: Driver Performance Test
DRI: Disability Rating Index
DRS: Dementia Rating Scale
DSM III-R: Diagnostic and Statistical Manual
DTVP-2: Developmental Test of Visual Perception II
EAE: Eligibility and Agency Evaluation (ED)
ECG: Electrocardiogram
EDSS: Kutzke Expanded Disability Status Scale
EDPA: Erhardt Developmental Prehension Assessment
EIDP: Early Intervention Developmental Profile
ELC: EPIC Lift Capacity Test
EMG: ElectroMyoGram
EPESE: Established Populations for Epidemiologic Studies of the Elderly
FAP: Functional Ambulation Profile; Functional Analysis Profile
FAQ: Functional Activities Questionnaire
FCE: Functional Capacity Evaluation
FDS: Framingham Disability Scale
FEFA: Frail Elderly Functional Assessment Questionnaire
FES: Falls Efficacy Scale
FHS: Functional Health Scale
FIM: Functional Independence Measure
FMA: Fugl-Meyer Assessment (stroke)
FSI: Functional Status Index
FSQ: Functional Status Questionnaire
GARS: Gait Abnormality Rating Scale
GAS: Goal Attainment Scale
GCS: Glasgow Coma Scale
GDS: Geriatric Depression Scale

GMFM: Gross Motor Function Measure
GOAT: Galveston Orientation and Amnesia Test
HAOF: Hospice Assessment of Occupational Function
HAQ: Health Assessment Questionnaire
HELP: Hawaii Early Learning Profile
HHD: Hand Held Dynamometer
HINT: Harris Infant Neuromotor Test
HR: Heart Rate
ILSE: Independent Living Skills Evaluation
INA: Infant Neuromotor Assessment
INFANIB: Infant Neurological International Battery
IQ: Intelligence Quotient
IWS: Isernhagen Work Systems
JPSA: Jacobs Prevocational Skills Assessment
JVD: Jugular Venous Distention
KELS: Kohlman Evaluation of Living Skills
KFCE: Key Functional Capacity Evaluation
KSHQ: Knickerbocker Sensorimotor History Questionnaire
LAP-R: Learning Accomplished Profile-Revised Edition
LCFS: Levels of Cognitive Function Scale
LCL: Low Cognitive Level Test
LEAP: Lower Extremity Activity Profile
LOCF: Rancho Los Amigos Levels of Cognitive Functioning
LORS-III: Level of Rehabilitation Scale–III
MABC: Movement Assessment Battery for Children
MACTAR: McMaster–Toronto Arthritis Patient Function Preference Questionnaire
MAI: Movement Assessment of Infants; Multilevel Assessment Instrument
MAI-ST: Movement Assessment of Infants-Screening Test
MAP: Miller Assessment for Preschoolers
MAS: Carr & Shepard Motor Assessment Scale
MBHI: The Million Behavioral Health Inventory
MDI: Maryland Disability Index (most commonly referred to as the Barthel Index)
MDS: Minimum Data Set (Medicare)
MEAMS: Middlesex Elderly Assessment of Mental State
MEAP: Multiphasic Environmental Assessment Procedure
MEDLS: Milwaukee Evaluation of Daily Living Skills
MEVEIET: Maximal Exercise to Volitional Exhaustion Incremental Exercise Test
MFAQ: Multidimensional Functional Assessment Questionnaire

MMPI: Minnesota Multiphasic Personality Inventory

MMSE: Mini-Mental State Exam

MMT: Manual Muscle Test

MOS-36: Measure of Self-Functioning

MPQ: McGill Pain Questionnaire

MRFA: Medical Rehab Follow Along

MRMT: Minnesota Rate of Manipulation

MSFAM: Measure System: Functional Autonomy Measuring System

MSQ: Mental Status Questionnaire

MVAS: The Million Visual Analog Scale (pain)

MVPT: Motor-Free Visual Perceptive Test

NAPFI: Neurological Assessment of the Pre-Term and Full-Term Infant

NBAS: Neonatal Behavioral Assessment Scale

NCS: Nerve Conduction Studies

NCSE: Neurobehavioral Cognitive Status Examination

NDDG: National Diabetes Data Group

NDS: Neck Disability Scale

NHANES: National Health and Nutrition Examination Survey

NIDCAP: Neonatal Individualized Developmental and Care Assessment Profile (also referred to as NONB)

NINDS: National Institute of Neurological Disorders and Stroke Myotatic Reflex Scale

NLTCS: National Long-Term Care Survey

NMES: National Medical Expenditure Survey

NNE: Neonatal Neurobehavioral Evaluation

NNHS: National Nursing Home Survey

NOMAS: Neonatal Oral-Motor Assessment Scale

NONB: Naturalistic Observation of Newborn Behavior (also referred to as NIDCAP)

NRS: Numerical Rating Scale

OARS: Older American Resources and Services–Multidimensional Functional Assessment Questionnaire (MFAQ)

OASIS: Outcomes and Assessment Information Set (Medicare)

ODQ: Oswestry Low Back Pain Disability Questionnaire

OGA: Observational Gait Assessment (amputee)

OWAS: Ovako Working Posture Analysis System

PACE: Program of All-Inclusive Care for the Elderly

PADL: Performance Activities of Daily Living

P-CTSIB: Pediatric Clinical Test of Sensory Integration for Balance

PCWP: Pulmonary Capillary Wedge Pressure

PDI: Physical Disability Index

PDMS: Peabody Developmental Motor Scales
PDS: Pain Discomfort Scale
PECS: Patient Evaluations Conference System
PEDI: Pediatric Evaluation of Disability Inventory
PEO: Portable Ergonomic Observation Method
PEQ: Prosthesis Evaluation Questionnaire
PFMAI: Posture and Fine Motor Skills Assessment of Infant
PFSDS(M): Modified Pulmonary Function Status and Dyspnea Questionnaire
PFT: Pulmonary Function Test
PGC: Philadelphia Geriatric Center Scale
PGCII: Philadelphia Geriatric Center Scale II
PILE: Progressive Isoinertial Lifting Evaluation
PLSI: Personal Lifting Safety Index
POE: Post-Occupancy Evaluation
PPA: Prosthetic Profile of the Amputee
PPME: Physical Performance and Mobility Examination
PPS: Preschool Play Scale
PPT: Physical Performance Test
PST: Postural Stress Test
PULSES: P = physical condition, U = upper limb function, L = lower limb function, S = sensory components, E = excretory function, S = support factors
QNST: Quick Neurological Screening Test
QST: Quantitative Somatosensory Thermostat
QUEST: Quality of Upper Extremity Skills Test
RAI: Resident Assessment Instrument
RAPs: Resident Assessment Protocols
RBMT: Rivermead Behavioral Memory Test
RCFT: Rey Complex Figure Test
REG: Rapid Exchange of Grip
RER: Respiratory Exchange Ratio
RLSI: Relative Lifting Scale Index
RMA: Rivermead Motor Assessment
RMI: Rivermead Mobility Index
RNL: Reintegration to Normal Living Index
ROM: Range of Motion
RPE: Rating of Perceived Exertion
RPM: Raven Progressive Matrices
RR: Respiratory Rate
RT: Reach Test
RTI: Routine Task Inventory
RULA: Rapid Upper Limb Analysis

SAFE: Safety and Functional ADL Evaluation
SAFER: Safety Assessment of Function and the Environment for Rehabilitation
SAFFE: Survey of Activities and Fear of Falling in the Elderly
SAILS: Structured Assessment of Independent Living Skills
SAQ: Services Assessment Questionnaire
SCT: Short Category Test
SCWT: Stroop Color and Word Test
SDMT: Symbol Digit Modalities Test
SDS: Zung Self-Rating Depression Scale
SFA: School Functional Assessment
SF-36: Self Functional Assessment (36 items)
SIB: Severe Impairment Battery
SIP: Sickness Impact Profile
SIPT: Sensory Integration and Praxis Test
SIT: Sensory Integration Test
SM: Sphygmomanometer
SNAP: Sensory Nerve Conduction Studies
SOA: National Health Interview Survey: Supplement on Aging
SOT: Sensory Organization Test
SOTOF: Structured Observational Test of Function
SPA: Sensorimotor Performance Analysis
SPADI: Shoulder Pain and Disability Index
SPIT: Sensorimotor Integration and Praxis Tests
SPMSQ: Short Portable Mental Status Questionnaire
SPSQ: Satisfaction with Performance Scaled Questionnaire
SSP: Short Sensory Profile
STREAM: Stroke Rehabilitation Assessment of Movement Measure
SWM: Semmes-Weinstein Monofilament Test
TEA: Test of Everyday Attention
TEMPA: Upper Extremity Performance Test for the Elderly
TGMD: Test of Gross Motor Performance
TIE: Touch Inventory for Elementary-School-Aged Children
TIME: Toddler and Infant Motor Evaluation, The In-Hand Manipulation Skills
TIMP: Test of Infant Motor Performance
TIP: Touch Inventory for Preschoolers
TMNF: Test of Motor and Neurological Functions
TMP: Timed Manual Performance
TORP: Test of Orientation for Rehabilitation Patients
TOWER: Testing Orientation Work Evaluation and Rehabilitation
TQSB: Teacher Questionnaire on Sensorimotor Behavior

TSI: Test of Sensory Integration (also called the DeGangi-Berk Test)
TUG: Timed Up and Go Test
TVMS: Test of Visual Motor Skills
TVPS: Test of Visual Perceptual Skills (nonmotor)
VAS: Visual Analogue Scale
VAT: Visual Analogue Thermometer
VCWS: VALPAR Component Work Samples
VMI: Developmental Test of Visual-Motor Integration
VOSP: Visual Object and Space Perception Test
VRS: Verbal Rating Scale (pain scale)
WAIS: Wechsler Adult Intelligence Scale
WAIS-R: Wechsler Adult Intelligence Scale–Revised
WCST: Wisconsin Card Sorting Test
WeeFIM: Functional Independence for Children
WEST II: Work Evaluation Systems Technologies II
WIRE: Work and Industrial Rehabilitation Evaluation
WNSP: Western Neurosensory Stimulation Profile
WOMAC: Western Ontario and McMaster University Arthritis Index
WPSI: Wechsler Preschool and Primary Scale of Intelligence
WUSPI: Wheelchair User's Shoulder Pain Index

Organization Acronyms

AA: Alcoholics Anonymous

AAA: Area Agencies on Aging

AAACE: American Association of Adult and Continuing Education

AAAS: American Association for the Advancement of Science

AACHP: American Association for Comprehensive Health Planning

AAFP: American Academy of Family Practitioners

AAHPERD: American Alliance for Health, Physical Education, Recreation, and Dance

AAMR: American Association on Mental Retardation

AAP: American Academy of Pediatrics

AAPC: American Association of Pastoral Counselors

AAPD: American Academy of Pediatric Dentists

AAPH: American Association of Partial Hospitalization

AARP: American Association for Retired Persons

AART: American Association for Respiratory Therapy; Association for the Advancement of Rehabilitation Technology

ABPTS: American Board of Physical Therapy Specialists

ACA: American Counseling Association

ACALD: Association for Children and Adults with Learning Disabilities

ACCD: American Coalition of Citizens with Disabilities

ACCH: Association for the Care of Children's Health

ACCP: American College of Chest Physicians

ACDD: Accreditation Council on Services for People with Developmental Disabilities

ACF: Administration for Children and Families

ACHCA: American College of Health Care Administrators

ACIP: Advisory Committee on Immunization Practices

ACRE: American Council on Rural Education

ACRM: American Congress of Rehabilitation Medicine

ACSM: American College of Sports Medicine

ACYF: Administration on Children, Youth, and Families

ADA: American Dietetic Association

ADD: Administration on Developmental Disabilities

ADED: Association of Driver Educators for the Disabled

ADHA: American Dental Hygienists Association
ADRDA: Alzheimer's Disease and Related Disorders Association
AERA: American Educational Research Association
AF: Arthritis Foundation
AGA: American Geriatric Association
AGHE: Association for Gerontology in Higher Education
AHA: American Hospital Association
AHCA: American Health Care Association
AHCPR: Agency for Health Care Policy and Research
AHEA: American Home Economics Association
AHPA: Arthritis Health Professional Association
AICPA: American Institute of Certified Public Accountants
AMA: American Medical Association
AMDA: American Medical Directors Association
AMH: Accreditation Manual for Hospitals (JCAHO)
ANA: American Nurses Association
ANSI: American National Standards Institute
AOA: Administration on Aging (DHHS); American Optometric Association; American Osteopathic Association
AOPA: American Orthotic and Prosthetic Association
AOTA: American Occupational Therapy Association
APA: American Psychiatric Association; American Psychological Association
APHA: American Public Health Association
APTA: American Physical Therapy Association
ARC: Association for Retarded Citizens
ARCA: American Rehabilitation Counseling Association
ARF: Association of Rehabilitation Facilities
ASA: American Society on Aging
ASAE: American Society of Association Executives
ASAHP: American Society of Allied Health Professions
ASLHA: American Speech-Language-Hearing Association
ASHT: American Society of Hand Therapists
ASI: Assessment Systems, Inc
ASPA: Association of Specialized and Professional Accreditors
BC/BC: Blue Cross/Blue Shield Association
BCPE: Board for Certification in Professional Ergonomics
BHP: Bureau of Health Professions (DHHS)
BLS: Bureau of Labor Statistics (DOL)
BOC: Board of Commissioners (JCAHO)
BPD: Bureau of Policy Development (HCFA)
BPO: Bureau of Operations (HCFA)

CAAHEP: Commission on Accreditation of Allied Health Education Programs

CAHEA: Committee on Allied Health Education and Accreditation (AMA)

CAPTE: Commission on Accreditation in Physical Therapy Education

CARF: Commission on Accreditation of Rehabilitation Facilities

CBO: Congressional Budget Office

CCB: Child Care Bureau

CCD: Consortium for Citizens with Disabilities

CCR&R: Child Care Resource and Referral Agency

CCY: Coalition for Children and Youth

CDC: Centers for Disease Control and Prevention

CEC: Council for Exceptional Children

CHF: Coalition for Health Funding

CHHA/CHS: Council of Home Health Agencies and Community Health Services (NLN)

CLEAR: Clearinghouse on Licenser, Enforcement, and Regulation

CME: Council on Medical Education (AMA)

CMS: Center for Medical and Medicaid Services (formerly HCFA)

COPA: Council on Postsecondary Accreditation

CORE: Commission on Rehabilitation Education

CSG: Council of State Governments

CSN: Children's Safety Network

CSS: Children's Specialty Services

CWLA: Child Welfare League of America

DAHEA: Division of Allied Health Education and Accreditation (AMA)

DAHP: Division of Associated Health Professions (DHHS)

DHHS: Department of Health and Human Services

DOE: Department of Education

DOL: Department of Labor

ECELS: Early Childhood Education Linkage System

EFA: Epilepsy Foundation of America

EHA: Education of Handicapped Act

FAHD: Forum on Allied Health Data

FAO: United Nations Food and Agriculture Organization

FDA: Food and Drug Administration (DHHS)

FEC: Federal Election Commission

FEHBP: Federal Employees Health and Benefits Program

FM: Financial Management Department

FTC: Federal Trade Commission

FUSA: Families United for Senior Action

GAO: Government Accounting Office
GMENAC: Graduate Medical Education National Advisory Committee
GSA: Gerontological Society of America
GU: Generations United
GWSAE: Greater Washington Society of Association Executives
HCFA: Health Care Financing Administration (DHHS) (Has been renamed CMS)
HCPAC: Health Care Professionals Advisory Committee (AMA)
HCPDG: Health Care Professionals Discussion Group
HFMA: Healthcare Financial Management Association
HIAA: Health Insurance Association of America
HMHB: Healthy Mothers, Healthy Babies Coalition
HMO: Health Maintenance Organization
HRSA: Health Resources and Services Administration (DHHS)
HSF: Health Services Foundation
HSQB: Health Standards and Quality Bureau (HCFA)
HTCC: Hand Therapy Certification Commission
IHS: Indian Health Service
IOM: Institute of Medicine
IRB: Institutional Review Board
IRS: Internal Revenue Service
IRSG: Insurance Rehabilitation Study Group
JCAHO: Joint Commission on Accreditation of Healthcare Organizations
LDA: Learning Disabilities Association
MCHB: Maternal and Child Health Bureau (DHHS)
MDAA: Muscular Dystrophy Association of America
MPI: Meeting Planners International
MRC: Medical Research Council
NAATRP: National Association of Activity Therapy and Rehabilitation Programs
NACCRRA: National Association of Child Care Resource and Referral Agencies
NACOSH: National Advisory Committee on Scouting for the Handicapped
NADT: National Association for Drama Therapy
NAEYC: National Association for Education of Young Children
NAHB/NRC: National Association of Home Builders/National Research Center
NAHC: National Association for Home Care
NAHHA: National Association of Home Health Agencies
NAMI: National Alliance for the Mentally Ill

NAMME: National Association of Medical Minority Educators
NAMT: National Association for Music Therapy
NAPHS: National Association of Psychiatric Health Systems
NAPNAP: National Association of Pediatric Nurse Associates and Practitioners
NAPSO: National Alliance of Pupil Service Organizations
NARA: National Association of Rehabilitation Agencies
NARC: National Association for Retarded Citizens
NARF: National Association of Rehabilitation Facilities
NASA: National Aeronautics and Space Agency
NASDSE: National Association of State Directors of Special Education
NASL: National Association for Long-term-care
NASMHPD: National Association of State Mental Health Program Directors
NASUA: National Association of State Units on Aging
NASW: National Association of Social Workers
NAVESP: National Association of Vocational Education Special Personnel
NCAHE: National Commission on Allied Health Education
NCBFE: National Center for a Barrier-Free Environment
NCCNHR: National Citizens Coalition for Nursing Home Reform
NCD: National Council on Disability
NCDPEH: National Coalition for Disease Prevention and Environmental Health
NCEMCH: National Center for Education in Maternal and Child Health
NCES: National Center for Education Statistics (DHHS)
NCHC: National Council on Health Care Technologists
NCHCA: National Commission for Health Certifying Agencies
NCHHA: National Council of Homemakers and Home Health Aides
NCHP: National Council for Health Planning
NCHS: National Center for Health Statistics (DHHS)
NCIL: National Council on Independent Living
NCMRR: National Center for Medical Rehabilitation Research
NCOA: National Council on Aging
NCSL: National Conference of State Legislatives
NDTA: Neurodevelopmental Treatment Association
NHC: National Health Council
NHLA: National Health Lawyers Association
NHO: National Hospice Organization
NHTSA: National Highway Traffic Safety Administration

NIA: National Institute on Aging

NIAAA: National Institutes on Alcohol Abuse and Alcoholism (Public Health Service)

NICCYD: National Information Center for Children and Youth with Disabilities

NIDA: National Institute of Drug Abuse

NIDRR: National Institute on Disability and Rehabilitation Research

NIH: National Institutes of Health

NIHR: National Institute of Handicapped Research

NIMH: National Institute of Mental Health

NLN: National League for Nursing

NLRB: National Labor Relations Board

NMHA: National Mental Health Association

NMSS: National Multiple Sclerosis Society

NPSRC: National Professional Standards Review Council

NRA: National Rehabilitation Association

NRC: National Research Council

NRCA: National Rehabilitation Counseling Association

NRTI: National Rehabilitation Training Institutes

NUCEA: National University Continuing Education Association

NVOILA: National Voluntary Organizations for Independent Living for the Aging

OCR: Office of Civil Rights

OE: Office of Education

OH: Office of the Handicapped

OIG: Office of the Inspector General

OMB: Office of Management and Budget (Executive Office of the President)

OPM: Office of Personnel Management

OPRR: Office for Protection from Research Risks (DHHS)

OSEP: Office of Special Education Programs

OSERS: Office of Special Education and Rehabilitation Services (DOE)

OSG: Office of the Surgeon General

OSHA: Occupational Safety and Health Administration

OVR: Office of Vocational Rehabilitation

OWH: Office of Women's Health (DHHS)

PAC-APTA: Political Action Committee-American Physical Therapy Association

PATH: Partners Appropriate Technology for the Handicapped

PCMA: Professional Convention Management Association

PCPD: President's Committee on People with Disabilities

PPO: Preferred Provider Organization
PROPAC: Prospective Payment Assessment Commission
PRRB: Provider Reimbursement Review Board
PRSA: Public Relations Society of America
PSRO: Professional Standards Review Organization
PTAC: Professional and Technical Advisory Committee (JCAHO)
PVA: Paralyzed Veterans of America
RSA: Rehabilitation Services Administration (DOE)
SAMHSA: Substance Abuse and Mental Health Services Administration (DHHS)
SISSC: Special Interest Section Steering Committee
SNAP: Society of National Association Publications
SSA: Social Security Administration (DHHS)
TASH: The Association for Persons with Severe Handicaps
TRB: Transportation Research Board
UCPA: United Cerebral Palsy Association
USDA: United States Department of Agriculture
VA: Department of Veterans Affairs
VA DM&S: Veterans Administration Department of Medicine and Surgery
VEWAA: Vocational Evaluation and Work Adjustment Association (NRA)
WCPT: World Confederation of Physical Therapists
WFOT: World Federation of Occupational Therapists
WHCOA: White House Conference on Aging
WHIF: Washington Health Issues Forum
WHO: World Health Organization
WIC: Women in Communication

American Physical Therapy Association
Code of Ethics

PREAMBLE

This *Code of Ethics* of the American Physical Therapy Association sets forth principles for the ethical practice of physical therapy. All physical therapists are responsible for maintaining and promoting ethical practice. To this end, the physical therapist shall act in the best interest of the patient/client. This *Code of Ethics*, adopted by the American Physical Therapy Association, shall be binding on all physical therapists.

PRINCIPLE 1

A physical therapist shall respect the rights and dignity of all individuals and shall provide comprehensive care.

PRINCIPLE 2

A physical therapist shall act in a trustworthy manner toward patients/clients and in all other aspects of physical therapy practice.

PRINCIPLE 3

A physical therapist shall comply with laws and regulations governing physical therapy and shall strive to effect changes that benefit patients/clients.

PRINCIPLE 4

A physical therapist shall exercise sound professional judgment.

PRINCIPLE 5

A physical therapist shall achieve and maintain professional competence.

PRINCIPLE 6

A physical therapist shall maintain and promote high standards for physical therapy practice, education, and research.

PRINCIPLE 7

A physical therapist shall seek only such remuneration as is deserved and reasonable for physical therapy services.

PRINCIPLE 8

A physical therapist shall provide and make available accurate and relevant information to patients/clients about their care and to the public about physical therapy.

PRINCIPLE 9

A physical therapist shall protect the public and the profession from unethical, incompetent, and illegal acts.

PRINCIPLE 10

A physical therapist shall endeavor to address the health needs of society.

PRINCIPLE 11

A physical therapist shall respect the rights, knowledge, and skills of colleagues and other health care professionals.

The Bylaws give the Ethics and Judicial Committee (EJC) responsibility for interpreting the APTA's ethical principles and standards. The EJC has adopted the *Guide for Professional Conduct*, which interprets the *Code of Ethics* and provides guidelines by which physical therapists may determine the propriety of their conduct. The EJC also has adopted the *Guide for Conduct of the Affiliate Member*, which provides corresponding guidance for physical therapist assistants with respect to the interpretation of the *Standards of Ethical Conduct for the Physical Therapist Assistant*. The EJC's two guides are public statements of the values and principles of the profession. The EJC made the most recent amendments to the *Guide for Professional Conduct* at its January 1999 meeting. The EJC also has compiled a *Compendium of Interpretations and Opinions* containing statements on various ethical issues.

The APTA has a process for handling charges that any of its members has violated the *Code of Ethics* or the *Standards of Ethical Conduct for the Physical Therapist Assistant*. Under the Bylaws, each of the APTA's chapters is responsible for investigating complaints of ethical violations in accordance with the procedures, prescribed by the APTA Board of Directors, in the *Procedural Document on Disciplinary Action* (BOD 03-96-04-07). These procedures are intended to enable the Association to act fairly in the performance of its responsibilities as a professional organization while safeguarding the rights of the member against whom ethics charges have been made. Under the *Procedural Document*, a Chapter Ethics Committee (CEC) has the responsibility of investigating charges referred by the Chapter President and deciding whether to dismiss the charges (subject to the EJC's review and approval) or to recommend to the EJC that it impose one of the four forms of disciplinary action: (i) reprimand, (ii) probation, (iii) suspension, or (iv) expulsion. When a CEC recommends a punishment, the EJC may impose the sanction recommended or impose a lesser sanction (or no sanction at all), but it may not impose a more severe punishment than that recommended by the CEC. The decision of the EJC is subject to appeal to the Board of Directors.

Reprinted with permission of the American Physical Therapy Association.

American Physical Therapy Association
Guide for Professional Conduct

PURPOSE

This *Guide for Professional Conduct* (*Guide*) is intended to serve physical therapists who are members of the American Physical Therapy Association (Association) in interpreting the *Code of Ethics* (*Code*) and matters of professional conduct. The *Guide* provides guidelines by which physical therapists may determine the propriety of their conduct. The *Code* and the *Guide* apply to all physical therapists who are Association members. These guidelines are subject to changes as the dynamics of the profession change and as new patterns of health care delivery are developed and accepted by the professional community and the public. This *Guide* is subject to monitoring and timely revision by the Ethics and Judicial Committee of the Association.

INTERPRETING ETHICAL PRINCIPLES

The interpretations expressed in this *Guide* are not to be considered all inclusive of situations that could evolve under a specific principle of the *Code* but reflect the opinions, decisions, and advice of the Judicial Committee. While the statements of ethical principles apply universally, specific circumstances determine their appropriate application. Input related to current interpretations, or situations requiring interpretation, is encouraged from Association members.

PRINCIPLE 1

Physical therapists respect the rights and dignity of all individuals.

1.1 Attitudes of Physical Therapists

A. Physical therapists shall recognize that each individual is different from all other individuals and shall respect and be responsive to those differences.

B. Physical therapists are to be guided at all times by concern for the physical, psychological, and socioeconomic welfare of those individuals entrusted to their care.

C. Physical therapists shall not engage in conduct that constitutes harassment or abuse of, or discrimination against, colleagues, associates, or others.

1.2 Confidential Information

A. Information relating to the physical therapist–patient relationship is confidential and may not be communicated to a third party not involved in that patient's care without the prior written consent of the patient, subject to applicable law.

B. Information derived from component-sponsored peer review shall be held confidential by the reviewer unless written permission to release the information is obtained from the physical therapist who was reviewed.

C. Information derived from the working relationships of physical therapists shall be held confidential by all parties.

D. Information may be disclosed to appropriate authorities when it is necessary to protect the welfare of an individual or the community. Such disclosure shall be in accordance with applicable law.

1.3 Patient Relations

Physical therapists shall not engage in any sexual relationship or activity, whether consensual or nonconsensual, with any patient while a physical therapist/patient relationship exists.

1.4 Informed Consent

Physical therapists shall obtain patient informed consent before treatment, to include disclosure of: (i) the nature of the proposed intervention, (ii) material risks of harm or complications, (iii) reasonable alternatives to the proposed intervention, and (iv) goals of treatment.

PRINCIPLE 2

Physical therapists comply with the laws and regulations governing the practice of physical therapy.

2.1 Professional Practice

Physical therapists shall provide consultation, evaluation, treatment, and preventive care, in accordance with the laws and regulations of the jurisdiction(s) in which they practice.

PRINCIPLE 3

Physical therapists accept responsibility for the exercise of sound judgment.

3.1 Acceptance of Responsibility

A. Upon accepting a patient/client for provision of physical therapy services, physical therapists shall assume the responsibility for examining, evaluating, and diagnosing that individual; prognosis and intervention; reexamination and modification of the plan of care; and maintaining adequate records of the case including progress reports. Physical therapists establish the plan of care and provide and/or supervise the appropriate intervention.

B. If the diagnostic process reveals findings that are outside the scope of the physical therapist's knowledge, experience, or expertise, the physical therapist shall so inform the patient/client and refer to an appropriate practitioner.

C. Regardless of practice setting, physical therapists shall maintain the ability to make independent judgments.

D. The physical therapist shall not provide physical therapy services to a patient while under the influence of a substance that impairs his or her ability to do so safely.

E. When the patient is referred from another practitioner, the physical therapist shall communicate the findings of the examination, the diagnosis, the proposed intervention, and reexamination findings (as indicated) to the referring practitioner and any other appropriate individuals involved in the patient's care, while maintaining standards of confidentiality.

3.2 Delegation of Responsibility

A. Physical therapists shall not delegate to a less qualified person any activity which requires the unique skill, knowledge, and judgment of the physical therapist.

B. The primary responsibility for physical therapy care rendered by supportive personnel rests with the supervising physical therapist. Adequate supervision requires, at a minimum, that a supervising physical therapist perform the following activities:

    1. Designate or establish channels of written and oral communication.

2. Interpret available information concerning the individual under care.
3. Examine, evaluate, and determine a diagnosis.
4. Develop plan of care, including short- and long-term goals.
5. Select and delegate appropriate tasks of plan of care.
6. Assess competence of supportive personnel to perform assigned tasks.
7. Direct and supervise supportive personnel in delegated tasks.
8. Identify and document precautions, special problems, contraindications, goals, anticipated progress, and plans for reevaluation.
9. Reevaluate, adjust plan of care when necessary, perform final evaluation, and establish follow-up plan.

3.3 Provision of Services

A. Physical therapists shall recognize the individual's freedom of choice in selection of physical therapy services.

B. Physical therapists' professional practices and their adherence to ethical principles of the Association shall take preference over business practices. Provisions of services for personal financial gain rather than for the need of the individual receiving the services are unethical.

C. When physical therapists judge that an individual will no longer benefit from their services, they shall so inform the individual receiving the services. Physical therapists shall avoid overutilization of their services.

D. In the event of elective termination of a physical therapist/patient relationship by the physical therapist, the therapist should take steps to transfer the care of the patient, as appropriate, to another provider.

E. Physical therapists shall recognize that third-party payer contracts may limit, in one form or another, provision of physical therapy services. Physical therapists shall inform patients of any known limitations. Third-party limitations do not absolve the physical therapist from adherence to ethical principles. Physical therapists shall avoid underutilization of their services.

3.4 Practice Arrangements

A. Participation in a business, partnership, corporation, or other entity does not exempt the physical therapist, whether employer, partner, or stockholder, either individually or collectively, from the obligation of promoting and maintaining the ethical principles of the Association.

B. Physical therapists shall advise their employer(s) of any employer practice which causes a physical therapist to be in conflict with the ethical principles of the Association. Physical therapist employees shall attempt to rectify aspects of their employment which are in conflict with the ethical principles of the Association.

PRINCIPLE 4

Physical therapists maintain and promote high standards for physical therapy practice, education, and research.

4.1 Continued Education

A. Physical therapists shall participate in educational activities which enhance their basic knowledge and provide new knowledge.

B. Whenever physical therapists provide continuing education, they shall ensure that course content, objectives, and responsibilities of the instructional faculty are accurately reflected in the promotion of the course.

4.2 Review and Self-Assessment

A. Physical therapists shall provide for utilization review of their services.

B. Physical therapists shall demonstrate their commitment to quality assurance by peer review and self-assessment.

4.3 Research

A. Physical therapists shall support research activities that contribute knowledge for improved patient care.

B. Physical therapists engaged in research shall ensure:

1. the consent of subjects;
2. confidentiality of the data on individual subjects and the personal identities of the subjects;

3. well-being of all subjects in compliance with facility regulations and laws of the jurisdiction in which the research is conducted;

4. the absence of fraud and plagiarism;

5. full disclosure of support received;

6. appropriate acknowledgment of individuals making a contribution to the research; and

7. that animal subjects used in research are treated humanely and in compliance with facility regulations and laws of the jurisdiction in which the research experimentation is conducted.

C. Physical therapists shall report to appropriate authorities any acts in the conduct or presentation of research that appear unethical or illegal.

4.4 Education

A. Physical therapists shall support quality education in academic and clinical settings.

B. Physical therapists functioning in the educational role are responsible to the students, the academic institutions, and the clinical settings for promoting ethical conduct in educational activities. Whenever possible, the educator shall ensure:

1. the rights of students in the academic and clinical setting;

2. appropriate confidentiality of personal information;

3. professional conduct towards the student during the academic and clinical education processes; and

4. assignment to clinical settings prepared to give the student a learning experience.

C. Clinical educators are responsible for reporting to the academic program student conduct which appears to be unethical or illegal.

PRINCIPLE 5

Physical therapists seek remuneration for their services that is deserved and reasonable.

5.1 Fiscally Sound Remuneration

A. Physical therapists shall never place their own financial interest above the welfare of individuals under their care.

B. Fees for physical therapy services should be reasonable for the service performed, considering the setting in which it is provided, practice costs in the geographic area, judgment of other organizations, and other relevant factors.

C. Physical therapists should attempt to ensure that providers, agencies, or other employers adopt physical therapy fee schedules that are reasonable and that encourage access to necessary services.

5.2 Business Practices/Fee Arrangements

A. Physical therapists shall not:

1. directly or indirectly request, receive, or participate in the dividing, transferring, assigning, or rebating of an unearned fee, and

2. profit by means of a credit or other valuable consideration, such as an unearned commission, discount, or gratuity in connection with furnishing of physical therapy services.

B. Unless laws impose restrictions to the contrary, physical therapists who provide physical therapy services in a business entity may pool fees and moneys received. Physical therapists may divide or apportion these fees and moneys in accordance with the business agreement.

C. Physical therapists may enter into agreements with organizations to provide physical therapy services if such agreements do not violate the ethical principles of the Association.

5.3 Endorsement of Equipment or Services

A. Physical therapists shall not use influence upon individuals under their care or their families for utilization of equipment or services based upon the direct or indirect financial interest of the physical therapist in such equipment or services. Realizing that these individuals will normally rely on the physical therapists' advice, their best interest must always be maintained as well as their right of free choice relating to the use of any equipment or service. While it cannot be considered unethical for physical therapists to own or have a financial interest in equipment companies or services, they must act in accordance with law and make full disclosure of their interest whenever such companies or services become the source of equipment or services for individuals under their care.

B. Physical therapists may be remunerated for endorsement or advertisement of equipment or services to the lay public, physical therapists, or other health professionals provided they disclose any financial interest in the production, sale, or distribution of said equipment or services.

C. In endorsing or advertising equipment or services, physical therapists shall use sound professional judgment and shall not give the appearance of Association endorsement.

5.4 Gifts and Other Considerations

A. Physical therapists shall not accept nor offer gifts or other considerations with obligatory conditions attached.

B. Physical therapists shall not accept nor offer gifts or other considerations that affect or give an objective appearance of affecting their professional judgment.

PRINCIPLE 6

Physical therapists provide accurate information to the consumer about the profession and about those services they provide.

6.1 Information about the Profession

Physical therapists shall endeavor to educate the public to an awareness of the physical therapy profession through such means as publication of articles and participation in seminars, lectures, and civic programs.

6.2 Information about Services

A. Information given to the public shall emphasize that individual problems cannot be treated without individualized evaluation and plans/programs of care.

B. Physical therapists may advertise their services to the public.

C. Physical therapists shall not use, or participate in the use of, any form of communication containing a false, plagiarized, fraudulent, misleading, deceptive, unfair, or sensational statement or claim.

D. A paid advertisement shall be identified as such unless it is apparent from the context that it is a paid advertisement.

PRINCIPLE 7

Physical therapists accept the responsibility to protect the public and the profession from unethical, incompetent, or illegal acts.

7.1 *Consumer Protection*

A. Physical therapists shall report any conduct which appears to be unethical, incompetent, or illegal.

B. Physical therapists may not participate in any arrangements in which patients are exploited due to the referring sources enhancing their personal incomes as a result of referring for, prescribing, or recommending physical therapy.

C. Physical therapists shall be obligated to safeguard the public from underutilization or overutilization of physical therapy services.

7.2 *Disclosure*

The physical therapist shall disclose to the patient if the referring practitioner derives compensation from the provision of physical therapy. The physical therapist shall ensure that the individual has freedom of choice in selecting a provider of physical therapy.

PRINCIPLE 8

Physical therapists participate in efforts to address the health needs of the public.

8.1 **Pro Bono** *Service*

Physical therapists should render *pro bono publico* (reduced or no fee) services to patients lacking the ability to pay for services, as each physical therapist's practice permits.

Issued by the Ethics and Judicial Committee
American Physical Therapy Association
October 1981
Last Amended January 1999
(current as of 4/99)

JANUARY 1999 AMENDMENTS TO *GUIDE FOR PROFESSIONAL CONDUCT*

The APTA's Ethics and Judicial Committee (EJC) made a number of amendments to the *Guide for Professional Conduct* at its January 1999 meeting. The amendments address three areas as to which the House of Delegates (in the Support Statement for RC 18-98) indicated that the document needed revision: (i) diagnosis by physical therapists; (ii) referral relationships, and the inappropriateness of using the term "prescribes" to characterize the role of a referring practitioner; and (iii) underutilization attributable to third-party limitations on the provision of physical therapy services (not including limitations that give the practitioner a financial incentive to limit or curtail services).

The EJC voted to amend the *Guide for Professional Conduct* by amending Section 3.1(A) to read as follows:

A. Upon accepting a patient/client for provision of physical therapy services, physical therapists shall assume the responsibility for examining, evaluating, and diagnosing that individual; prognosis and intervention; reexamination and modification of the plan of care; and maintaining adequate records of the case including progress reports. Physical therapists establish the plan of care and provide and/or supervise the appropriate intervention.

This change makes explicit that physical therapists are responsible for making diagnoses, consistent with *Diagnosis by Physical Therapists* (HOD 06-97-06-19). The change makes the *Guide for Professional Conduct* more consistent with the terminology of the APTA's *Guide to Physical Therapist Practice*.

The Committee voted to amend the *Guide for Professional Conduct* by deleting Section 3.1(B) and replacing it with the following language:

B. If the diagnostic process reveals findings that are outside the scope of the physical therapist's knowledge, experience, or expertise, the physical therapist shall so inform the patient/client and refer him or her to an appropriate practitioner.

This change makes explicit that physical therapists are responsible for making diagnoses, consistent with *Diagnosis by Physical Therapists* (HOD 06-97-06-19). The replacement language derives largely from the *Guide to Physical Therapist Practice* (page 1 to 7, under the heading "Diagnosis").

The Committee voted to amend the *Guide for Professional Conduct* by adding the following new Section 3.1(E):

E. When the patient is referred from another practitioner, the physical therapist shall communicate the findings of the examination, the diagnosis, the proposed intervention, and reexamination findings (as indicated) to the referring practitioner and any other appropriate individuals involved in the patient's care, while maintaining standards of confidentiality.

This addition requires the physical therapist to engage in some communication with referring practitioners (and others, as appropriate). Communicating reexamination findings to the referring practitioner is required only where that practitioner has so indicated. This change should be understood in conjunction with the Committee's deletion of former Section 3.4 (Referral Relationships), a Section which infelicitously used the term "prescribes" to characterize the role of the referring practitioner. See *Position on Term "Prescription"* (BOD 03-93-22-59).

The Committee voted to amend the *Guide for Professional Conduct* by deleting clause 3 in Section 3.2(B) and replacing it with the following language:

  3.   Examine, evaluate, and determine a diagnosis.

This change makes explicit that physical therapists are responsible for making diagnoses, consistent with *Diagnosis by Physical Therapists* (HOD 06-97-06-19). The change makes the *Guide for Professional Conduct* more consistent with the terminology of the *Guide to Physical Therapist Practice*.

The Committee voted to amend the *Guide for Professional Conduct* by adding a new Section 3.3(E) to read as follows:

  E.   Physical therapists shall recognize that third-party payer contracts may limit, in one form or another, provision of physical therapy services. Physical therapists shall inform patients of any known limitations. Third-party limitations do not absolve the physical therapist from adherence to ethical principles. Physical therapists shall avoid underutilization of their services.

This new Section 3.3(E) begins to address the ethical implications of limitations by payers on the provision of physical therapy services. In the Committee's view, the new language extends to limitations on the number of visits or length of treatment for which the third party will pay, but it does not extend to situations in which a limitation takes the form of the physical therapist's having a financial incentive to limit or curtail services. Therefore, the new language does not require a physical therapist to inform the patient of a limitation attributable to a capitation or other arrangement that gives the physical therapy service a financial incentive to limit or curtail therapy.

The Committee voted to amend the *Guide for Professional Conduct* by deleting Section 3.4 (Referral Relationships) in its entirety, and by renumbering current Section 3.5 (Practice Arrangements) as Section 3.4.

The deletion of this Section eliminates a problematic use of the term "prescribes" in relation to the role of the referring practitioner. See *Position on Term "Prescription"* (BOD 03-93-22-59).

Reprinted with permission of the American Physical Therapy Association.

American Physical Therapy Association *Standards of Ethical Conduct for the Physical Therapist Assistant*

PREAMBLE

Physical therapist assistants are responsible for maintaining and promoting high standards of conduct. These *Standards of Ethical Conduct for the Physical Therapist Assistant* shall be binding on physical therapist assistants who are affiliate members of the Association.

STANDARD 1

Physical therapist assistants provide services under the supervision of a physical therapist.

STANDARD 2

Physical therapist assistants respect the rights and dignity of all individuals.

STANDARD 3

Physical therapist assistants maintain and promote high standards in the provision of services, giving the welfare of patients their highest regard.

STANDARD 4

Physical therapist assistants provide services within the limits of the law.

STANDARD 5

Physical therapist assistants make those judgments that are commensurate with their qualifications as physical therapist assistants.

STANDARD 6

Physical therapist assistants accept the responsibility to protect the public and the profession from unethical, incompetent, or illegal acts.

Adopted by House of Delegates
June 1982
Amended June 1991

Reprinted with permission of the American Physical Therapy Association.

American Physical Therapy Association
Guide for Conduct of the Affiliate Member

PURPOSE

This *Guide* is intended to serve physical therapist assistants who are affiliate members of the American Physical Therapy Association in the interpretation of the *Standards of Ethical Conduct for the Physical Therapist Assistant*, providing guidelines by which they may determine the propriety of their conduct. These guidelines are subject to change as new patterns of health care delivery are developed and accepted by the professional community and the public. This *Guide* is subject to monitoring and timely revision by the Ethics and Judicial Committee of the Association.

INTERPRETING STANDARDS

The interpretations expressed in this Guide are not to be considered all inclusive of situations that could evolve under a specific standard of the *Standards of Ethical Conduct for the Physical Therapist Assistant* but reflect the opinions, decisions, and advice of the Judicial Committee. While the statements of ethical standards apply universally, specific circumstances determine their appropriate application. Input related to current interpretations, or situations requiring interpretation, is encouraged from APTA members.

STANDARD 1

Physical therapist assistants provide services under the supervision of a physical therapist.

1.1 Supervisory Relationships

Physical therapist assistants shall work under the supervision and direction of a physical therapist who is properly credentialed in the jurisdiction in which the physical therapist assistant practices.

1.2 Performance of Service

A. Physical therapist assistants may not initiate or alter a treatment program without prior evaluation by and approval of the supervising physical therapist.

B. Physical therapist assistants may modify a specific treatment procedure in accordance with changes in patient status.

C. Physical therapist assistants may not interpret data beyond the scope of their physical therapist assistant education.

D. Physical therapist assistants may respond to inquiries regarding patient status to appropriate parties within the protocol established by a supervising physical therapist.

E. Physical therapist assistants shall refer inquiries regarding patient prognosis to a supervising physical therapist.

Standard 2

Physical therapist assistants respect the rights and dignity of all individuals.

2.1 Attitudes of Physical Therapist Assistants

A. Physical therapist assistants shall recognize that each individual is different from all other individuals and respect and be responsive to those differences.

B. Physical therapist assistants shall be guided at all times by concern for the dignity and welfare of those patients entrusted to their care.

C. Physical therapist assistants shall not engage in conduct that constitutes harassment or abuse of, or discrimination against, colleagues, associates, or others.

2.2 Request for Release of Information

Physical therapist assistants shall refer all requests for release of confidential information to the supervising physical therapist.

2.3 Protection of Privacy

Physical therapist assistants must treat as confidential all information relating to the personal conditions and affairs of the persons whom they serve.

2.4 Patient Relations

Physical therapist assistants shall not engage in any sexual relationship or activity, whether consensual or nonconsensual, with any patient while a physical therapist assistant/patient relationship exists.

STANDARD 3

Physical therapist assistants maintain and promote high standards in the provision of services, giving the welfare of patients their highest regard.

3.1 Information about Services

A. Physical therapist assistants may provide consumers with information regarding provision of services within the protocol established by a supervising physical therapist.

B. Physical therapist assistants may not use, or participate in the use of any form of, communication containing a false, fraudulent, misleading, deceptive, unfair, or sensational statement or claim.

3.2 Organizational Employment

Physical therapist assistants shall advise their employer(s) of any employer practice which causes them to be in conflict with the *Standards of Ethical Conduct for the Physical Therapist Assistant.*

3.3 Endorsement of Equipment

Physical therapist assistants may not endorse equipment or exercise influence on patients or families to purchase or lease equipment except as directed by a physical therapist acting in accord with the stipulation in paragraph 5.3.A. of the *Guide for Professional Conduct.*

3.4 Financial Considerations

Physical therapist assistants shall never place their own financial interest above the welfare of their patients.

3.5 Exploitation of Patients

Physical therapist assistants shall not participate in any arrangements in which patients are exploited. Such arrangements include situations where referring sources enhance their personal incomes as a result of referring for, delegating, prescribing, or recommending physical therapy services.

STANDARD 4

Physical therapist assistants provide services within the limits of the law.

4.1 Supervisory Relationships

Physical therapist assistants shall comply with all aspects of the law. Regardless of the content of any law, physical therapist assistants shall provide services only under the supervision and direction of a physical therapist who is properly credentialed in the jurisdiction in which the physical therapist assistant practices.

4.2 Representation

Physical therapist assistants shall not hold themselves out as physical therapists.

STANDARD 5

Physical therapist assistants make those judgments that are commensurate with their qualifications as physical therapist assistants.

5.1 Patient Treatment

Physical therapist assistants shall report all untoward patient responses to a supervising physical therapist.

5.2 Patient Safety

A. Physical therapist assistants may refuse to carry out treatment procedures that they believe to be not in the best interest of the patient.

B. The physical therapist assistant shall not provide physical therapy services to a patient while under the influence of a substance that impairs his or her ability to do so safely.

5.3 Qualifications

Physical therapist assistants may not carry out any procedure that they are not qualified to provide.

5.4 Discontinuance of Treatment Program

Physical therapist assistants shall discontinue immediately any treatment procedures which in their judgment appears to be harmful to the patient.

5.5 Continued Education

Physical therapist assistants shall continue participation in various types of educational activities which enhance their skills and knowledge and provide new skills and knowledge.

STANDARD 6

Physical therapist assistants accept the responsibility to protect the public and the profession from unethical, incompetent, or illegal acts.

6.1 Consumer Protection

Physical therapist assistants shall report any conduct which appears to be unethical, incompetent, or illegal.

Issued by Ethics and Judicial Committee
American Physical Therapy Association
October 1981
Last Amended January 1996
(current as of 4/99)

Reprinted with permission of the American Physical Therapy Association.

American Physical Therapy Association
Standards of Practice for Physical Therapy and the Accompanying Criteria

PREAMBLE

The physical therapy profession is committed to providing an optimum level of service delivery and to striving for excellence in practice. The House of Delegates of the American Physical Therapy Association, as the formal body that represents the profession, attests to this commitment by adopting and promoting the following *Standards of Practice for Physical Therapy*. These *Standards of Practice for Physical Therapy* are the profession's statement of conditions and performances which are essential for the provision of high-quality physical therapy. The *Standards* provide a foundation for assessment of physical therapy practice.

I. LEGAL/ETHICAL CONSIDERATIONS

A. Legal Considerations

The physical therapist complies with all the legal requirements of the jurisdictions regulating the practice of physical therapy.

The physical therapist assistant complies with all the legal requirements of the jurisdictions regulating the work of the assistant.

B. Ethical

The physical therapist practices according to the *Code of Ethics* of the American Physical Therapy Association.

The physical therapist assistant complies with the *Standards of Ethical Conduct for the Physical Therapist Assistant* of the American Physical Therapy Association.

II. ADMINISTRATION OF THE PHYSICAL THERAPY SERVICE

A. Statement of Mission, Purposes, and Goals

The physical therapy service has a statement of mission, purposes, and goals that reflect the needs and interests of the individuals served, and the physical therapy personnel affiliated with the service.

CRITERIA

The statement:
- Defines scope and limitation of service.
- Lists objectives and goals of service provided.
- Is reviewed annually.

B. Organizational Plan

The physical therapy service has a written organizational plan.

CRITERIA

The plan:
- Describes the relationships within the service, where the physical therapy service is part of a larger organization, between the physical therapy service and other components of the organization.
- Ensures that the service is directed by a physical therapist.
- Defines supervisory structures within the service.
- Reflects current personnel functions.

C. Policies and Procedures

The physical therapy service has written policies and procedures that reflect the operation of the service and that are consistent with the mission, purposes, and goals of the service.

CRITERIA

The policies and procedures, which are reviewed regularly and revised as necessary, address pertinent information including (but not limited to) the following:
- Clinical education.
- Clinical research.
- Interdisciplinary collaboration.
- Criteria for access to, initiation of, continuation of, and termination of care.
- Equipment maintenance.
- Environmental safety.
- Fiscal management.
- Infection control.
- Job/position descriptions.
- Competency assessment.
- Medical emergencies.

- Patient/client/client care policies and protocols.
- Patient/client/client rights.
- Personnel-related policies.
- Quality/performance assurance and improvement.
- Documentation.
- Staff orientation.

The policies and procedures meet the requirements of state law and external agencies.

D. Administration

A physical therapist is responsible for the direction of the physical therapy service.

CRITERIA

- Ensures compliance with local, state, and federal requirements.
- Ensures compliance with current APTA documents, including *Standards of Practice for Physical Therapy, Guide for Professional Conduct,* and *Guide for Conduct of the Affiliate Member.*
- Ensures that services provided are consistent with the mission, purposes, and goals of the service.
- Ensures that the service is provided in accordance with established policies and procedures.
- Reviews and updates policies and procedures as appropriate.
- Provides appropriate education, training, and review of physical therapy support personnel.
- Provides for continuous in-service training on safety issues and for periodic safety inspection of equipment by qualified individuals.

E. Fiscal Management

The director of the physical therapy service, in consultation with staff and appropriate administrative personnel, is responsible for planning for, and allocation of, resources. Fiscal planning and management of the physical therapy service are based upon sound accounting principles.

CRITERIA

- Preparation and monitoring of a budget that provides for optimum use of resources.
- Accurate recording and reporting of financial information.

- Conformance with legal requirements.
- Cost-effective utilization of resources.
- A fee schedule that is consistent with cost of services and that is within customary norms of fairness and reasonableness.

F. Quality/Performance Improvement

The physical therapy service has a written plan for continuous improvement of the performance of services provided.

CRITERIA

The plan:
- Provides evidence of ongoing review and evaluation of the service.
- Provides a mechanism for documentation of performance improvement.
- Is consistent with requirements of external agencies, if applicable.

G. Staffing

The physical therapy personnel affiliated with the physical therapy service have demonstrated competence and are sufficient to achieve the mission, purposes, and goals of the service.

CRITERIA

The service:
- Meets all legal requirements regarding licensure and/or certification of appropriate personnel.
- Provides staff expertise that is appropriate to the patients/clients served.
- Provides for appropriate staff-to-patient/client ratios.
- Provides for appropriate ratios of support staff to professional staff.

H. Staff Development

The physical therapy service has a written plan that provides for appropriate ongoing staff development.

CRITERIA

The plan:
- Provides for consideration of self-assessments, individual goal setting, and organization needs in directing continuing education and learning activities.

- Includes strategies for long-term learning and professional development.

I. Physical Setting

The physical setting is designed to provide a safe, accessible environment that facilitates fulfillment of the mission and achievement of the purposes and goals of the physical therapy service. The equipment is safe and sufficient to achieve the purposes and goals of physical therapy.

CRITERIA

The physical setting:
- Meets all applicable legal requirements for health and safety.
- Meets space needs appropriate for the number and type of patient/clients served.

The equipment:
- Meets all applicable legal requirements for health and safety.
- Is inspected routinely.

J. Interdisciplinary Collaboration

The physical therapy service collaborates with all appropriate disciplines.

CRITERIA

The collaboration includes:
- An interdisciplinary team approach to patient/client care.
- Interdisciplinary patient/client and family education.
- Interdisciplinary staff development and continuing education.

III. PROVISION OF CARE

A. Informed Consent

The physical therapist has the sole responsibility for providing information to the patient/client and for obtaining the patient's/client's informed consent in accordance with jurisdictional law before initiating physical therapy.

CRITERIA

The information provided to the patient/client should include the following:
- A clear description of the proposed intervention/treatment.

- A statement of material (decisional) risks associated with the proposed intervention/treatment.
- A statement of expected benefits of the proposed intervention/treatment.
- A comparison of the benefits and risks possible both with and without intervention/treatment.
- An explanation of reasonable alternatives to the recommended intervention/treatment.

Informed consent requires:
- Consent by a competent adult.
- Consent by a parent/legal guardian as the surrogate decision maker when the adult patient/client is not competent or when the patient/client is a minor.
- The patient's/client's acknowledgment of understanding and consent before the intervention/treatment proceeds.

B. *Initial Examination and Evaluation*

The physical therapist performs and documents an initial examination and evaluates the results to identify problems and determine the diagnosis prior to intervention/treatment.

CRITERIA

The examination:
- Is documented, dated, and signed by the physical therapist who performed the examination.
- Identifies the physical needs of the patient/client.
- Incorporates appropriate objective tests and measures to facilitate outcome measurement.
- Documents sufficient data to establish a plan of care.
- May result in recommendations for additional services to meet the needs of the patient/client.

C. *Plan of Care*

The physical therapist establishes and provides a plan of care for the individual based on the results of the examination and evaluation and on patient/client needs.

The physical therapist involves the patient/client and appropriate others in the planning, implementation, and assessment of the intervention/treatment program.

The physical therapist, in consultation with appropriate disciplines, plans for discharge of the patient/client taking into consideration goal achievement, and provides for appropriate follow-up or referral.

<small>CRITERIA</small>

The plan of care includes:
- Realistic goals and expected functional outcomes.
- Intervention/treatment, including its frequency and duration.
- Documentation that is dated and signed by the physical therapist who established the plan of care.

D. Intervention/Treatment

The physical therapist provides, or delegates and supervises, the physical therapy intervention/treatment consistent with the results of the examination and evaluation and plan of care.

The physical therapist documents, on an ongoing basis, services provided, responses to services, and changes in status relative to the plan of care.

<small>CRITERIA</small>

The intervention/treatment is:
- Provided under the ongoing personal care or supervision of the physical therapist.
- Provided in such a way that delegated responsibilities are commensurate with the qualifications and legal limitations of the physical therapy personnel involved in the intervention/treatment.
- Altered in accordance with changes in individual response or status.
- Provided at a level that is consistent with current physical therapy practice.
- Interdisciplinary when necessary to meet the needs of the patient/client.

Documentation of the services provided includes:
- Date and signature of the physical therapist and/or of the physical therapist assistant when permissible by law.

E. Reexamination and Reevaluation

The physical therapist reexamines and reevaluates the individual continually and modifies or discontinues the plan of care accordingly.

CRITERIA

The physical therapist:
- Periodically documents, dates, and signs the patient/client reexamination and modifications of the plan of care.

F. Discharge/Discontinuation of Treatment or Intervention

The physical therapist discharges the patient/client from physical therapy intervention/treatment when the goals or projected outcomes for the patient/client have been met.

Physical therapy intervention/treatment shall be discontinued when the goals are achieved, the patient/client declines to continue care, the patient/client is unable to continue, or the physical therapist determines that intervention/treatment is no longer warranted.

CRITERIA

Discharge documentation shall include:
- The patient's/client's status at discharge and functional outcomes/goals achieved.
- Dating and signing of the discharge summary by the physical therapist.
- When a patient/client is discharged prior to goal achievement, the patient's/client's status and the rationale for discontinuation.

IV. EDUCATION

The physical therapist is responsible for individual professional development. The physical therapist assistant is responsible for individual career development.

The physical therapist participates in the education of physical therapist students, physical therapist assistant students, and students in other health professions. The physical therapist assistant participates in the education of physical therapist assistant students and other student health professionals.

The physical therapist educates and provides consultation to consumers and the general public regarding the purposes and benefits of physical therapy.

The physical therapist educates and provides consultation of consumers and the general public regarding the roles of the physical therapist and the physical therapist assistant.

Criteria

The physical therapist educates and provides consultation of consumers and the general public regarding the roles of the physical therapist, the physical therapist assistant, and other support personnel.

V. RESEARCH

The physical therapist applies research findings to practice and encourages, participates in, and promotes activities that establish the outcomes of physical therapist patient/client management.

The physical therapist supports collaborative and interdisciplinary research.

VI. COMMUNITY RESPONSIBILITY

The physical therapist demonstrates community responsibility by participating in community and community agency activities, educating the public, formulating public policy, or providing *pro bono* physical therapy services.

Criteria

The physical therapist demonstrates community responsibility by participating in community and community agency activities, educating the public, formulating public policy, or providing *pro bono* physical therapy services.

Standards:
Adopted by the House of Delegates
June 1980
Amended June 1985, June 1991, June 1996

Criteria:
Adopted by the Board of Directors
March 1993
Amended November 1994, March 1995

Reprinted with permission of the American Physical Therapy Association.

American Physical Therapy Association
Guidelines for Physical Therapy Documentation

PREAMBLE

The American Physical Therapy Association (APTA) is committed to meeting the physical therapy needs of society, to meeting the needs and interests of its members, and to developing and improving the art and science of physical therapy, including: practice, education, and research. To help meet these responsibilities, the APTA Board of Directors has approved the following guidelines for physical therapy documentation. It is recognized that these guidelines do not reflect all of the unique documentation requirements associated with the many specialty areas within the physical therapy profession. Applicable for both handwritten and electronic documentation systems, these guidelines are intended to be used as a foundation for the development of more specific documentation guidelines in specialty areas, while at the same time providing guidance for the physical therapy profession across all practice settings.

OPERATIONAL DEFINITIONS

Guidelines: APTA defines "guidelines" as approved, non-binding statements of advice.

Documentation: Any entry into the client record, such as: consultation report, initial examination report, progress note, flow sheet/checklist that identifies the care/service provided, reexamination, or summation of care.

Authentication: The process used to verify that an entry is complete, accurate, and final. Indications of authentication can include original written signatures and computer "signatures" on secured electronic record systems.

I. GENERAL GUIDELINES

A. All documentation must comply with the applicable jurisdictional/regulatory requirements.

   1. All handwritten entries shall be made in ink and will include original signatures. Electronic entries should be made with appropriate security and confidentiality provisions.

2. Informed consent: As required by the APTA *Standards of Practice for Physical Therapy and the Accompanying Criteria.*

   2.1 The physical therapist has sole responsibility for providing information to the patient and for obtaining the patient's informed consent in accordance with jurisdictional law before initiating physical therapy.

   2.2 Those deemed competent to give consent are competent adults. When the adult is not competent, and in the case of minors, a parent or legal guardian consents as the surrogate decision maker.

   2.3 The information provided to the patient should include the following: (a) a clear description of the treatment ordered or recommended, (b) material (decisional) risks associated with the proposed treatment, (c) expected benefits of treatment, (d) comparison of the benefits and risks possible with and without treatment, and (e) reasonable alternatives to the recommended treatment. The physical therapist should solicit questions from the patient and provide answers. The patient should be asked to acknowledge understanding and consent before treatment proceeds.

Examples of ways in which to accomplish this documentation:

Ex 2.3.1 Signature of patient/guardian on long or short consent form.

Ex 2.3.2 Notation/entry of what was explained by the physical therapist or the physical therapist assistant in the official record.

Ex 2.3.3 Filing of a completed consent checklist signed by the patient.

3. Charting errors should be corrected by drawing a single line through the error and initialing and dating the chart or through the appropriate mechanism for electronic documentation that clearly indicates that a change was made without deletion of the original record.

4. Identification.

   4.1 Include patient's full name and identification number, if applicable, on all official documents.

   4.2 All entries must be dated and authenticated with the provider's full name and appropriate designation (eg, PT, PTA).

4.3 Documentation by students (SPT/SPTA) shall be authenticated by a licensed physical therapist.

4.4 Documentation by graduates (GPT/GPTA) or others pending receipt of an unrestricted license shall be authenticated by a licensed physical therapist.

5. Documentation should include the manner in which physical therapy services are initiated.

Ex 5.1 Self-referral/direct access.

Ex 5.2 Attachment of the referral/consultation request by a qualified practitioner.

Ex 5.3 File copy of correspondence to referral source as acknowledgment of the referral.

II. Initial Examination and Evaluation/Consultation

A. Documentation is required at the outset of each episode of physical therapy care.

B. Elements include:

1. Obtaining a history and identifying risk factors:

1.1 History of the presenting problem, current complaints, and precautions (including onset date).

1.2 Pertinent diagnoses and medical history.

1.3 Demographic characteristics, including pertinent psychological, social, and environmental factors.

1.4 Prior or concurrent services related to the current episode of physical therapy care.

1.5 Comorbidities that may affect goals and treatment plan.

1.6 Statement of patient's knowledge of problem.

1.7 Goals of patient (and family members, or significant others, if appropriate).

2. Selecting and administering tests and measures to determine patient status in a number of areas. The following is a partial list of these areas, with illustrative tests and measures.

2.1 Arousal, mentation, and cognition.

Examples include objective findings related, but not limited to the following areas:

Ex 2.1.1 Level of consciousness.

Ex 2.1.2 Ability to process commands.

Ex 2.1.3 Alertness.

Ex 2.1.4 Gross expressive and receptive language deficits.

    2.2 Neuromotor development and sensory integration.

Examples include objective findings related, but not limited, to the following areas:

Ex 2.2.1 Gross and fine motor skills.

Ex 2.2.2 Reflex and movement patterns.

Ex 2.2.3 Dexterity, agility, and coordination.

    2.3 Range of motion.

Examples include objective findings related, but not limited, to the following areas:

Ex 2.3.1 Extent of joint motion.

Ex 2.3.2 Pain and soreness of surrounding soft tissue.

Ex 2.3.3 Muscle length and flexibility.

    2.4 Muscle performance.

Examples include objective findings related, but not limited, to the following areas:

Ex 2.4.1 Strength.

Ex 2.4.2 Power.

Ex 2.4.3 Endurance.

    2.5 Ventilation, respiration, and circulation.

Examples include objective findings related, but not limited, to the following areas:

Ex 2.5.1 Vital signs.

Ex 2.5.2 Breathing patterns.

Ex 2.5.3 Heart sounds.

    2.6 Posture.

Examples include objective findings related, but not limited, to the following areas:

Ex 2.6.1 Static posture.

Ex 2.6.2 Dynamic posture.

    2.7 Gait, locomotion, and balance.

Examples include objective findings related, but not limited, to the following areas:

Ex 2.7.1 Characteristics of gait.

Ex 2.7.2 Functional ambulation.

Ex 2.7.3 Characteristics of balance.

    2.8 Self-care and home management status.

Examples include objective findings related, but not limited, to the following areas:

Ex 2.8.1 Activities of daily living.

Ex 2.8.2 Functional capacity.

Ex 2.8.3 Static and dynamic strength.

2.9 Community and work (job/school/play).

Examples include objective findings related, but not limited, to the following areas:

Ex 2.9.1 Instrumental activities of daily living.

Ex 2.9.2 Functional capacity.

Ex 2.9.3 Adaptive skills.

3. Evaluation (a dynamic process in which the physical therapist makes clinical judgments based on data gathered during the examination).

4. Diagnosis (a label encompassing a cluster of signs and symptoms, syndromes, or categories that reflects the information obtained from the examination).

5. Goals.

5.1 Patient (and family members or significant others, if appropriate) is involved in establishing goals.

5.2 All goals are stated in measurable terms.

5.3 Goals are linked to problems identified in the examination.

5.4 Short- and long-term goals are established when applicable (may include potential for achieving goals).

6. Intervention plan or recommendation requirements:

6.1 Shall be related to realistic goals and expected functional outcomes.

6.2 Should include frequency and duration to achieve the stated goals.

6.3 Should include patient and family/caregiver educational goals.

6.4 Should involve appropriate collaboration and coordination of care with other professionals/services.

7. Authentication and appropriate designation of physical therapist.

III. DOCUMENTATION OF THE CONTINUUM OF CARE

A. Intervention or service provided.

1. Documentation is required for each patient visit/encounter. Authentication is required for every note by the physical therapist or the physical therapist assistant providing the service under the supervision of the physical therapist.

Examples include:

Ex 1.1 Checklist.

Ex 1.2 Flow sheet.

Ex 1.3 Graph.

Ex 1.4 Narrative.

   2. Elements may include:

   2.1 Identification of specific interventions provided.

   2.2 Equipment provided.

B. Patient status, progress, or regression.

   1. Documentation is required for each patient visit/encounter. Authentication is required for every note by the physical therapist or the physical therapist assistant providing the service under the supervision of the physical therapist.

   2. Elements may include:

   2.1 Subjective status of patient.

   2.2 Changes in objective and measurable findings as they relate to existing goals.

   2.3 Adverse reaction to treatment.

   2.4 Progression/regression of existing therapeutic regimen, including patient education and adherence.

   2.5 Communication/consultation with providers/patient/family/significant other.

   2.6 Authentication and appropriate designation of either a physical therapist or a physical therapist assistant.

C. Reexamination and reevaluation.

   1. Documentation is required monthly for patients seen at intervals of a month or less; if the patient is seen less frequently, documentation is required for every visit or encounter.

   2. Elements include:

   2.1 Documentation of elements as identified in III.B.2.1 through III.B.2.5 to update patient's status.

   2.2 Interpretation of findings and, when indicated, revision of goals.

   2.3 When indicated, revision of treatment plan, as directly correlated with documented goals.

   2.4 Authentication and appropriate designation of physical therapist.

IV. Summation of Care

A. Documentation is required following conclusion of the current episode in the physical therapy care sequence.

B. Elements include:

1. Reason for discontinuation of service.

Examples include:

Ex 1.1 Satisfactory goal achievement.

Ex 1.2 Patient declines to continue care.

Ex 1.3 Patient is unable to continue to work toward goals due to medical or psychosocial complications.

2. Current physical/functional status.

3. Degree of goal achievement and reasons for goals not being achieved.

4. Discharge plan that includes written and verbal communication related to the patient's continuing care.

Examples include:

Ex 4.1 Home program.

Ex 4.2 Referrals for additional services.

Ex 4.3 Recommendations for follow-up physical therapy care.

Ex 4.4 Family and caregiver training.

Ex 4.5 Equipment provided.

5. Authentication and appropriate designation of physical therapist.

References

1. *Direction, Delegation, and Supervision in Physical Therapy Services.* HOD 06-96-30-4.

2. *Comprehensive Accreditation Manual for Hospitals.* Oakbrook Terrace, Ill: Joint Commission on Accreditation of Healthcare Organizations; 1996.

3. *Glossary of Terms Related to Information Security.* Schamburg, Ill: Computer-Based Patient Record Institute; 1996.

4. *Guidelines for Establishing Information Security Policies at Organizations Using Computer-Based Patient Records.* Schamburg, Ill: Computer-Based Patient Record Institute; 1995.

Adopted by the Board of Directors
March 1997
American Physical Therapy Association

American Physical Therapy Association Mission and Goal Statements

MISSION STATEMENT

The mission of the American Physical Therapy Association (APTA), the principle membership organization representing and promoting the profession of physical therapy, is to further the profession's role in the prevention, diagnosis, and treatment of movement dysfunction and the enhancement of the physical health and functional abilities of members of the public.

POLICY ON APTA MISSION STATEMENT

To fulfill the American Physical Therapy Association's (APTA) Mission to meet the needs and interests of its members and to promote physical therapy as a vital professional career, the Association shall:

- Promote physical therapy care and services through the establishment, maintenance, and promotion of ethical principles and quality standards for practice, education, and research;
- Influence policy in the public and private sectors;
- Enable physical therapy practitioners to improve their skills, knowledge, and operation in the interest of furthering the profession;
- Develop and improve the art and science of physical therapy, including practice, education, and research;
- Facilitate a common understanding and appreciation for the diversity of the profession, the membership, and the communities we serve; and
- Maintain a stable and diverse financial base from which to fund the programs, services, and operations that support this mission.

GOALS THAT REPRESENT THE
2001 PRIORITIES OF THE ASSOCIATION

Goal I: Participate actively in shaping the current and emerging health care environment to promote the development of high-quality, cost effective health care services and to further the recognition of and support for the profession of physical therapy and the role of physical therapists.

Goal II: Stimulate innovation in the practice of physical therapy that supports physical therapists and physical therapist assistants.

Goal III: Qualify and interpret the demand for, the need for, and the access to physical therapy services.

Goal IV: Stimulate innovation in physical therapy education and professional development at all levels to ensure currency with the changing environments in health care and education and with student and professional needs.

Goal V: Stimulate research to further the science of physical therapy, to influence current and emerging health care policies, and to advance the profession.

Goal VI: Increase APTA's responsiveness to the needs of current and future members.

These goals are based on the priorities that have been adopted annually by the House of Delegates since 1988 to provide direction to the APTA Board of Directors, and have been established based on education, practice, and research being the highest priorities of the Association. The Association's awareness of cultural diversity, its commitment to expanding minority representation and participation in physical therapy, and its commitment to equal opportunity for all members permeate these goals.

American Physical Therapy Association
House of Delegates 2002
Mission and Goals

Historical Practitioners Influential in the Genesis of Physical Therapy

Note: These important individuals in the evolution of the field of physical therapy practice are not listed in alphabetical order, but rather from a historical perspective, more or less ordered according to the timing of their emergence in the profession.

MARY LIVINGSTON MCMILLAN

Boston-born and British-educated, Mary "Mollie" McMillan was at the forefront of the physical therapy movement launched in the first decades of the 20th century. She was the first president and generally considered the founder of the American Physical Therapy Association (APTA). McMillan was assigned to the Walter Reed Hospital as the head reconstruction aide in 1918, and there founded the first organized physical therapy department in the U.S. Army. She taught at Reed College in Oregon, where the graduates of this and other emergency programs were prepared to handle the peak load of patients in 1919 during World War I. In 1921, McMillan established and became the founding president of the American Physiotherapy Association. She authored the first text on physical therapy entitled *Massage and Therapeutic Exercises*. During World War II, she volunteered her services at the Army Hospital in Manila in 1941 and was subsequently interred as a prisoner-of-war by the Japanese. The Mary McMillan Scholarship Award was established in 1963 to acknowledge and honor outstanding physical therapy students and funded through a provision in her will upon her death in 1959. The Mary McMillan Lectureship, established in 1963 to pay tribute to her, is the highest honor for physical therapists invited to speak at each annual APTA conference. McMillan was the guiding spirit of the profession of physical therapy and led the way toward higher standards in treatment and academic preparation of physical therapists.

DUDLEY ALLEN SARGENT

Sargent, a physician, founded the Sargent School in Boston in 1881, which offered physical education students postgraduate courses in anatomy, physiology, activity skills, anthropometry, body mechanics, nutrition, physical diagnosis, and the study of mind-body interactions. This was the first educational program to place "physical educators" in clinical settings.

MARIE MARCELLIN LUCAS-CHAMPIONNIÈRE

Lucas-Championnière, a French surgeon, was the first to explicate the benefits of massage as a follow-up to orthopedic surgery and "bonesetting." In 1889, Lucas-Championnière published a report regarding the faster healing rate and stronger bone resulting from not immobilizing an upper extremity fracture. This was published in *Massage and Mobilization in the Treatment of Fractures*.

SIR ROBERT JONES

Jones was an influential orthopedic physician who purported the use of movement and massage, as opposed to immobilization, as a more beneficial mode of intervention to speed healing following a fracture. Mary McMillan worked with Jones in Liverpool, England, during her first professional clinical position. Jones is credited with mentoring James Mennell as well. Jones became the director of orthopedics for the British Military Service during World War I and implemented the use of physical rehabilitation in the treatment of amputations, fractures, and other war-related disabilities. Jones was also responsible for inaugurating the use of the Thomas splint (which his uncle invented).

ROBERT W. LOVETT

A respected Boston orthopedist, Lovett was known for his physical rehabilitation orientation in treating scoliosis and polio. He practiced at Boston Children's Hospital and accepted a faculty appointment to Dudley Allen Sargent's postgraduate program. Lovett was one of four orthopedic physicians who initiated the use of plaster jackets in the treatment of spinal deformities and was known for the "Vermont Plan," a unique approach to intervention in polio victims.

WILHELMINE WRIGHT

Wright managed Robert Lovett's "gymnasium" clinic at Boston Children's Hospital as senior assistant and published extensively on muscle training. She taught a new examination technique called *manual muscle testing*, grading individual muscles from totally paralyzed to normal, and applied the results of this in tailoring intervention to increase function. Wright published this pioneering work in 1928 in a text entitled *Muscle Function*, which "stands as one of the true benchmarks in the history of physical therapy."[1]

MARJORIE BOUVÉ

Bouvé was the director of the Boston School of Physical Education (currently Boston Bouvé of Northeastern University), which, in 1914, was the third institution to initiate a 2-year professional program for specialization in physical education in a clinic setting.

MARGUERITE SANDERSON

Appointed by the U.S. Army Surgeon General's Office in 1917 to train and supervise the reconstruction aides during World War I, Sanderson taught corrective physical education at the Boston School of Physical Education (a "War Emergency Training Center"). She conceived the notion of the educational program at the Boston School, and with classmates Marjorie Bouvé and Mary Florence Stratton, their vision became a reality. The very first applicant to the program was Mary McMillan.

JAMES B. MENNELL

Mennell authored the text, *Physical Treatment by Movement, Manipulation and Massage*, which was published in 1917. The book, currently in its 5th edition, is still being studied by students of physical medicine in the United States. Mennell was an influential and effectual leader in the use of movement, manipulation, and massage in the early 1990s. Mennell, along with Lucas-Championnière, pioneered the principles of "early movement" following injury to enhance healing and prevent disability.

CHARLES LOWMAN

Lowman popularized the use of warm-water exercises, which he called *hydrogymnastics*. He founded the Los Angeles Orthopedic Hospital in 1919 and became the director of the physical therapy program at the University of Southern California.

JOHN STANLEY CATILTER

With Catilter's guidance, standards for accreditation of educational facilities were developed in 1928 by the American Physiotherapy Association.

ELIZABETH "SISTER" KENNY

An Australian nurse, Kenny came to the United States in 1940 and revolutionized traditional polio intervention through aggressive treatment from the onset of the disease. She initiated the use of passive exercise, massage, and moist heat treatments to areas of involvement. Her treatment techniques were challenged by the physical therapy community due to the lack of scientific scrutiny, and ultimately her approach was proven to be potentially harmful. She can be credited with ruffling many feathers and establishing the need for "evidence-based" practice.

CATHERINE WORTHINGHAM

Worthingham was the 11th president of the American Physiotherapy Association, serving from 1940 to 1944. She coauthored the landmark texts *Muscle Testing* (1946) and *Therapeutic Exercise* (1957) with Lucille Daniels. Worthingham was the first physical therapist to hold a doctoral degree (in anatomy). She led the way for establishing degree granting programs in physical therapy. She served as the president of the National Foundation for Infantile Paralysis for 16 years. Her "Study of Physical Therapy Education," evaluating 42 physical therapy schools, was a major instrument in the evolution of physical therapy education, making it more relevant to contemporary needs and standards. Worthingham delivered the second Mary McMillan Lecture in 1965. An APTA award is named the Catherine Worthingham Fellows Award, a membership category established in 1980 for individuals "whose work, like the distinguished woman honored in this action, has resulted in lasting and significant advances in science, education, and the practice of the profession."[1]

EMMA "EMMY LOU" VOGEL

Vogel, another frontrunner in physical therapy, succeeded Mary McMillan at Walter Reed Hospital as chief head aide in the department of physiotherapy. She was appointed to direct a 4-month-long training program for physical therapists, which provided the army with a continued source of skilled physical therapists. She established the first postwar course for civilian physical therapists. Through legislative efforts, Vogel secured rights, privileges, and benefits for physical therapists in keeping with that of army nurses. In 1944, her efforts gained insurance, through the Bolton Bill, for full commissioned status, advancing the profession of physical therapy and of women. She was the first physical therapist to be granted the status of Major in the army and became the first chief of the Women's Medical Specialists Corps. Vogel delivered the Mary McMillan Lecture in 1967.

IDA MAY HAZENHYER

Hazenhyer was the author of the first formal history of the APTA, which appeared in four issues of the *PT Review* in 1946.

HERMAN KABAT

Kabat was a neurophysiologist and physician who hypothesized that "all kinds of deficient or pathological neuromuscular mechanisms and their resulting limitations of movement might be reversed through the facilitating effects of physical therapy."[1] Kabat's theories, initially called *neuromuscular reeducation*, were the basis for proprioceptive neuromuscular facilitation techniques developed in concert with Margaret Knott.

MARGARET (MAGGIE) KNOTT

Working with Herman Kabat, and later with Dorothy Voss, Knott developed the therapeutic intervention that we know as proprioceptive neuromuscular facilitation. She and Dorothy Voss published the first textbook on PNF in 1956, entitled *Proprioceptive Neuromuscular Facilitation*. Knott gave the McMillan Lecture in 1972.

HENRY O. AND FLORENCE PETERSON KENDALL

Challenged by the controversy over Elizabeth "Sister" Kenny's methods of polio evaluation and intervention, the Kendalls sought to establish a scientific basis for techniques employed. Their well-crafted article entitled "Orthopedic and Physical Therapy Objectives in Poliomyelitis Treatment" in *PT Review* [1947;27(3)], based on extensive research of testing flexibility and strength in children and adults, established the basis for the publication of *Muscles, Testing and Function*, first published in 1949. This text, in its 4th edition (1993), is still a staple in every physical therapy program around the world. Florence Kendall delivered the Mary McMillan Lecture in 1980. The APTA Henry O. and Florence P. Kendall Award, established in 1981 (2 years after Henry's death), was developed "to recognize excellence in clinical practice,"[1] and honors the many contributions that the Kendalls have made to the field of physical therapy practice.

MARGARET "ROODY" ROOD

Rood was a neurophysiological innovator who is credited with establishing the importance of the sensory system in sensory-motor behavior and the importance of the autonomic nervous system as the basis for normal movement and function. Rood was certified in occupational therapy in 1933, and after World War II gained her master's degree and certification in physical therapy. Rood's thesis was that, because fundamental reflex patterns were the basis for normal movement, overriding abnormal sensory input repeatedly could potentially result in normal movement in individuals with brain damage. Her therapeutic approaches are still taught and utilized today. Rood delivered the Mary McMillan Lecture in 1969.

LUCY BLAIR

A crusader for quality, research-based care in polio after-care, Blair served as a Lieutenant with the Women Appointed for Voluntary Emergency Service (WAVES) at Navy hospitals in California, Oregon, and New York before joining the APTA's staff. Blair occupied every senior staff position during her many years (1950 to 1969) of service to the APTA. During the polio epidemic in the early 1950s, Blair directed the role of the APTA and the profession in evaluating the efficacy of gamma globulin and, later, the polio vaccine. In 1959, she became the executive director, a position that she held until her retirement in 1969. Blair delivered the Mary McMillan Lecture in 1971. The Lucy Blair Award was established in 1969 to honor those therapists who, like Blair, serve the profession with unrelenting commitment, selfless contributions, genuine interest and concern for every individual they meet, and dedicated service to the field of physical therapy.

MILDRED ELSON

The first executive director of the APTA (1944 to 1956) and the first president of the World Confederation for Physical Therapy (1951 to 1955), Elson also served the profession as editor-in-chief of the *PT Review* (1936 to 1944) and as a consultant on physical therapy to the US Army and Veteran's Bureau.[1] Elson delivered the first Mary McMillan Lecture in 1964.

ELEANOR JANE CARLIN

The 19th president of the APTA, Carlin was an influential educator in the field of physical therapy at the University of Pennsylvania. In 1949, she served as education secretary for the National Foundation of Infantile Paralysis and was the editor of the APTA journal from 1950 to 1956. She substantiated the need for "record keeping" (1957) and "documentation" (1958) in a series of editorials in the *PT Review*. Carlin was the first woman to advance to the rank of Brigadier General, serving as an officer in the Women's Medical Specialist Corps of the Women's Army Corps. Carlin delivered the Mary McMillan Lecture in 1976. The Dorothy Baethke–Eleanor J. Carlin Award, granted by the APTA, was established in 1981 to recognize "excellence in academic teaching."

DOROTHY BAETHKE

An influential educator in the field of physical therapy teaching at the University of Pennsylvania, Baethke was a pioneer in physical therapy education. The Dorothy Baethke–Eleanor J. Carlin Award, granted by the APTA, was established in 1981 to recognize "excellence in academic teaching."

DOROTHY VOSS

Teaming with Margaret Knotts, Voss coauthored the classic text, *Proprioceptive Neuromuscular Facilitation*, and developed continuing education curriculum for PNF. She was fondly known as a "teacher's teacher." Voss later joined the APTA staff and taught at Northwestern University, where she was involved in formulating the renowned study of motor behavior known as *NU-STEP*. She was the editor of the APTA journal from 1958 to 1962. In 1982, Voss was honored as a Mary McMillan Lecturer.

BERTA "BERTI" AND KAREL BOBATH

Coming to the United States in 1958, Berta Bobath, a physical therapist trained in Germany, and Karel Bobath, a German neurologist, developed a reputation for success in treating children with spastic cerebral palsy and later in managing spasticity related to cerebrovascular accidents. The Bobaths' approach of early intervention (before the individual "perfected his handicap") established that spasticity was not unalterable. The Bobath techniques were based on "the inhibition of released and exaggerated abnormal reflex action, the counteraction of abnormal patterns, and the facilitation of more normal automatic and voluntary movement."[1] The system the Bobaths developed is now called *neurodevelopmental treatment*, or *NDT*.

HELEN J. HISLOP

Instrumental in establishing credentialing of academic programs in physical therapy through a series of articles on the inadequacy of educational programs in the *PT Review*, Hislop was appointed editor of the APTA journal in 1963. She is credited with reformatting the journal and expanding its quality and breadth. A visionary, in 1964, she wrote that, as a profession we must abandon our passive resistance to technological change and "accept responsibility for designing its methods and adapting these changing concepts to physical therapy's uses..."[1] She was one of the first to write about the role of computers for storing, analyzing, and synthesizing data collected through clinical testing and to predict outcomes.[1] Hislop delivered the Mary McMillan Lecture in 1975, focusing on the topic of "specialization" and advanced academic degrees. The Helen J. Hislop Award for Outstanding Contributions to Professional Literature, established in 1975, honors Hislop's contributions to the quality and clarity of written material in PT journals and texts.

GERTRUDE BEARD

Beginning her career as a surgical nurse during World War I, Beard went on to become a physical therapist in 1920. She taught at Northwestern University and was the fourth president of the American Physiotherapy Association (1926 to 1928). She is credited with enhancing *PT Review* and changing its name to *Physiotherapy Review*. She wrote *Foundations for Growth*, a history of the first four decades of the Association in 1961, a classic review of the growth of the organization since its inception in 1921 by Mary McMillan.

SIGNE BRUNNSTRÖM

In 1970, Brunnström's book, *Movement Therapy in Hemiplegia*, was published. She brought to light the basic reflex behaviors of the nervous system and the "Brunnström approach," incorporating the sequential changes in motor function that typically occur following a stroke dependent on the region of the brain that is injured. She also coauthored the text *Training of the Lower Extremity Amputee* with Donald Kerr in 1956 and wrote *Clinical Kinesiology* in 1962 (still in circulation as a standard academic text on the mechanics of body motion). Brunnström has been honored many times by the APTA for her contributions to physical therapy. She was presented the first Marian Williams Award in 1965 for her contributions to the study of locomotion and exercise in stroke and amputations. She twice declined the prestigious Mary McMillan Lectureship, though was honored with the invitations. In 1988, the APTA established the Brunnström Award for Excellence in Clinical Teaching, recognizing her as "an outstanding early pioneer in physical therapy... well-known author, educator, researcher, humanitarian, and clinician who has dedicated 50 years of her life to the profession of physical therapy."[1]

MAJORIE IONTA

The first recipient of the National Foundation of Infantile Paralysis scholarship, Ionta attended the Harvard Medical School Course for Physical Therapy, graduating in 1946 and distinguishing herself as a major contributor to the physical therapy profession. When Margaret Knott died in 1978, Ionta assisted Dorothy Voss in the writing of the 3rd edition of *Proprioceptive Neuromuscular Facilitation*, which was published in 1985.

MARGARET L. MOORE

Moore made sustained and exceptional contributions to the APTA, serving early in her career as the educational consultant on the APTA staff, later serving in the elected office of secretary from 1961 to 1964, and then as the Speaker of the House from 1964 to 1967. Throughout her career, she was a driving force in promoting and fostering legislative contacts and involvement for physical therapy. Her 2-year grant for the study of clinical education improved and changed the quality of education in physical therapy. As Moore fostered the development and potential of many new faculty members during her years as director of the division of physical therapy at the University of North Carolina, her mentorship inspired in her associates the true meaning of becoming a "member of the academy" and a productive member of the physical therapy profession. The Margaret L. Moore Award for Outstanding New Academic Faculty Member was established in 1989 to recognize excellence in research and teaching by a new faculty member. Moore delivered the 1978 Mary McMillan Lecture.

DOROTHY BRIGGS

Briggs was an outstanding educator and an active investigator at the University of Wisconsin, where she received a doctoral degree in physiology. Briggs' exceptional contributions to the Association include serving as chairman of the editorial board of *Physical Therapy*, serving as a charter member of the committee on research, and as a diligent member of the section on research. Briggs' desire and dedication were unstintingly directed toward the improvement of physical therapy, and through her efforts, a significant number of physical therapists learned the methods of scientific inquiry. In 1969, the Dorothy Briggs Memorial Scientific Inquiry

Award was established to give recognition to a physical therapist member of the APTA for an outstanding article in *Physical Therapy* prepared while a student.

MARIAN WILLIAMS

Williams' life was dedicated to promoting the profession of physical therapy through teaching, writing, and research. Her research interests and scholarly publications covered the areas of kinesiology and electromyography; she coauthored books on biomechanics, muscle testing, and therapeutic exercise. She is credited with initiating one of the first post-baccalaureate master's programs in physical therapy. Her superb teaching skills enabled students to understand very complex concepts, and her skills as a mentor fostered analytical thinking in her students. In 1963, the Marian Williams Award for Research in Physical Therapy was established to acknowledge an individual who has made significant contributions to physical therapy through excellence in research, as exemplified by the professional and research career of Williams.

EUGENE MICHELS

Michels served as APTA's associate executive vice president for Research and Education and as executive director. He provided the major impetus in the Association's plans to foster research in physical therapy. He served as APTA president for two terms from 1967 to 1973, as APTA treasurer from 1964 to 1967, as president of the World Confederation for Physical Therapy from 1974 to 1982, and has been an active member of the section on research. The annual Eugene Michels Researcher's Forum was established in his honor in 1982, and the Foundation for Physical Therapy, Inc established the Eugene Michels Fund for Educational Research in his honor in 1984. In 1989, the Eugene Michels New Investigator Award was established to recognize physical therapists engaged in independent research. The leadership and vision of Michels has been and continues to be a driving force in the development and improvement of the profession of physical therapy.

REFERENCES

1. Murphy W. *Healing the Generations: A History of Physical Therapy and the American Physical Therapy Association*. Fairfax, Va: American Physical Therapy Association; 1995:35,142,165,170,174,181,182,242.

Past Presidents of the
American Physical Therapy Association

Mary McMillan, Boston, Massachusetts	1921 to 1923
Inga Lohne, Boston, Massachusetts	1923 to 1924
Dorothea M. Beck, Montclair, New Jersey	1924 to 1926
Gertrude Beard, Chicago, Illinois	1926 to 1928
Hazel E. Furscott, San Francisco, California	1928 to 1930
Edith Monro, Boston, Massachusetts	1930 to 1932
Margaret S. Campbell, Chicago, Illinois	1932 to 1934
Sarah U. Colby, Los Angeles, California	1934 to 1936
Constance K. Greene, Boston, Massachusetts	1936 to 1938
Helen L. Kaiser, Cleveland, Ohio	1938 to 1940
Catherine Worthingham, Stanford, California	1940 to 1944
Jessie L. Stevenson, New York, New York	1944 to 1946
Susan G. Roen, Los Angeles, California	1946 to 1948
Lois Ransom, Washington, DC	1948 to 1949
Marguerite Irvine, Seattle, Washington	1949 to 1950
Mary Clyde Singleton, Durham, North Carolina	1950 to 1952
Harriet S. Lee, Washington, DC	1952 to 1954
Mary E. Nesbitt, Boston, Massachusetts	1954 to 1956
Eleanor Jane Carlin, Jenkintown, Pennsylvania	1956 to 1958
Agnes P. Snyder, San Antonio, Texas	1958 to 1961
Mary Elizabeth Kolb, Leetsdale, Pennsylvania	1961 to 1967
Eugene Michels, Philadelphia, Pennsylvania	1967 to 1973
Charles M. Magistro, Pomona Valley, California	1973 to 1976
Robert C. Bartlett, Durham, North Carolina	1976 to 1979
Don W. Wortley, Salt Lake City, Utah	1979 to 1982
Robert W. Richardson, Pittsburgh, Pennsylvania	1982 to 1985
Jane S. Matthews, Gloucester, Massachusetts	1985 to 1991
Marilyn Moffet, Locust Valley, New York	1991 to 1997
Jan K. Richardson, Durham, North Carolina	1997 to 2000
Ben F. Massey, Jr., Durham, North Carolina	2000 to 2003

Directory of State Licensure Boards and State Physical Therapy Associations

Alabama
Alabama State Board of Physical Therapy
100 N Union Street, Suite 627
Montgomery, AL 36130-5040
Phone: 334-242-4064
Fax: 334-240-3288

Practice Act
www.legislature.state.al.us/codeofalabama/1975/coatoc.htm

Alabama Chapter of the APTA
PO Box 11628
Montgomery, AL 36111-0628
Phone: 334-272-5668
Fax: 334-272-7128

Alaska
State Physical Therapy and Occupational Therapy Board Division
of Occupational Licensing
Department of Commerce and Economic Development
333 Willoughby Avenue, 9th Floor
State Office Building
Juneau, AK 99801
Phone: 907-465-2534
Fax: 907-465-2974

Practice Act
www.touchngo.com/lglcntr/akstats/Statutes/Title08/Chapter84.
htm

Alaska Chapter of the APTA
8970 Northwood Park Circle
Eagle River, AK 99577

Arizona
Arizona State Board of Physical Therapy
1400 W. Washington, Suite 230
Phoenix, AZ 85007
Phone: 602-542-3095
Fax: 602-542-3093

Practice Act
www.sosaz.com/public_services/Title_04/4-24.htm

Arizona Chapter of the APTA
4035 E Fanfol
Phoenix, AZ 85028
Phone: 602-569-9101
Fax: 602-996-3966

Arkansas
Arkansas State Board of Physical Therapy
9 Shackleford Plaza, Suite 3
Little Rock, AR 72211
Phone: 501-228-7100
Fax: 501-228-0294

Practice Act
www.arkleg.state.ar.us/lpbin/lpext.dll?f=file[browse-h.htm]

Arkansas Chapter of the APTA
PO Box 2068
Conway, AR 72033-2068
Phone: 501-269-8247
Fax: 501-327-1370

California
California State Board of Physical Therapy
1418 Howe Avenue, Suite 16
Sacramento, CA 95825
Phone: 916-263-2550 or 916-561-8200
Fax: 916-263-2560

Practice Act
www.leginfo.ca.gov

California Chapter of the APTA
2520 Venture Oaks Way, Suite 150
Sacramento, CA 95833-4228
Phone: 916-929-2782
Fax: 916-646-5960

Colorado
Colorado State Board of Physical Therapy Licensure
1560 Broadway, Suite 1340
Denver, CO 80202-5146
Phone: 303-894-2440
Fax: 303-894-7802

Practice Act
www.dora.state.co.us/Physical-Therapy/PTact.html

Colorado Chapter of the APTA
7853 E. Arapahoe Court, Suite 2100
Englewood, CO 80112-1361
Phone: 303-694-4728
Fax: 303-694-4869

Connecticut
Connecticut Department of Public Health
410 Capital Avenue, MS #12APP
PO Box 340308
Hartford, CT 06134-0308
Phone: 860-509-7562
Fax: 860-509-8457

Practice Act
www.dph.state.ct.us

Connecticut Chapter of the APTA
330 Main Street, 3rd Floor
Hartford, CT 06106-5408
Phone: 860-246-4414
Fax: 860-541-6484

Delaware

Division of Professional Regulation
Examining Board of Physical Therapists
Cannon Building
861 Silver Lake Boulevard, Suite 203
Dover, DE 19904-2467
Phone: 302-744-4500
Fax: 302-739-2711

Practice Act
http://198.187.128.2/delaware/lpext.dll?f=templates&fn=fs-main.
htm&20

Delaware Chapter of the APTA
Phone: 302-456-0677

District of Columbia

DC Board of Physical Therapy
Dept. of Consumer or Reg. Affairs
Occupational and Professional Licensing Administration
825 N Capital Street
Washington, DC 20002
Phone: 202-442-4778
Fax: 202-442-4830

DC Chapter of the APTA
6981 32nd Street, NW
Washington, DC 20015
Phone: 202-723-2819
Fax: 202-537-1388

Florida

Department of Health, Medical Therapies/Psychology
Board of Physical Therapy
4052 Bald Cypress Way
Bin #C05
Tallahassee, FL 32399-3255
Phone: 850-488-0595
Fax: 850-414-6860

Practice Act
www.flsenate.gov/statutes/index.cfm?App_mode=Display_Statut
es&URL=CH0486/title0486.htm

Florida Chapter of the APTA
1705 South Gadsden Street
Tallahassee, FL 32301
Phone: 580-222-1243
Fax: 852-224-5281

Georgia
Georgia Board of Physical Therapy
237 Coliseum Drive
Macon, GA 31217-3858
Phone: 478-207-1620

Practice Act
www.sos.state.ga.us/plb/pt

Georgia Chapter of the APTA
1260 Winchester Parkway, Suite 205
Smyrna, GA 30080
Phone: 770-433-2418
Fax: 770-433-2907

Hawaii
Department of Commerce and Consumer Affairs
Professional and Vocational Licensing Division
Board of Physical Therapy
1010 Richards Street, PO Box 3469
Honolulu, HI 96801
Phone: 808-586-2696
Fax: 808-586-2874

Practice Act
www.capitol.hawaii.gov/hrscurrent/vol10_ch436-471/hrs461j

Hawaii Chapter of the APTA
1360 S Bertania Street, Suite 301
Honolulu, HI 96814
Phone: 808-528-2782
Fax: 808-523-7809

Idaho
Idaho Board of Medicine
1755 Westgate Drive
PO Box 83720
Boise, ID 83720
Phone: 208-327-7000
Fax: 208-327-7005

Practice Act
www3.state.id.us/idstat/TOC/54022KTOC.html

Idaho Chapter of the APTA
PO Box 1273
Boise, ID 83701-1273
Phone: 208-342-6647

Illinois
Illinois State Board of Physical Therapy
Department of Professional Regulation
320 W Washington Street, 3rd Floor
Springfield, IL 62786
Phone: 217-782-0218
Fax: 217-782-7645

Practice Act
www.legis.state.il.us/ilcs/ch225/ch225act90.htm

Illinois Chapter of the APTA
1010 Jorie Boulevard, Suite 134
Oak Brook, IL 60523
Phone: 630-571-1400 or 800-552-4782 (IL residents only)
Fax: 630-571-1406

Indiana
Indiana Physical Therapy Committee
Health Professions Bureau
Attn: Physical Therapy Committee
402 W Washington Street, Room W041
Indianapolis, IN 46204
Phone: 317-232-2960
Fax: 317-233-4236
website: www.in.gov/hpb/boards/ptc

Practice Act
www.ai.org/legislative/ic/code/title25/ar27/ch1.html

Indiana Chapter of the APTA
PO Box 26692
Indianapolis, IN 46226-0692
Phone: 317-823-3681
Fax: 317-823-3681

Iowa
Iowa Department of Health
Board of Physical and Occupational Therapy Examiners
Lucas State Office Building
321 E 12th Street
Des Moines, IA 50319-0075
Phone: 515-281-4413
Fax: 515-281-3121

Practice Act
www2.legis.state.ia.us/IACODE/1999/148A/

Iowa Chapter of the APTA
1228 8th Street, Suite 106
West Des Moines, IA 50265-2624
Phone: 515-222-9838 or 800-925-3064
Fax: 515-222-9839

Kansas

Kansas State Board of Healing Arts
Kansas State Board of Physical Therapy
235 SW Topeka Boulevard
Topeka, KS 66603-3068
Phone: 785-296-7413
Fax: 785-296-0852

Practice Act
www.kumc.edu/kpta/practice.html

Kansas Chapter of the APTA
214 SW 6th Street, Suite 300
Topeka, KS 66603-3719
Phone: 785-233-5400
Fax: 785-290-0476

Kentucky

Kentucky State Board of Physical Therapy
9110 Leesgate Road, Suite 6
Louisville, KY 40222
Phone: 502-327-8497
Fax: 502-423-0934

Practice Act
www.lrc.state.ky.us/KRS/327-00/CHAPTER.htm

Kentucky Chapter of the APTA
225 Capital Avenue
Frankfort, KY 40601-2832
Phone: 800-482-5782
Fax: 502-226-6383

Louisiana

Louisiana State Board of Physical Therapy Examiners
714 E Kaliste Saloom Road, Suite D2
Lafayette, LA 70508
Phone: 318-262-1043
Fax: 318-262-1054

Practice Act
www.laptboard.org/PracticeActRulesReg.htm

Louisiana Chapter of the APTA
8550 United Plaza Boulevard, Suite 1001A
Baton Rouge, LA 70809-2256
Phone: 225-922-4614
Fax: 225-922-4611

Maine
Maine State Board of Examiners in Physical Therapy
Physical Therapy Board
#35 State House Station
Augusta, ME 04333
Phone: 207-624-8600
Fax: 207-624-8637

Practice Act
http://janus.state.me.us/legis/statutes/32/title32ch45-Asec0.html

Maine Chapter of the APTA
PO Box 1783
Portland, ME 04104-1783
Phone: 207-799-1584
Fax: 207-799-1584

Maryland
Board of Physical Therapy Examiners
4201 Patterson Avenue, #318
Baltimore, MD 21215-2299
Phone: 410-764-4752
Fax: 410-358-1183

Maryland Chapter of the APTA
PO Box 1099
Laurel, MD 20715-1099
Phone: 800-306-5596
Fax: 800-675-9438

Massachusetts
Massachusetts Board of Allied Health Professionals
239 Causeway Street
Boston, MA 02114
Phone: 617-727-3071
Fax: 617-727-2669

Practice Act
www.state.ma.us/reg/boards/ah

Massachusetts Chapter of the APTA
34 Atlantic Street
Gloucester, MA 01930-1625
Phone: 978-281-5393
Fax: 978-282-4384

Michigan
Michigan State Board of Physical Therapy
Department of Commerce—BOPR/Health Services
PO Box 30670
Lansing, MI 48909
Phone: 517-373-9102
Fax: 517-373-2179

Practice Act
http://michiganlegislature.org/mileg.asp?page=getObject&objNa
me=mcl-368-1978-15-178&highlight=

Michigan Chapter of the APTA
PO Box 21236
Lansing, MI 48989-1236
Phone: 800-242-8131 or 517-347-0880
Fax: 517-347-4720

Minnesota
Minnesota State Board of Medical Practice
Physical Therapy Advisory Council
2829 University Avenue, SE, Suite 315
Minneapolis, MN 55414
Phone: 612-627-5406
Fax: 612-627-5403

Minnesota Chapter of the APTA
1711 West County Road B
Suite 102 South
Roseville, MN 55113-4036
Phone: 612-635-0902
Fax: 612-635-0903

Mississippi
Mississippi State Department of Health
Professional Licensure Division—Physical Therapy
PO Box 1700
Jackson, MS 39215-1700
Phone: 601-987-4153
Fax: 601-987-3784

Mississippi Chapter of the APTA
921 N. Congress Street
Jackson, MS 39202-2554
Phone: 601-354-3629
Fax: 601-355-1506

Missouri
Missouri Advisory Commission for Professional Physical Therapists
3605 Missouri Boulevard
PO Box 4
Jefferson City, MO 65102
Phone: 573-751-0098
Fax: 573-751-3166

Practice Act
www.moga.state.mo.us/statutes/c334.htm

Missouri Chapter of the APTA
205 East Capital, Suite 100
Jefferson City, MO 65101
Phone: 573-556-6730 or 888-222-6782
Fax: 573-556-6731

Montana
Department of Commerce—Division of Public Safety
Board of Physical Therapy Examiners
Lower Level, Arcade Building
Helena, MT 59620-0513

Practice Act
www.discoveringmontana.com/dli/bsd/license/bsd_boards/ptp
_board/statutes.htm

Montana Chapter of the APTA
PO Box 4553
Missoula, MT 59806-4553
Phone: 406-251-5232
Fax: 406-251-5270

Nebraska
Department of Health Bureau of Examining Boards
Nebraska State Board of Physical Therapy
Credentialing Division
PO Box 94986
301 Centennial Mall South
Lincoln, NE 68509
Phone: 402-471-0547
Fax: 402-471-3577

Practice Act
www.hhs.state.ne.us/reg/t172.htm

Nebraska Chapter of the APTA
PO Box 540427
Omaha, NE 68154-0427
Phone: 402-491-3660
Fax: 402-491-1372

Nevada
Nevada State Board of Physical Therapy Examiners
Executive Director
810 Durango Drive, Suite 109
Las Vegas, NV 89145
Phone: 702-876-5535
Fax: 702-876-2097

Practice Act
www.leg.state.nv.us/NRS/NRS-640.html

Nevada Chapter of the APTA
PMB 105
8665 West Flamingo Road, Suite 131
Las Vegas, NV 89147
Phone: 702-571-1535
Fax: 702-888-1674

New Hampshire
New Hampshire State Board of Registration in Medicine
Allied Health Board
2 Industrial Park Drive
Concord, NH 03301
Phone: 603-271-8389
Fax: 603-271-6702

Practice Act
http://gencourt.state.nh.us/rsa/html/indexes/328-A.html

New Hampshire Chapter of the APTA
PO Box 978
Manchester, NH 03105-0978
Phone: 603-627-7970
Fax: 603-627-3970

New Jersey
New Jersey State Board of Physical Therapy
PO Box 45014
Newark, NJ 07101
Phone: 973-504-6455
Fax: 973-648-3536

Practice Act
www.njleg.state.nj.us/cgi-bin/om_isapi.dll?clientID=19874
&depth=2&expandheadings=on&headingsw

New Jersey Chapter of the APTA
1100 US Highway 130, Suite 3
Robbinsville, NJ 08691-1108
Phone: 609-208-0200
Fax: 609-208-1000

New Mexico
New Mexico Physical Therapists Licensing Board
2055 S. Pacheco, Suite 400
Santa Fe, NM 87505
Phone: 505-476-7117
Fax: 505-476-7095
website: www.governor.state.nm.us/boards/pboards/physical
therapists.htm

New Mexico Chapter of the APTA
5125 Highlands
McKinney, TX 75070
Phone: 469-247-1134
Fax: 972-540-1895

New York
State Board for Physical Therapy
Phone: 518-474-3817
Fax: 518-474-1449
website: www.op.nysed.gov/ptb.htm

Practice Act
http://assembly.state.ny.us/leg/?cl=30&a=129

New York Chapter of the APTA
5 Palisades Drive, Suite 330
Albany, NY 12205
Phone: 800-459-4489 or 518-459-4499
Fax: 518-459-8953

North Carolina
North Carolina Board of Physical Therapy Examiners
18 W. Colony Place, Suite 140
Durham, NC 27705
Phone: 919-490-6393
Fax: 919-490-5106

Practice Act
www.mcptboard.org/rules/practiceact.html

North Carolina Chapter of the APTA
316 West Millbrook Road, #105
Raleigh, NC 27609
Phone: 919-841-0268 or 800-948-2672
Fax: 919-841-0269

North Dakota
North Dakota Examining Committee for Physical Therapists
West 6th Street
Grafton, ND 58237
Phone: 701-352-4553
Fax: 701-352-1270

Practice Act
www.state.nd.us/lr/cencode/CCT43.pdf

North Dakota Chapter of the APTA
Department of Physical Therapy
UND School of Medicine
Grand Forks, ND 58202
Phone: 701-777-3873
Fax: 701-777-4199

Ohio
Ohio Occupational Therapy, Physical Therapy, and Athletic Trainers Board
77 S. High Street, 16th Floor
Columbus, OH 43215-6108
Phone: 614-466-3774
Fax: 614-995-0816

Practice Act
www.state.oh.us/pyt/pdfs/PTLawsRules.pdf

Ohio Chapter of the APTA
2066 West Henderson Road, Suite 202
Columbus, OH 43220-2452
Phone: 614-538-9612
Fax: 614-538-9614

Oklahoma
Oklahoma State Board of Medical Licensure and Supervision
5104 N. Francis, Suite C
Oklahoma City, OK 73118
Phone: 405-848-6841
Fax: 405-848-8240

Practice Act
www.osbmls.state.ok.us

Oklahoma Chapter of the APTA
223 West Ridgewood
Shawnee, OK 74801
Phone: 405-275-7588
Fax: 405-275-7588

Oregon
Oregon Physical Therapist Licensing Board
800 N.E. Oregon Street, Suite 407
Portland, OR 97232
Phone: 503-731-4047
Fax: 503-731-4207

Practice Act
http://landru.leg.state.or.us/ors/688.html

Oregon Chapter of the APTA
147 SE 102nd
Portland, OR 97216
Phone: 877-452-4919
Fax: 503-253-9172

Pennsylvania
Pennsylvania State Board of Physical Therapy
PO Box 2649
Harrisburg, PA 17105-2649
Phone: 717-783-7134
Fax: 717-787-7769

Pennsylvania Chapter of the APTA
4701 Devonshire Road, Suite 106
Harrisburg, PA 17109
Phone: 717-541-9169
Fax: 717-541-9182

Puerto Rico
Office of Regulation and Certification of the Profession of Health
Puerto Rico Board of Physical Therapy
Call Box 10200
Santurce, PR 00908
Phone: 787-725-8161 x209 or 787-725-7904
Fax: 787-725-7903

Puerto Rico Chapter of the APTA
PO Box 1142
Manati, PR 00674
Phone: 787-854-3700 ext 1279

Rhode Island
Rhode Island Board of Examiners in Physical Therapy
Rhode Island Department of Health—Division of Professional Regulation
3 Capitol Hill
104 Cannon Health Building
Providence, RI 02908-5097
Phone: 401-222-2827 x106
Fax: 401-222-1272

Practice Act
www.rilin.state.ri.us/statutes/TITLE5/5-40/INDEX.HTM

Rhode Island Chapter of the APTA
PO Box 1409
Kingston, RI 02881-0492
Phone: 401-874-5391
Fax: 401-874-5630

South Carolina
South Carolina State Board of Physical Therapy Examiners
PO Box 11329
Columbia, SC 29211-1329
Phone: 803-896-4655
Fax: 803-896-4719

Practice Act
www.llr.state.sc.us/PT/ptpact.htm

South Carolina Chapter of the APTA
3650-A Center Circle
Fort Mill, SC 29715
Phone: 803-802-5450
Fax: 803-371-1499

South Dakota
South Dakota State Board of Medical & Osteopathic Examiners
1323 S. Minnesota Avenue
Sioux Falls, SD 57105
Phone: 605-334-8343
Fax: 605-336-0270

Practice Act
http://198.187.128.12/southdakota/lpext.dll?f=templates&fn=fs-main.htm&20

South Dakota Chapter of the APTA
PO Box 88033
Sioux Falls, SD 57109-0033
Phone: 605-339-4839
Fax: 605-357-8780

Tennessee
Board of Occupational and Physical Therapy Examiners
Health Related Board
425 5th Ave N
1st Floor Cordell Hull Building
Nashville, TN 37247-1010
Phone: 615-532-3202
Fax: 615-741-2491

Practice Act
www.state.tn.us/health

Tennessee Chapter of the APTA
PO Box 23071
Nashville, TN 37202
Phone: 615-269-5312
Fax: 615-297-5852

Texas
Texas Board of Physical Therapy Examiners
333 Guadalupe, Suite 2-510
Austin, TX 78701-3942
Phone: 512-305-6900
Fax: 512-305-6951

Practice Act
www.ecptote.state.tx.us/pt/rules.html

Texas Chapter of the APTA
800 Brazos Street, Suite 430
Austin, TX 78701
Phone: 512-477-1818
Fax: 512-477-1434

Utah
Utah Health Professions Licensing Occupational & Professional
Licensing Division
160 E. 300 S.
Salt Lake City, UT 84114-6741
Phone: 801-530-6628
Fax: 801-530-6511

Practice Act
www.le.state.ut.us/

Utah Chapter of the APTA
2101 East 3780 South
Salt Lake City, UT 84109
Phone: 801-278-4016
Fax: 801-278-2752

Vermont
Vermont State Board of Physical Therapy
Office of Professional Regulation
Licensing and Registration Division
Redstone Building
26 Terrace Street
Drawer 09
Montpelier, VT 05609-1101
Phone: 802-828-2390
Fax: 802-828-2496

Practice Act
www.leg.state.vt.us/statutes/title26/chap038.htm

Vermont Chapter of the APTA
1878 Mountain Road, Suite 1
Stowe, VT 05672-4775
Phone: 802-253-2273
Fax: 802-253-7754

Virginia
Virginia State Board of Physical Therapy
Department of Health Professions—Board of Medicine
6606 W. Broad Street, 5th Floor
Richmond, VA 23230-1712
Phone: 804-662-9924
Fax: 804-662-9523

Practice Act
http://leg1.state.va.us/031/lst/LH203087.htm

Virginia Chapter of the APTA
1111 N. Fairfax Street
Alexandria, VA 22314-1541
Phone: 800-999-2782 x3235
Fax: 703-706-8578

Washington
Washington Department of Health
PO Box 47868
1300 S.E. Quince Street
Olympia, WA 98504-7868
Phone: 360-753-3132
Fax: 360-753-0657

Practice Act
www.leg.wa.gov/pub/rcw/RCW%20%2018%20%20TITLE/RCW
%20%2018%20.%2074%20%20CHAPTER

Washington PT Association
208 Rogers Street NW
Olympia, WA 98502-4940
Phone: 360-352-7290
Fax: 206-352-7298

West Virginia
West Virginia Board of Physical Therapy
153 W. Main Street, Suite 103
Clarksburg, WV 26301
Phone: 304-627-2251
Fax: 304-627-2253

Practice Act
http://129.71.161.254/scripts/as_web.exe?\state_code\finished-data\chap30.ask+F

West Virginia Chapter of the APTA
2110 Kanawha Boulevard E, Suite 220
Charleston, WV 25311
Phone: 304-345-6808
Fax: 304-344-4139

Wisconsin
Wisconsin State Board of Physical Therapy
Department of Regulation and Licensing
PO Box 8935
Madison, WI 53708-8935
Phone: 608-266-0483
Fax: 608-267-0644

Practice Act
http://folio.legis.state.wi.us/cgi-bin/om_isapi.dll?clientID=81158
&infobase=stats.nfo&j1-448.50&jump

Wisconsin Chapter of the APTA
802 W Broadway, Suite 208
Madison, WI 53713
Phone: 608-221-9191
Fax: 608-221-9697

Wyoming
Wyoming State Board of Physical Therapy
2020 Carey Avenue, Suite 201
Cheyenne, WY 82002
Phone: 307-777-3507
Fax: 307-777-3508

Practice Act
http://legisweb.state.wy.us/statutes/titles/title33/chapter.htm

Wyoming Chapter of the APTA
1347 Wisconsin
Casper, WY 82609
Phone: 307-235-3910
Fax: 307-266-2891

THE AMERICAN PHYSICAL THERAPY ASSOCIATION SECTIONS AND ASSEMBLIES

Please contact the American Physical Therapy Association at
The American Physical Therapy Association
1111 N. Fairfax Street
Alexandria, VA 22314
Phone: 703-684-2782 or 800-999-APTA x3124
Fax: 703-684-7343
for more information on the following sections and assemblies.

- Acute Care
- Administration
- Cardiopulmonary
- Clinical Electrophysiology*
- Community Home Health
- Education
- Geriatrics
- Hand Rehabilitation
- Health Policy, Legislation, and Regulation
- Neurology
- Oncology
- Orthopaedics
- Pediatrics
- Private Practice
- Research
- Sports Physical Therapy
- Veterans Affairs
- Women's Health

ASSEMBLY CONTACTS

National Assembly
1111 N. Fairfax Street
Alexandria, VA 22314-1436
Phone: 800-999-2782, ext 3231
Fax: 703-706-8578

STUDENT ASSEMBLY

1111 N. Fairfax Street
Alexandria, VA 22314-1436
Phone: 800-999-2782, ext 3254
Fax: 703-706-8578

DIRECTORY OF STATE PRACTICE ACTS

Alabama
(Title 35, Article 5)

Alaska
(Title 8, Chapter 84)

Arizona
(Title 32, Chapter 19)

Arkansas
(Title 17, Chapter 93)

California
(Business & Professions Code,
Div. 2 Chapter 5.7)

Colorado
(Title 12, Article 41)

Connecticut
(Title 20, Section 20)

Delaware
(Title 24, Chapter 26)

District of Columbia
(Unavailable)

Florida
(Chapter 486)

Georgia
(Title 43, Chapter 33)

Hawaii
(Chapter 461J)

Idaho
(Title 54, Chapter 22)

Illinois
(225 ILCS 90)

Indiana
(Title 25, Article 27)

Iowa
(Title 4, Chapter 148A)

Kansas
(Chapter 65, Article 29)

Kentucky
(KRS Title 26, Chapter 327)

Louisiana
(LIV)

Maine
(Title 32, Chapter 45-A)

Maryland
(gbo)

Massachusetts
(Chapter 122, Section 23 A to D)

Michigan
(Act 368, Part 178)

Minnesota
(MN statutes 148.65 to 148.78)

Mississippi
(Title 73, Chapter23)

Missouri
(Title 12, Chapter 334.5 to 685)

Montana
(Title 37, Chapter 11)

Nebraska
(Title 172, Chapter 137)

Nevada
(Title 54, Chapter 328A)

New Hampshire
(Title 30 Chapter 328A)

New Jersey
(Title 45:9-37.11)

New Mexico
(Chapter 61-12D)

New York
(Article 136)

North Carolina
(Unavailable)

North Dakota
(Chapter 43-26)

Ohio
(4755.02-.56 ORC)

Oklahoma
(59-887.1-.59-887)

Oregon
(Chapter 668)

Pennsylvania
(PL 383)

Puerto Rico
(Unavailable)

Rhode Island
(Chapter 5-40)

South Carolina
(Title 40, Chapter 45)

South Dakota
(Chapter 36-10)

Tennessee
(Title 63, Chapter 13)

Texas
(Article 4512e)

Utah
(Title 58, Chapter 24a)

Washington
(Chapter 18.74 rcw)

Vermont
(Title 26, Chapter 38)

West Virginia
(Chapter 30, Article 20)

Virginia
(54-1.2900-2993)

Wisconsin
(Chapter 448.50)

Virgin Islands
(Unavailable)

Wyoming
(Title 35, Chapter 25)

STATES THAT PERMIT PHYSICAL THERAPY EVALUATION WITHOUT REFERRAL

1. Alaska
2. Arizona
3. Arkansas
4. California
5. Colorado
6. Connecticut
7. Delaware
8. Florida
9. Georgia
10. Hawaii
11. Idaho
12. Illinois
13. Iowa
14. Kansas
15. Kentucky
16. Louisiana
17. Maine
18. Maryland
19. Massachusetts
20. Michigan
21. Minnesota
22. Mississippi
23. Montana
24. Nebraska
25. Nevada
26. New Hampshire
27. New Jersey
28. New Mexico
29. New York
30. North Carolina
31. North Dakota
32. Oklahoma
33. Oregon
34. Pennsylvania
35. Rhode Island
36. South Carolina
37. South Dakota
38. Tennessee
39. Texas
40. Utah
41. Vermont
42. Virginia
43. Washington
44. Washington, DC
45. West Virginia
46. Wyoming
47. Wisconsin

STATES THAT PERMIT PHYSICAL THERAPY TREATMENT WITHOUT REFERRAL

1. Alaska (1986)
2. Arizona (1983)
3. Arkansas (1997)
4. California (1968)
5. Colorado (1988)
6. Delaware (1993)
7. Florida (1992)
8. Idaho (1987)
9. Illinois (1988)
10. Iowa (1988)
11. Kentucky (1987)
12. Maine (1991)
13. Maryland (1979)
14. Massachusetts (1984)
15. Minnesota (1988)
16. Montana (1987)
17. Nebraska (1957)
18. Nevada (1985)
19. New Hampshire (1988)
20. New Mexico (1989)
21. North Carolina (1985)
22. North Dakota (1989)
23. Oregon (1993)
24. Rhode Island (1992)
25. South Carolina (1998)
26. South Dakota (1986)
27. Texas (1991)
28. Utah (1985)
29. Vermont (1988)
30. Virginia
31. Washington (1988)
32. West Virginia (1984)
33. Wisconsin (1989)

STATES WITHOUT DIRECT ACCESS

1. Alabama
2. Indiana
3. Missouri
4. Ohio

as of: 3/9/03

World Wide Web Sites in Rehabilitation

Physical Therapy Associations

American Physical Therapy Association

www.apta.org
An Internet site for physical therapists, physical therapist assistants, and students. It features physical therapy news, continuing education information, practice guidelines, research information, and membership/association information. It is also an excellent resource for general information in the educational field, accreditation, and contains links to schools and related publications.

APTA Chapters and Section Home Pages

www.apta.org/components
Contains information and newsletters regarding state chapter and APTA section activities. (Note: A password is needed in order to gain access.)

Exercise, Fitness, and Sports Medicine

www.hsls.pitt.edu/guides/internet/fitness
An extensive list of links to physical therapy, exercise, and sports medicine resources. Includes links to practice guidelines, electronic newsletters, mailing lists, patient information sites, and more. This site is maintained by the Health Sciences Library System, University of Pittsburgh, Pa.

Physical Therapist Online

www.physicaltherapist.com
This is an extensive and interactive site for individuals involved in the field of physical therapy/physiotherapy.

Physical Therapy and Rehabilitation Resources

www.ketthealth.com/medlib
This site is designed to link individuals to Internet web sites for physical therapists, occupational therapists, and others in rehabilitation. It is maintained by the Kettering Medical Center.

Private Practice Section of the APTA

www.ppsapta.org
This site is maintained by the Private Practice Section of the APTA and contains section newsletters and valuable information about the section.

PT Central

www.ptcentral.com
Presents news, events, and job information on the physical therapy profession. Also includes consumer health and wellness materials, continuing education opportunities in physical therapy, and more.

PT WWW Pages

www.mindspring.com/~wbrock/ptcnts.htm
This site includes a history and introduction of physical therapy, information on specialization, and general conditions that respond to physical therapy.

Section on Geriatrics of the APTA

www.geriatricspt.org
This site is maintained by the Section on Geriatrics of the APTA and contains *GeriNotes* and *Issues on Aging*. It also provides interactive communication with section executive officers and board of directors and current information on reimbursement, legislation, and policy issues affecting geriatric physical therapy.

Web Physical Therapy

www.webpt.com
This site contains advertising, equipment/supplier databases, employment databases, service databases, university research links, and seminar events and schedules.

OTHER ASSOCIATIONS

American College of Sports Medicine

www.acsm.org

American Congress of Rehabilitation Medicine

www.acrm.org
News and general information about the ACRM.

American Medical Association

www.ama-assn.org
News and general information about the AMA.

American Occupational Therapy Association

www.aota.org
AOTA's home page provides both professional and consumer information.

American Speech-Language-Hearing Association

www.asha.org

Centers for Medicare and Medicaid Services

http://cms.hhs.gov
Information on the government agency that regulates Medicare and Medicaid.

Gerontological Society of America

www.geron.org

GOVERNMENT-RELATED SITES

Americans with Disabilities Act Home Page

www.usdoj.gov/crt/ada
Description of ADA, links to ADA Info Line, enforcement, settlement information, technical assistance program, etc, from the Department of Justice.

Agency for Healthcare Research and Quality (United States Department of Health and Human Services)

www.ahcpr.gov
This site contains practical health care information, research findings, and data regarding health care issues.

Healthfinder

www.healthfinder.gov
Maintains links to government agencies and provides a catalog of online health care resources maintained by the United States government.

Minimum Data Set

www.cms.hhs.gov/medicaid/mds20/default.asp
This site contains information regarding the MDS, which is the assessment tool used under the skilled nursing facility prospective payment system.

National Athletic Trainers' Association

www.nata.org

National Health Information Center

www.health.gov/nhic
Health information resource database.

National Institutes of Health

www.nih.gov
Scientific resources, grants and contracts, health information, and links to all branches of the NIH.

National Library of Medicine

http://igm.nlm.nih.gov
Offers assisted searching in MEDLINE and other NLM databases.

National Rehabilitation Information Center

www.naric.com
Information clearinghouse containing over 46,000 documents related to disabilities and rehabilitation.

Occupational Safety and Health Administration

www.osha.gov
OSHA establishes and enforces protective standards for the workplace.

Office of the Inspector General

www.ed.gov/offices/OIG/index.html
This site contains OIG fraud and abuse sanction reports, current investigations, and enforcement and compliance.

Society for Neuroscience

http://apu.sfn.org
Home page and information.

World Health Organization

www.who.int/en
News and information about the organization, its projects, and updated WHO classifications for International Classification of Impairments, Disabilities, and Handicaps codes.

JOURNALS

Physical Therapy Journal

www.ptjournal.org
This site provides access to current and past issues of the official research journal of the APTA, as well as indexing by author and subject.

PT Magazine

www.apta.org/PTmagazine
Links user to recent *PT Magazine* issues with a keyword search mechanism that provides articles of specific topics in the field of physical therapy and related areas.

MISCELLANEOUS

Community Information & Referral

www.cirs.org
CIR is an organization that gathers and provides information of vital concern in order to assist people in need.

ErgoWeb, Inc

www.ergoweb.com
News, reference room, marketplace, and more.

Hosford Muscle Tables: Skeletal Muscles of the Human Body

www.ptcentral.com/muscles
This web site is an index containing detailed information about the skeletal muscles of the human body.

Neurosciences on the Internet

www.lm.com/~nab

Includes a searchable index of resources for neuroscience.

World Health Organization Classifications

INTERNATIONAL CLASSIFICATION OF IMPAIRMENT, DISABILITY, AND HANDICAP

Impairments	Activities	Participation	Contextual Factors
LEVEL OF FUNCTIONING			
Body (body parts)	Person (person as a whole)	Society (relationships with society)	Environmental (external influences on functioning)
CHARACTERISTICS			
Body function and structure	Person's daily activities	Involvement in the situation	Feature of the physical, social, and attitudinal world
POSITIVE ASPECT			
Functional and structural integrity	Activity	Participation	Facilitators
NEGATIVE ASPECT			
Impairment	Activity limitation	Participation restriction	Barriers/hindrances
QUANTIFIERS			
• Severity • Localization • Duration	• Degree of difficulty • Assistance • Duration • Outlook	• Extent of participation • Facilitators or barriers in the environment	• None

Reprinted with permission from the World Health Organization.

WORLD HEALTH ORGANIZATION CLASSIFICATIONS RELATING TO THE CONSEQUENCES OF DISEASES

Classification	Definition	Assessment Level
Handicap	A disadvantage for a given individual, resulting from an impairment or a disability, that limits or prevents the fulfillment of a role that is normal (depending on age, sex, and social and cultural factors) for the individual	Role performance
Disability	Any restriction or lack resulting from impairment of ability to perform an activity in the manner or within the range considered normal for a human being	Occupational performance
Impairment	Any loss or abnormality of psychological, physiological, or anatomical structure or function	Performance components

Reprinted with permission from the World Health Organization.

Diseases, Pathologies, and Syndromes Defined

achlorhydria: A condition resulting in the absence of hydrochloric acid in the gastric juice.

acquired immunodeficiency syndrome (AIDS): AIDS is characterized by progressive destruction of cell-mediated (T cell) immunity (as well as humoral immunity), resulting in susceptibility to opportunistic diseases. It is a syndrome caused by the human immunodeficiency virus that renders immune cells ineffective, permitting opportunistic infections, malignancies, and neurologic diseases to develop; it is transmitted sexually or through exposure to contaminated blood.

acromegaly: A disease that develops after closure of the epiphyses of the long bones affecting the bones of the face, jaw, hands, and feet. Acromegaly (ie, hyperpituitarism) occurs as a result of excessive secretion of growth hormone after normal completion of body growth. It results in increased bone thickness and hypertrophy of the soft tissues due to growth hormone-secreting adenomas of the anterior pituitary gland.

Adams-Stokes syndrome: A condition characterized by sudden attacks of unconsciousness, with or without convulsions. It frequently accompanies heart block.

Addison's disease: A disease characterized by a bronze-like pigmentation of the skin, severe prostration, progressive anemia, low blood pressure, diarrhea, and digestive disturbance. It is due to disease (hypofunction) of the adrenal glands and is usually fatal.

adhesive capsulitis: Also known as *periarthritis* or *frozen joints*, it is characterized by diffuse joint pain and loss of motion in all directions, often with a positive painful arc test and limited joint accessory motions.

adult respiratory distress syndrome (ARDS): ARDS is a group of symptoms that accompany acute respiratory failure following a systemic or pulmonary insult. It is also called *shock lung, wet lung, stiff lung, adult hyaline membrane disease, posttraumatic lung,* or *diffuse alveolar damage (DAD)*.

allergy: *See* hypersensitivity disorder.

Alzheimer's disease (AD): Alzheimer's disease is a progressive dementia characterized by a slow decline in memory, language, visuospatial skills, personality, cognition, and motor skills. It is a disabling neurological disorder that may be characterized by memory loss; disorientation; paranoia; hallucinations; violent changes of mood; loss of the ability to read, write, eat, or walk; and, finally, dementia. It usually affects people over the age of 65 and has no known cause or cure.

amyotrophic lateral sclerosis (ALS): ALS is a progressive motor neuron disease in which degeneration and scarring of the motor neurons in the lateral aspect of the spinal cord, brainstem, and cerebral cortex result in progressive weakness and profound limitation of movement. ALS attacks the upper motor neurons of the medulla oblongata and the lower neurons of the spinal cord. It is also called *Lou Gehrig disease.*

anemia: Anemia is a reduction in the oxygen-carrying capacity of the blood owing to an abnormality in the quantity or quality of erythrocytes (RBC). Hemoglobin is < 14 g/dL for men and < 12 g/dL for women. Hematocrit is < 41% for men and < 37% for women.

anencephaly: The most severe form of neural tube defect in which there is no development above the brainstem; absence of the brain.

aneurysm: A condition in which there is an abnormal stretching (dilation) in the wall of an artery, a vein, or the heart. The dilation can weaken to the point of rupture.

ankylosing spondylitis: Ankylosing spondylitis is an inflammatory arthropathy of the axial skeleton, including the sacroiliac joints, apophyseal joints, costovertebral joints, and the intervertebral disk articulations. It results in the dissolution of a vertebrae.

anorexia nervosa: Anorexia nervosa is an eating disorder in which the individual refuses to eat. It is characterized by severe weight loss in the absence of physical cause and attributed to emotions such as anxiety, irritation, anger, and fear. It is characterized by distortion of body image and the fear of becoming fat. The individual does not eat enough to maintain appropriate weight (maintenance of weight 15% below normal for age, height, and body type is indicative of anorexia). It most often occurs in adolescent girls and young women.

anterior cerebral artery syndrome: Infarction in the territory of the anterior cerebral artery is uncommon, but when it occurs, it results in profound abulia, or a delay in verbal and motor response with paraplegia.

anterior cord syndrome: Damage to the anterior and anterolateral aspect of the cord results in bilateral loss of motor function, pain, and temperature sensation due to interruption of the anterior and lateral spinothalamic tracts and corticospinal tract. It is frequently associated with flexion injuries.

anterior inferior cerebellar artery syndrome: A stroke-related syndrome in which the principle symptoms include ipsilateral deafness, facial weakness, vertigo, nausea and vomiting, nystagmus (or rhythmic oscillations of the eye), and ataxia. Horner's syndrome ptosis, miosis (ie, constriction of the pupil), and loss of sweating over the ipsilateral side of the face may also occur. A paresis of lateral gaze may be seen. Pain and temperature sensation are lost on the contralateral side of the body.

anterograde amnesia: A disorder of recent memory in which there is failure of new learning.

anxiety disorder: A generalized emotional state of fear and apprehension that is usually associated with a heightened state of physiologic arousal, such as elevation in heart rate and sweat gland activity.

aortic stenosis: Progressive valvular calcification of the bicuspid valve.

appendicitis: Inflammation of the vermiform appendix that often results in necrosis and perforation with subsequent localized or generalized peritonitis.

Arnold-Hilgartner hemophilic arthropathy: A condition in hemophilic individuals beginning with soft tissue swelling of the joints, osteoporosis, and overgrowth of epiphysis with no erosion or narrowing of cartilage space; leading to subchondral bone cysts, squaring of the patella, significant cartilage space narrowing; and ending in fibrous joint contracture, loss of joint cartilage space, marked enlargement of the epiphyses, and substantial disorganization of the joints.

arrhythmia: Disturbance of heart rate or rhythm caused by an abnormal rate of electrical impulse generation by the sinoatrial (SA) node or the abnormal conduction of impulses. Sinus arrhythmia is an irregularity in rhythm that may be a normal variation or may be caused by an alteration in vagal stimulation. Atrial fibrillation, or involuntary, irregular muscular contractions of the atrial myocardium, is the most common chronic arrhythmia; it occurs in rheumatic heart disease, dilated cardiomyopathy, atrial septal defect, hypertension, mitral valve prolapse, and hypertrophic cardiomyopathy. Ventricular fibrillation, or involuntary contractions of the ventricular muscle, is a frequent cause of cardiac arrest. Heart block is a disorder of the heartbeat caused by an interruption in the passages of impulses through the heart's electrical system. Causes include CAD, hypertension, myocarditis, overdose of cardiac medications (such as digitalis), and aging.

arteriosclerosis (obliterans): Atherosclerosis in which proliferation of the intima has caused complete obliteration of the lumen of the artery. Arteriosclerosis represents a group of diseases characterized by thickening and loss of elasticity of the arterial walls, often referred to as *hardening of the arteries*.

arteritis: A vasculitis primarily involving multiple sites of the temporal and cranial arteries.

arthrogryposis multiplex congenita (AMC): A nonprogressive neuromuscular syndrome in which multiple congenital contractures, either in flexion or extension, are present at birth. There are three types of AMC: contracture syndromes, amyoplasia (ie, lack of muscle formation or development), and distal arthrogryposis, primarily affecting the hands and feet. The child is born with stiff joints and weak muscles.

ascites: An abnormal accumulation of serous (edematous) fluid within the peritoneal cavity, the potential space between the lining of the liver, and the lining of the abdominal cavity. It is most often caused by cirrhosis, but other diseases associated with ascites include heart failure, constrictive pericarditis, abdominal malignancies, nephrotic syndrome, and malnutrition.

asthma: An inflammatory condition of the lungs with secondary bronchospasm marked by recurrent attacks of dyspnea, with wheezing due to the spasmodic constriction of the bronchi.

atelectasis: The collapse of normally expanded and aerated lung tissue at any structural level (eg, lung parenchyma, alveoli, pleura, chest wall, bronchi) involving all or part of the lung.

atherosclerosis: This condition represents a group of diseases characterized by thickening and loss of elasticity of the arterial walls, often referred to as *hardening of the arteries*.

athetoid cerebral palsy (Vogt's syndrome): A type of cerebral palsy characterized by continuous, slow, twisting motions of the upper and lower extremities and facial and trunk musculature.

attention deficit disorder (ADD): Characterized by an inability to focus attention and impulsiveness; often diagnosed in children.

attention deficit hyperactivity disorder (ADHD): Characterized by an inability to focus attention, impulsiveness, and hyperactivity; often diagnosed in children.

autism: Developmental disorder characterized by a severely reduced ability to communicate and emotionally relate to other people; self-absorption.

autoimmune disease: Autoimmune diseases fall into a category of conditions in which the cause involves immune mechanisms directed against self-antigens. The body fails to distinguish self from nonself, causing the immune system to direct immune responses against normal (ie, self) tissue and become self-destructive.

avascular necrosis (AVN): Death of bone and/or cartilaginous tissue as a result of having a poor or absent blood supply (*see also* osteonecrosis).

bacterial infection(s): An infection process in which a bacterial organism establishes a parasitic relationship with its host.

Barlow's syndrome: Mitral valve prolapse. A slight variation in the shape or structure of the mitral valve causes prolapse. This syndrome is also referred to as *floppy valve syndrome* or *click-murmur syndrome*.

basal cell carcinoma: A slow-growing surface epithelial skin tumor originating from undifferentiated basal cells contained in the epidermis. This type of carcinoma rarely metastasizes beyond the skin and does not invade blood or lymph vessels but can cause significant local damage.

basilar artery syndrome: Atheromatous lesions along the basilar trunk resulting in ischemia as a result of occlusion affect the brainstem, including the corticospinal tracts, corticobulbar tracts, medial and superior cerebellar peduncles, spinothalamic tracts, and cranial nerve nuclei. If the basilar artery is occluded, the brainstem symptoms are bilateral. When a branch of the basilar artery is occluded, the symptoms are unilateral, involving sensory and motor aspects of the cranial nerves.

Bell's palsy: Facial paralysis due to a functional disorder of the seventh cranial nerve. A condition in which the facial nerve is unilaterally affected. Etiology is uncertain, although it is suggested that it occurs as an inflammatory response in the auditory canal. Any agent that causes inflammation and swelling creates a compression that initially causes demyelination.

benign prostatic hyperplasia (BPH): An age-related, nonmalignant enlargement of the prostate gland.

biliary cirrhosis: Primary biliary cirrhosis is one type of cirrhosis characterized by chronic, progressive, inflammatory liver disease. Secondary biliary cirrhosis can occur with prolonged, partial, or complete obstruction of the common bile duct or its branches.

boil: A painful nodule, formed in the skin by inflammation of the dermis and subcutaneous tissue, enclosing a central slough or "core;" also called *furuncle*.

botulism: Classified as a bacterial infection, botulism is a rare paralytic disease that has a predilection for the cranial nerves and then progresses caudally and symmetrically to the trunk and extremities. It is often caused by the ingestion of neurotoxins in food that resist gastric digestion and proteolytic enzymes and are readily absorbed into the blood from the proximal small intestine.

brain abscess: Brain abscesses occur when microorganisms reach the brain and cause a local infection.

brainstem syndrome: This syndrome reflects lesions of cranial nerves III through XII at the root, nuclear, or bulbar level. Common symptoms are gaze palsies, a loss of active control of eye movement; nystagmus, involving rhythmic tremor of the eye; and dysarthria, abnormal speech resulting from poor control of the muscles of speech. It is commonly associated with multiple sclerosis.

breast cancer: Breast cancer is the most common malignancy of females in the United States. Most breast carcinomas are adenocarcinomas derived from the glandular epithelium of the terminal duct lobular unit.

bronchiectasis: This is a form of obstructive lung disease that is actually an extreme form of bronchitis. There is chronic dilation of the bronchi and bronchioles that develops when the supporting structures (ie, bronchial walls) are weakened by chronic inflammatory changes associated with secondary infection.

bronchiolitis: Bronchiolitis is a commonly occurring acute, diffuse, and often severe inflammation of the lower airways (bronchioles) caused by a viral infection.

Brown-Séquard's syndrome: A set of symptoms, caused by a primary intraspinal tumor, in which there is nerve root pain followed by motor weakness and wasting of muscle supplied by the nerve. This syndrome involves motor changes of extramedullary lesions beginning with segmental weakness at the lesion site and progressing to damage of half of the spinal cord. There is paralysis of motion on one side of the body and loss of sensation on the other side, depending on the site of the lesion involving one side of the spinal cord.

Buerger's disease: Also called *thromboangiitis obliterans*, this condition is a vasculitis that causes inflammatory lesions of the peripheral blood vessels accompanied by thrombus formation and vasospasm occluding blood vessels. The pathogenesis of Buerger's disease is unknown; however, it is generally considered an inflammatory process.

bulimarexia: An eating disorder in which anorexia nervosa and bulimia nervosa coexist. This is characterized by a period of starving to lose weight, alternating with periods of bingeing and purging.

bulimia nervosa: Bulimia nervosa is a compulsive eating disorder characterized by episodic binge eating (ie, consuming large amounts of food at one time) followed by purging behavior, such as self-induced vomiting, fasting, laxative and diuretic abuse, and excessive exercising.

burns: Injuries that result from direct contact or exposure to any thermal, chemical, electrical, or radiation source. The depth of injury is a function of temperature or source of energy and duration of exposure.

cachexia: A state of ill health, malnutrition, and wasting. It may occur in many chronic diseases, such as Alzheimer's disease; certain malignancies; and advanced pulmonary tuberculosis.

cancer: *Cancer* is a term that refers to a large group of diseases characterized by uncontrolled growth and spread of abnormal cells. Other terms used interchangeably for cancer are *malignant neoplasm, tumor, malignancy,* and *carcinoma.* Cancer in its various forms is a genetic disease characterized by deviations of the normal genetic mechanisms that regulate cell growth.

Caplan's syndrome: A condition associated with pneumoconiosis (*see* pneumoconiosis) and characterized by the presence of rheumatoid nodules in the periphery of the lung.

carbuncle: A circumscribed inflammation of the skin and deeper tissues that terminates in a slough and suppuration or boil. It results in a painful node that is covered by tight, reddened skin and contains pus.

carcinoma: A new growth or malignant tumor enclosing epithelial cells in connective tissue and tending to infiltrate and give rise to metastases. It may affect almost any organ or part of the body and spread by direct extension or through lymphatics or the blood stream.

cardiomyopathy (CM): A group of conditions affecting the heart muscle so that contraction and relaxation of myocardial muscle fibers are impaired.

carpal tunnel syndrome (CTS): Entrapment and compression of the median nerve within the carpal tunnel of the wrist. It is characterized by pain, tingling, numbness, and paresthesia, progressing to muscular weakness in the distribution of the median nerve.

celiac disease: This describes the condition that is a symptom complex including steatorrhea (ie, fat in feces), general malnutrition, abdominal distention, and secondary vitamin deficiencies. The disease is defined by an inability to digest gluten, one of the proteins found in wheat, barley, rye, and oats.

central cord syndrome: A result of damage to the central aspect of the spinal cord, often caused by hyperextension injuries in the cervical region. Characteristically, there is more severe neurologic involvement in the upper extremities than in the lower extremities. Function is typically retained in the thoracic, lumbar, and sacral regions, including the bowel, bladder, and genitals as peripherally located fibers are not affected.

cerebellar syndrome: Cerebellar syndrome deficits are usually symmetrical with all four limbs involved. Manifestations of cerebellar lesions are ataxia hypotonia and truncal weakness causing postural and movement disorders. Dysarthria of cerebellar origin (scanning speech, producing a prolonged, monotone sound) is common.

cerebral palsy (CP): A nonhereditary and nonprogressive lesion of the cerebral cortex resulting in a group of neuromuscular disorders of posture and voluntary movement, including lack of voluntary control; spasticity; impaired speech, vision, hearing, and perceptual functions; seizure disorder; hydrocephalus; microcephaly; or mental retardation. Damage to the motor area of the brain occurs during fetal life, birth, or infancy.

cerebral syndrome: Characterized by optic neuritis, the manifestation of demyelination of the optic nerve seen in multiple sclerosis and associated with visual field defects, decreased color vision, and reduced clarity of vision.

cerebrovascular accident (CVA): *See* stroke.

cerebrovascular disease: Intrinsic damage to the vessels of the brain caused by atherosclerosis, lipohyalinosis, inflammation, amyloid deposition, arterial dissection, developmental malformation, aneurysm, or venous thrombosis resulting in a stroke.

Charcot-Marie-Tooth disease: This is a peroneal muscular atrophy that is an inherited autosomal dominant disorder affecting motor and sensory nerves. Initially, the disorder involves the peroneal nerve and affects muscles in the foot and lower leg. It later progresses to the hands and forearms.

childhood disintegrative disorder: Marked regression in multiple areas of functioning following a period of at least 2 years of apparently normal development. The onset of the disorder takes place before the age of 10. Loss of previously acquired skills in at least two of the following areas: expressive or receptive language, social skills or adaptive behavior, bowel or bladder control, play, or motor skills.

cholangitis: Sclerosing cholangitis is an inflammatory disease of the bile ducts that has been linked to altered immunity, toxins, and infectious agents and is thought to be of genetic etiology.

cholecystitis: Inflammation of the gallbladder as a result of impaction of gallstones in the cystic duct causing painful distention of the gall bladder.

choledocholithiasis: Calculi in the common bile duct in persons with gallstones.

cholelithiasis (gallstones): Cholelithiasis is the formation or presence of gallstones that remain in the lumen of the gallbladder or are ejected with bile into the cystic duct.

chondrosarcoma: Chondrosarcoma is a tumor in which the neoplastic cells produce cartilage rather than the osteoid seen with the osteosarcoma.

chronic fatigue syndrome (CFS): CFS is a combination of symptoms hypothesized to be an autoimmune system response to stress. It is associated with severe and prolonged fatigue, low-grade fever, sore throat, painful lymph nodes, muscle weakness, discomfort or myalgia, sleep disturbances, headaches, migratory arthralgias without joint swelling or redness, photophobia, forgetfulness, irritability, confusion, depression, transient visual scotomata, difficulty in thinking, and inability to concentrate.

chronic obstructive bronchitis: This condition is clinically defined as a condition of productive cough lasting for at least 3 months per year for 2 consecutive years. The primary distinction between chronic obstructive bronchitis and chronic obstructive pulmonary disease is the chronic cough.

chronic obstructive pulmonary disease (COPD): Also called *chronic obstructive lung disease*, this condition refers to a number of disorders that affect movement of air in and out of the lungs, particularly within the small airways. There is blockage of air and abnormalities of the lungs, causing an effect on expiratory flow. The most important of these disorders are obstructive bronchitis, emphysema, and asthma.

chronic pain disorder (syndrome): Chronic pain has been recognized as pain that persists part of the normal healing time. Chronic pain is often associated with depressive disorders, whereas acute pain appears to be associated with anxiety disorders.

chronic renal failure (CRF): The loss of nephrons results in progressive deterioration of glomerular filtration, tubular reabsorption, and endocrine functions of the kidneys. This ultimately leads to failure of the kidneys and affects all other body systems.

cirrhosis: Cirrhosis of the liver is a group of chronic end-stage diseases of the liver resulting from a variety of chronic inflammatory, toxic, metabolic, or congestive damage most commonly associated with alcohol abuse.

click-murmur syndrome: *See* Barlow's syndrome or mitral valve prolapse.

cluster headache: Cluster headaches are severe unilateral headaches of relatively short duration. The episodic cluster headache is defined as the period of susceptibility to headache, called *cluster periods*, alternating with periods of remission. *Chronic cluster headache* is a term used when remissions have not occurred for at least 12 months.

coal workers' pneumoconiosis: Lung disease resulting from inhalation of coal dust.

colitis: An irritable bowel syndrome in which there is a suppression of normal gastrointestinal flora, the bacteria normally residing in the lumen of the intestines, allowing yeasts and molds to flourish.

collagen vascular disease: Also called *connective tissue disease*, this condition is associated with pulmonary manifestations, including exudative pleural effusion, pulmonary nodules, rheumatoid nodules, interstitial fibrosis, and pulmonary vasculitis.

congenital heart disease: An anatomic defect in the heart that develops in utero during the first trimester and is present at birth. There are two categories: cyanotic defects resulting from obstruction of blood flow to the lungs or mixing of desaturated blue venous blood with fully saturated red arterial blood within the chambers of the heart; and acyanotic defects primarily involving left-to-right shunting of blood through an abnormal opening.

congenital hip dysplasia: Developmental dysplasia of the hip that is unilateral or bilateral and occurs in three forms: unstable hip dysplasia in which the hip is positioned normally but can be dislocated by manipulation, subluxation or complete dislocation in which the femoral head remains intact with the acetabulum but the head of the femur is partially displaced or uncovered, and complete dislocation in which the femoral head is totally outside the acetabulum.

congestive heart failure (CHF): A heart condition in which the heart is unable to pump sufficient blood to supply the body's needs. Congestive heart disease represents a group of clinical manifestations caused by inadequate pump performance from either the cardiac valves or the myocardium. There is excessive or abnormal accumulation of blood (congestion) in the heart. It causes mechanical or functional inadequacy to fully empty the blood from the heart, due to hypertrophic cardiac muscle changes.

connective tissue disease: A rheumatoid disease, such as systemic lupus erythematosus (SLE), scleroderma, or polymyositis (*see* systemic lupus erythematosus (SLE), scleroderma, and polymyositis).

Conn's syndrome: Conn's syndrome, or primary aldosteronism, is a metabolic disorder that occurs when an adrenal lesion results in hypersecretion of aldosterone, the most powerful of the mineralocorticoids (aldosterone's primary role is to conserve sodium, and it also promotes potassium excretion). There is an excess of sodium in the blood (ie, hypernatremia), indicating water loss exceeding sodium loss, and fluid volume excess (ie, hypervolemia), leading to an increase in the volume of circulating fluid or plasma in the body; low blood levels of potassium (ie, hypokalemia), and metabolic alkalosis. All of these factors lead to blood pressure increases.

constipation: A condition in which fecal matter is too hard to pass easily or in which bowel movements are so infrequent that discomfort and other symptoms interfere with activities of daily living.

contact dermatitis: An acute or chronic skin inflammation caused by exposure to a chemical, mechanical, physical, or biological agent.

conversion disorder: A psychodynamic phenomenon rather than a behavioral response to illness or injury defined as a transformation of an emotion into a physical manifestation.

coronary heart (or artery) disease (CAD): Blockage of the coronary arteries of the heart leading to myocardial infarction, arrhythmias, or failure.

cor pulmonale: Also called *pulmonary heart disease* in which there is an enlargement of the right ventricle secondary to pulmonary hypertension that occurs in diseases of the thorax, lung, and pulmonary circulation. It is a term that describes the pathologic effects of lung dysfunction as it affects the right side of the heart. There is hypertrophy or failure of the right ventricle. Heart disease is secondary to disease of the lungs or of the lungs' blood vessels.

corticospinal syndrome: This syndrome involves the corticospinal tract and dorsal column and results in stiffness, slowness, and weakness of the limbs.

Creutzfeldt-Jakob disease: Presenile dementia that is chronic in nature. It is a rapidly dementing disease thought to be activated by a slow virus of genetic predisposition. It results in memory deficits and electroencephalographic changes, and myoclonus is prevalent. Involves the frontal lobe with symptoms of apathy, lack of personal care, and the display of psychomotor retardation. Motor symptoms include incontinence and seizures.

Crohn's disease: Crohn's disease is a chronic lifelong inflammatory disorder of the bowel that can affect any segment of the intestinal tract and even tissues in other organs. It is characterized by exacerbations and periods of remission.

Cushing's syndrome: A metabolic disorder, also referred to as *hypercortisolism* (ie, hyperfunction of the adrenal gland), in which there is increased secretion of cortisol by the adrenal cortex, resulting in liberation of amino acids from muscle tissue with resultant weakening of protein structures. The end results include a protuberant abdomen with striae ("stretch marks"), poor wound healing, generalized muscle weakness, and marked osteoporosis.

cystic fibrosis (CF): An inherited disease of the exocrine glands affecting the hepatic, digestive, male reproductive (the vas deferens is functionally disrupted in nearly all cases), and respiratory systems. The majority of morbidity and mortality is caused by lung disease and almost all persons develop obstructive lung disease associated with chronic infection that leads to progressive loss of pulmonary function. Cystic fibrosis is a chronic, progressive disorder characterized by abnormal mucous secretion in the glands of the pancreas and lungs. It is usually diagnosed early in life due to frequent respiratory infections or failure to thrive.

cystitis: Lower urinary tract infection.

cystocele: A herniation of the urinary bladder into the vagina.

cytomegalovirus (CMV): A commonly occurring DNA herpes virus infection occurring congenitally, peri- or postnatally, or disseminated in immunocompromised persons. This infection increases in frequency with age.

dactylitis: Painful swelling of the hands or feet that occurs as a result of clot formation. Occurs most often in those individuals affected by sickle cell disease.

degenerative intervertebral disk disease: A degenerative joint process that applies to any synovial joint, including the facet joints, or any intervertebral disk articulation of the spinal column. Events leading to disk degeneration include impaired cellular nutrition, reduced cellular viability, cellular senescence, accumulation of degraded matrix macromolecules, or fatigue failure of the matrix.

dehydration: Removal or loss of water from the body or a tissue; water deficit; severe dehydration may lead to acidosis, accumulation of waste products in the body (ie, uremia), and fatal shock.

dementia: Irrecoverable deteriorative mental state, the common end result of many entities.

depression: A morbid sadness, dejection, or a sense of melancholy, distinguished from grief, which is a normal response to a personal loss.

dermatitis: Infection of the skin. *Eczema* and *dermatitis* are terms that are used interchangeably. A superficial inflammation of the skin due to irritant exposure, allergic sensitization (delayed hypersensitivity), or genetically determined idiopathic factors (eg, eczema, atopic dermatitis, seborrheic dermatitis, etc).

dermatomyositis: Diffuse, inflammatory myopathies that produce symmetrical weakness of striated muscle, primarily the proximal muscles of the shoulder and pelvic girdles, neck, and pharynx. This inflammatory disorder is related to the family of rheumatic diseases and has periods of exacerbations and remissions.

dermatophytoses: Fungal infections, such as ringworm, that are caused by a group of fungi that invade the stratum corneum, hair, and nails. These are superficial infections that live on, not in, the skin and are confined to the dead keratin layers, unable to survive in the deeper layers.

diabetes insipidus: Diabetes insipidus, a rare disorder, involves a physiologic imbalance of water secondary to antidiuretic hormone (ADH) deficiency. Injury or loss of function of the hypothalamus, the neurohypophysial tract, or the posterior pituitary gland can result in diabetes insipidus.

diabetes mellitus (DM): A metabolic disorder in which the pancreas is unable to produce insulin, a substance the body needs to metabolize glucose as an energy source. A chronic, systemic disorder characterized by hyperglycemia (ie, excess glucose in the blood) and disruption of the metabolism of carbohydrates, fats, and proteins. Insufficient insulin is produced in the pancreas, resulting in high blood glucose levels. Over time, DM results in small- and large-vessel vascular complications and neuropathies.

diarrhea: Frequent, watery stools; results in poor absorption of water, nutritive elements, and electrolytes; fluid volume deficit; and acidosis as a result of potassium depletion. Other systemic effects of prolonged diarrhea are dehydration, electrolyte imbalance, and weight loss.

diplopia: Damage to the third cranial nerve, causing double vision.

discitis: A spinal infection affecting the disk, discitis can range from a self-limiting inflammatory process to a pyogenic infection. It may involve the intervertebral disk, vertebral end plates, or both.

discoid lupus erythematosus: A condition marked by chronic skin eruptions that, if left untreated, can lead to scarring and permanent disfigurement. Evidence suggests that this is an autoimmune defect.

disseminated intravascular coagulation (DIC): Sometimes referred to as *consumption coagulopathy*, it is a thrombotic disease caused by overactivation of the coagulation cascade. It is an acquired disorder of platelet function, with diffuse or widespread coagulation occurring within arterioles and capillaries all over the body.

diverticular disease: *Diverticular disease* is the term used to describe diverticulosis (uncomplicated disease) and diverticulitis (disease complicated by inflammation). *Diverticulosis* refers to the presence of outpouchings (diverticula) in the wall of the colon or small intestine, a condition in which the mucosa and submucosa herniate through the muscular layers of the colon to form outpouchings containing feces.

Down syndrome: A genetic disorder attributed to a chromosomal aberration referred to as *trisomy 21*. Down syndrome is characterized by muscle hypotonia, cognitive delay, abnormal facial features, and other distinctive physical abnormalities. Distinct physical characteristics include a large tongue, poor muscle tone, a flat face, and heart problems.

Duchenne's muscular dystrophy: Progressive fatal disorder of the skeletal muscles beginning in early childhood caused by a hereditary sex-linked gene on the X chromosome.

Dupuytren's contracture: A finger deformity characterized by the formation of a flexion contracture and thickening band of palmar fascia, usually involving the third and fourth digits accompanied by pain and decreased extension. Characterized by progressive fibrosis (increase in fibrous tissue) of the palmar aponeurosis, resulting in the shortening and thickening of the fibrous bands that extend from the aponeurosis to the bases of the phalanges. These fibrous bands pull the digits into such marked flexion at the metacarpophalangeal joints that they cannot be straightened.

dysphagia: Difficulty swallowing. It may be caused by neurologic conditions, local trauma and muscle damage, or mechanical obstruction.

dysplasia: A general diagnostic category that indicates a disorganization of cells in which an adult cell varies from its normal size, shape, or organization.

dystonia: A neurologic syndrome dominated by sustained muscle contractions frequently causing twisting and repetitive movements or abnormal postures often exacerbated by active voluntary movements. Dystonia is both a symptom and the name for a collection of neurologic disorders characterized by these movements and postures.

ectopic pregnancy: A pregnancy marked by the implantation of a fertilized ovum outside the uterine cavity.

eczema: *See* dermatitis.

edema: Excessive accumulation of interstitial fluid (fluid that bathes the cells) that may be localized or generalized.

emphysema: Emphysema is defined as a pathologic accumulation of air in tissues, particularly in the lungs. Distention of tissues is caused by gas or air in the interstices. In chronic pulmonary disease, there is a characteristic increase beyond the normal in the size of air spaces distal to the terminal bronchiole with destructive changes in the alveolar sac walls.

encephalitis: An acute inflammatory disease of the brain caused by direct viral invasion or hypersensitivity initiated by a virus.

encephalocele: Hernia protrusion of brain substance and meninges through a congenital or traumatic opening in the skull.

encephalocystocele: Hernia protrusion of the brain distended by fluid.

enchondroma: A common, benign tumor that arises from residual cartilage in the metaphysis of bone. The hand, femur, and humerus are common sites.

endocarditis: Infective, or bacterial, endocarditis is an infection of the endocardium, the lining inside the heart, including the heart valves.

endometriosis: A condition marked by functioning endometrial tissue found outside the uterus, resulting in ectopic pregnancy.

entrapment syndromes: Entrapment or compression of peripheral nerves resulting from their proximity to bony, muscular, and vascular structures (*see* specific disorders: carpal tunnel syndrome, sciatica, Bell's palsy, tardy ulnar palsy, thoracic outlet syndrome, Saturday night palsy).

ependymoma: A neoplasm derived from the ependymal cell lining of the ventricular system and the central canal of the spinal cord. It is usually reddish, lobulated, and well circumscribed, resembling a cauliflower in shape.

epilepsy: Defined as a chronic disorder of various causes characterized by recurrent seizures due to excessive discharge of cerebral neurons.

Epstein-Barr virus (EBV): Also known as *infectious mononucleosis*, it is an acute infectious disease caused by EBV, a member of the herpes virus group.

Erb's palsy: A paralysis of the upper limb resulting from a traction injury to the brachial plexus at birth. Erb-Duchenne palsy affects the C5 to C6 nerve roots, whole-arm palsy affects C5 to T1, and Klumpke's palsy affects the C8 and T1 (lower plexus) nerve roots.

Ewing's sarcoma: A malignant primary bone tumor. The pelvis and lower extremity are the most common sites. This malignant bone tumor often attacks the shaft of the long bones.

facioscapulohumeral dystrophy: A mild form of muscular dystrophy beginning with weakness and atrophy of the facial muscles and shoulder girdle. The inability to close the eyes may be the earliest sign; the face is expressionless when laughing or crying, forward shoulders and scapular winging develop, and the person has difficulty raising the arms overhead.

factitious disorder: A psychophysiologic disorder characterized by somatic symptom production that is intentional or self-induced for the purpose of gaining attention by deceiving health care personnel or for personal gain.

fecal incontinence: Inability to control bowel movements. Psychological factors include anxiety, confusion, disorientation, and depression. Physiologic causes include neurologic sensory and motor impairment, anal distortion secondary to traumatic childbirth, sexual assault, hemorrhoids, and hemorrhoidal surgery; altered levels of consciousness; and severe diarrhea.

fibromyalgia: Fibromyalgia or fibromyalgia syndrome, often mislabeled or misdiagnosed as fibrocytis, fibromyositis, nonarticular arthritis, myofascial pain, chronic fatigue syndrome, or systemic lupus erythematosus, is a chronic muscle pain syndrome with no known cause and no known cure. Fibromyalgia has been defined as pain that is widespread with multiple tender points.

fibrositis: A term that means inflammation of the fibrous connective tissue, although muscle biopsy studies have failed to demonstrate an inflammatory process.

floppy valve syndrome: *See* mitral valve prolapse.

Friedreich's ataxia: A disease involving neurologic degeneration due to cell loss in the dorsal root ganglia and secondary degeneration in the ascending and descending posterior columns and spinocerebellar tracts. It is primarily a disorder of movement with ataxic gait the most common presenting symptom.

frontal lobe syndrome: Lesions affecting the frontal lobe result in change from the premorbid personality in terms of a person's character and temperament, slowness in processing information, lack of judgment based on known consequences, withdrawal, and irritability. Disinhibition and apathy are common clinical dysfunctions of the frontal lobe. The person may lack insight into the deficits; therefore, behavior can be difficult to control.

fulminant hepatitis: A rare form of hepatitis (occurs in less than 1% of persons with acute viral hepatitis) is defined as hepatic failure with stage III or IV encephalopathy (confusion, stupor, and coma) as a result of massive hepatic necrosis.

furuncle: *See* boil.

furunculosis: Persistent sequential occurrence of boils (furnucles) over a period of weeks of months.

gallstone(s): Gallstones, also called *cholelithiasis*, is the formation or presence of gallstones that remain in the lumen of the gallbladder or are ejected with bile into the cystic duct. Gallstones are stone-like masses called *calculi* (singular: calculus) that form in the gallbladder as a result of changes in the normal components of bile.

gangrene: Death of body tissue usually associated with loss of vascular (nutritive, arterial circulation) supply, and followed by bacterial invasion and putrefaction. The three major types of gangrene are dry, moist, and gas. Dry and moist gangrene result from loss of blood circulation due to various causes; gas gangrene occurs in wounds infected by anaerobic bacteria, leading to gas production and tissue breakdown.

gastric adenocarcinoma: A malignant neoplasm arising from the gastric mucosa, it constitutes more than 90% of the malignant tumors of the stomach.

gastritis: Inflammation of the lining of the stomach (gastric mucosa). It is not a single disease but represents a group of the most common stomach disorders.

gastroesophageal reflux disease (GERD): Also called *esophagitis*, it may be defined as an inflammation of the esophagus, which may be the result of reflux (backward flow) of gastric juices, infections, chemical irritants, involvement by systemic diseases, or physical agents, such as radiation and nasogastric intubation.

gigantism: An overgrowth of the long bones resulting from growth hormone-secreting adenomas of the anterior pituitary gland. Gigantism develops in children before the age when epiphyses of the bones close and results in generalized "largeness," with heights often reaching 8 to 9 feet.

gliomas: Primary tumors of the brain, gliomas are the most prevalent and are tumors of the glial cells, the group of cells that support, insulate, and metabolically assist the neurons.

goiter: An enlargement of the thyroid gland that may be the result of lack of iodine, inflammation, or tumors (benign or malignant). Enlargement may also appear in hyperthyroidism, especially Graves' disease.

gout: Gout represents a heterogeneous group of metabolic disorders marked by an elevated level of serum uric acid and the deposition of urate crystals in the joints, soft tissues, and kidneys. Primary gout refers to hyperuricemia in the absence of other disease. Secondary gout refers to hyperuricemia resulting from an antecedent disease.

grand mal seizure: Grand mal or tonic-clonic seizure is the archetypal seizure, which means total loss of control. The seizure begins with a sudden loss of consciousness, generalized rigidity (tonic) followed by jerking movements (clonic), incontinence of bowel and bladder. In the tonic phase, respiration can cease briefly.

Graves' disease: Hyperthyroidism, the excess secretion of thyroid hormone, creates a generalized elevation of body metabolism that is manifested in almost every system. Graves' disease, which increases T4 production, accounts for 85% of hyperthyroidism. The classic symptoms of Graves' disease are mild symmetrical enlargement of the thyroid (goiter), nervousness, heat intolerance, weight loss despite increased appetite, sweating, diarrhea, tremor, and palpitations.

Guillain-Barré syndrome (GBS): Guillain-Barré syndrome, also called *acute inflammatory demyelinating polyradiculoneuropathy* (AIDP), which describes the syndrome, is an immune-mediated disorder. Viral and bacterial infections, surgery, and vaccinations have been associated with AIDP. There is increased sensitivity response in the peripheral nervous system and inflammation of the spinal nerve roots, peripheral nerves, and occasionally the cranial nerves. It also results in rapid paralysis of the limbs, accompanied by sensory loss and muscle atrophy.

Gulf War syndrome: Occurring in individuals who served in the Persian Gulf War, symptoms include fatigue, skin rash, headache, muscle and joint pain, memory loss, shortness of breath, sleep disturbances, diarrhea and other gastrointestinal symptoms, and depression. There is no known cause, but possible causes include chemical or biologic weapons, insecticides, Kuwaiti oil well fires, parasites, pills protecting against nerve gas, and inoculations against petrochemical exposure.

heart block: *See* arrhythmias.

heartburn: A burning sensation in the esophagus usually felt in the midline below the sternum in the region of the heart. It is often a symptom of indigestion and occurs when acidic contents of the stomach move backward or regurgitate into the esophagus. Also called *dyspepsia, pyrosis,* or *indigestion.*

hemophilia: A bleeding disorder inherited as a sex-linked autosomal recessive trait in two-thirds of all cases. It is a coagulation (blood-clotting) disorder and caused by an abnormality of plasma-clotting proteins necessary for blood coagulation.

hemorrhoids: Hemorrhoids, or piles, are varicose veins in the perianal region and may be internal or external.

hemostasis: The arrest of bleeding after blood vessel injury involving the interaction between the blood vessel wall, the platelets, and the plasma coagulation proteins. Disorders of hemostasis are caused by defects in platelet number or function or problems in the formation of a blood clot, resulting in a bleeding or clotting disorder.

hemothorax: Blood in the pleural cavity following chest trauma.

hepatic encephalopathy: Also termed *hepatic coma,* it refers to a variety of neurologic signs and symptoms in persons with chronic liver failure or in whom portal circulation is impaired.

hepatitis: An acute or chronic inflammation of the liver caused by a virus, a chemical, a drug reaction, or alcohol abuse.

hernia: An acquired or congenital abnormal protrusion of part of an organ or tissue through the structure normally containing it.

herpes simplex: An acute virus disease marked by groups of watery blisters on the skin; mucous membranes, such as the borders of the lips or the nose; or the mucous surface of the genitals. It often accompanies fever. Also known as *cold sores.*

herpes zoster: Also called *shingles,* it is a local disease brought about by the reactivation of the same virus that causes the systemic disease called *varicella* (chickenpox). The disease is brought on by an immunocompromised state.

hiatal hernia: A hiatal or diaphragmatic hernia occurs when the cardiac (lower esophagus) sphincter becomes enlarged, allowing the stomach to pass through the diaphragm into the thoracic cavity.

hip dysplasia: *See* congenital hip dysplasia.

Hodgkin's disease: A neoplastic disease of lymphoid tissue with the primary histologic finding of giant Reed-Sternberg cells in the lymph nodes. These cells are part of the tissue macrophage system and have twin nuclei and nucleoli that give it the appearance of "owl eyes."

Horner's syndrome: Horner's syndrome includes ptosis (drooping of the upper eyelid), miosis (constriction of the pupil), and loss of sweating over the ipsilateral side of the face following an anterior inferior cerebellar artery stroke.

human immunodeficiency virus (HIV): A retrovirus that predominantly infects human T4 (helper) lymphocytes, the major regulators of the immune response, and destroys or activates them (see also acquired immunodeficiency syndrome [AIDS]).

Huntington's disease (HD): A progressive hereditary disease of the basal ganglia characterized by abnormalities of movement, abnormal posture, postural reactions, trunk rotation, distribution of tone, extraneous movements, personality disturbances, and progressive dementia. Often associated with choreic movement, which is brief, purposeless, involuntary, and random. The disease slowly progresses, and death is usually due to an intercurrent infection. Also called *Huntington's chorea.*

hyaline membrane disease: A respiratory disease of unknown cause in newborn infants, especially if premature, characterized by an abnormal membrane of protein lining the alveoli of the lungs.

hydrocephalus: The increased accumulation of cerebrospinal fluid within the ventricles of the brain. Results from interference with normal circulation and with absorption of fluid, and especially, from destruction of the foramina of Magendie and Luschka.

hyperparathyroidism: A metabolic disorder caused by overactivity of one or more of the four parathyroid glands that disrupts calcium, phosphate, and bone metabolism.

hyperpituitarism: An oversecretion of one or more of the hormones secreted by the pituitary gland, especially growth hormone, resulting in gigantism or acromegaly. It is primarily caused by a hormone-secreting pituitary tumor, typically a benign adenoma. Other syndromes associated with hyperpituitarism include Cushing's disease, amenorrhea (absence of the menstrual cycle), and hyperthyroidism.

hypersensitivity disorder: An exaggerated or inappropriate immune response, overreaction to a substance, or hypersensitivity, this disorder is often referred to as an *allergic response*. Although the term *allergy* is widely used, the term *hypersensitivity* is more appropriate. Hypersensitivity designates an increased immune response to the presence of an antigen that results in tissue destruction.

hypertension (HTN): Hypertension, or high blood pressure, is defined by the World Health Organization (WHO) as a persistent elevation of systolic blood pressure above 140 mmHg and of diastolic pressure above 90 mmHg measured on at least two separate occasions at least 2 weeks apart.

hyperthyroidism: An excessive secretion of thyroid hormone. It is sometimes referred to as *thyrotoxicosis*, a term used to describe the clinical manifestations that occur when the body tissues are stimulated by increased thyroid hormone. Excessive thyroid hormone creates a generalized elevation of body metabolism, the effects of which are manifested in almost every system.

hypochondriasis: A marked preoccupation with one's health; exaggeration of normal sensations and minor complaints into a serious illness.

hypoparathyroidism: Hyposecretion, hypofunction, or insufficient secretion of the parathyroid hormone (PTH) results in hypocalcemia, as the parathyroid's primary role is to regulate calcium balance. The most significant clinical consequence is neuromuscular irritability producing tetany.

hypopituitarism: Also called *panhypopituitarism* and *dwarfism*, it results from decreased or absent hormonal secretion by the anterior pituitary gland. It is a generalized condition in which all six of the pituitary's vital hormones (adrenocorticotropic hormone, thyroid-stimulating hormone, luteinizing hormone, follicle-stimulating hormone, human growth factor, and prolactin) are inadequately produced or absent.

hypotension: Decrease of systolic and diastolic blood pressure below normal due to a deficiency in tonus or tension (*see also* orthostatic hypotension).

hypothyroidism: Refers to a deficiency of thyroid hormone that results in a generalized slowed body metabolism. In primary hypothyroidism, the loss of thyroid tissue leads to a decreased production of thyroid hormone, and the thyroid gland responds by enlarging to compensate for the deficiency (*see* goiter). Secondary hypothyroidism is most commonly the result of failure of the pituitary to synthesize adequate amounts of thyroid-stimulating hormone (TSH).

iatrogenic immunodeficiency: A condition induced by immunosuppressive drugs, radiation therapy, or splenectomy in which the immune system is weakened by the intervention.

ichthyosis: A group of skin disorders characterized by dryness, roughness, and scaliness of the skin, resulting in thickening of the skin. It is sometimes referred to as *alligator skin*, *fish skin*, *crocodile skin*, or *porcupine skin*.

immune complex disease: Normally, excessive circulating antigen-antibody complexes called *immune complexes* are effectively cleared by the reticuloendothelial system. When circulating immune complexes successfully deposit in tissue around small blood vessels, they activate the complement cascade and cause acute inflammation and local tissue injury. This results in vasculitis, which can affect skin, causing an allergic reaction; synovial joints, such as in rheumatoid arthritis; kidneys, causing nephritis; the pleura, causing pleuritis; and the pericardium, causing pericarditis.

impotence: Impotence is a general term that expresses a problem with libido, penile erection, ejaculation, or orgasm. The contemporary diagnostic term is erectile dysfunction.

incontinence: Inability to retain urine, semen, or feces through loss of sphincter control (*see also* fecal incontinence and urinary incontinence).

infection: A process in which an organism establishes a parasitic relationship with its host. This invasion and multiplication of microorganisms produce signs and symptoms, as well as an immune response.

infectious diseases: Clinical manifestations of infectious disease are many and varied depending upon the etiologic agent (eg, viruses, bacteria, etc) and the system affected (eg, respiratory, central nervous system, gastrointestinal, genitourinary, etc). Systemic symptoms can include fever and chills, sweating, malaise, and nausea and vomiting. There may be changes in blood composition, such as an increased number of white blood cells (ie, leukocytes).

inflammatory bowel disease (IBD): Refers to two inflammatory conditions: Crohn's disease (CD) and ulcerative colitis (UC) (*see* Crohn's disease and ulcerative colitis).

insulin resistance syndrome: A syndrome of insulin resistance that is associated with hypertension, carbohydrate intolerance, abdominal obesity, dyslipidemia, and accelerated atherosclerosis associated with noninsulin dependent diabetes mellitus (NIDDH).

internal carotid artery syndrome: The clinical picture of internal carotid occlusion varies, depending on whether the cause of ischemia is thrombus, embolus, or low flow. The cortex supplied by the middle cerebral territory is most often affected (*see* middle cerebral artery syndrome). Occasionally, the origins of both the anterior (*see* anterior cerebral artery syndrome) and middle cerebral arteries are occluded at the top of the carotid artery. Symptoms consistent with both syndromes result.

intestinal ischemia: Results from embolic occlusions of the visceral branches of the abdominal aorta, generally in people with valvular heart disease, atrial fibrillation, or left ventricular thrombus. Symptoms include acute abdominal cramps or steady epigastric or periumbilical abdominal pain combined with high leukocyte count. It is sometimes called *intestinal angina* as it is the result of atherosclerotic plaque-induced ischemia. Intermittent back pain at the thoracolumbar junction, particularly with exertion, is also a common complaint.

intracerebral hemorrhage: It is bleeding from an arterial source into brain parenchyma (therefore is often referred to as an *interparenchymal hemorrhage*) and is widely regarded as the most deadly of stroke subtypes. It is characterized by spontaneous bleeding in the absence of an identifiable precipitant and usually associated with hypertension and/or aging.

irritable bowel syndrome (IBS): A group of symptoms that represent the most common disorder of the gastrointestinal system. IBS is referred to as *nervous indigestion, functional dyspepsia, spastic colon, nervous colon,* and *irritable colon,* but because of the absence of inflammation, it should not be confused with colitis or other inflammatory diseases of the intestinal tract. IBS is a functional disorder of motility as a response to diet or stress.

ischemic heart disease: Narrowing or blockage of the coronary arteries causing ischemia in the heart muscle supplied by that artery. Infarction may result (*see also* coronary heart [artery] disease).

Kaposi's sarcoma (KS): A malignancy of angiopoietic tissue that presents as a skin lesion. Growth of this tumor is promoted with a suppressed immune system and is an opportunistic infection associated with AIDS. It is characterized by raised, nontender, purplish lesions.

Kawasaki disease: A cardiovascular pathology also known as *mucocutaneous lymph node syndrome*, it is an acute systemic vasculitis that can occur in any ethnic group but seems most prevalent in Asian populations. There is extensive inflammation of the arterioles, venules, and capillaries initially, then progressing to the main coronary arteries and larger veins. Vessels develop scarring, intimal thickening, calcification, and formation of thrombi. This syndrome is characterized by high fever, swollen lymph nodes in the neck, rashes, irritated eyes and mucous membranes, with damage to the cardiovascular system. Synonym: Kawasaki's syndrome.

keratitis: Inflammation of the cornea.

Klebsiella pneumoniae: An organism closely similar to *Aerobacter aerogenes*, but occurring in patients/clients with lobar pneumonia and other infections of the respiratory tract.

Klinefelter's syndrome: Syndrome characterized by the presence of an extra X chromosome in males causing failure to develop secondary sex characteristics, enlarged breasts, poor musculature development, and infertility.

Klippel-Feil syndrome: Condition in which one or more vertebrae are fused together in the neck area, causing shortening of the cervical spine.

Korsakoff's psychosis: A chronic subcortical disorder caused by prolonged vitamin B_1 deficiency, which is usually caused by alcoholism.

kyphoscoliosis: Also called *Scheuermann's disease*, *juvenile kyphosis*, and *vertebral epiphysitis*, it is a condition of anteroposterior curvature of the spine affecting adolescents between the ages of 12 and 16. Growth retardation or vascular disturbance in the vertebral epiphyses are the two most common theories of pathogenesis of this structural deformity. This condition can also develop with advancing age and is associated with osteoporosis, endocrine disorders, Paget's disease, tuberculosis, poor posture, osteochondritis, and disk degeneration.

lacunar syndrome: Lacunar syndrome appears when a stroke (CVA) occurs in the deep areas of the brain and is representative of the area of infarct in which the lacunae are predominant. If the posterior limb of the internal capsule is affected, a pure motor deficit may result; in the anterior limb of the internal capsule, weakness of the face and dysarthria may occur. If the posterior thalamus is affected, there is a pure sensory stroke. When the lacunae occur predominantly in the pons, ataxia, clumsiness, and weakness may be seen.

Laënnec's cirrhosis: Alcoholic cirrhosis (*see* cirrhosis).

Landau-Kleffner syndrome: Acquired epileptic aphasia characterized by an acquired aphasia secondary to epileptic seizures in the absence of other neurological abnormalities.

lateral sclerosis: A rare form of involvement in ALS that results in neuronal loss in the cortex. Signs of corticospinal tract involvement include hyperactivity of tendon reflexes with spasticity causing difficulty in active movement. Weakness and spasticity of specific muscles represent the level and progression of the disease along the corticospinal tracts. There is no muscle atrophy, and fasciculations are not present.

Legg-Calvé-Perthes disease: Also known as *coxa plana* and *osteochondritis deformans juvenilis*, this disease is avascular necrosis of the proximal femoral epiphysis with flattening of the head of the femur caused by vascular interruption and ischemic necrosis (affects boys aged 3 to 12).

legionnaires' disease: An acute respiratory infection, often with pneumonia, caused by bacteria (*Legionella pneumophila*) that may contaminate water or soil. It was named after an outbreak of the illness at an American Legion convention in July 1976.

Lennox-Gastaut syndrome: A syndrome that occurs with epilepsies of infancy and childhood usually between ages 1 and 6 years of age. The most common seizures are atonic-akinetic, resulting in loss of postural tone. Violent falls occur suddenly with immediate recovery and resumption of activity, the attack lasting less than 1 second. Tonic attacks consist of sudden flexion of the head and trunk and consciousness is clouded.

leukemia: A malignant neoplasm of the blood-forming cells, specifically replacement of the bone marrow by a malignant clone (genetically identical cell) of lymphocytic or granulocytic cells. Acute leukemia is an accumulation of neoplastic, immature lymphoid, or myeloid cells in the bone marrow and peripheral blood; tissue invasion by these cells; and associated bone marrow failure. Chronic leukemia is a neoplastic accumulation of mature lymphoid or myeloid elements of the blood that usually progresses more slowly than an acute leukemic process.

leukocytosis: A condition in which there is an increase in number of leukocytes (above $10,000/mm^3$) in the blood, generally caused by the presence of infection. Leukocytosis may occur in response to bacterial infections, inflammation or tissue necrosis, metabolic intoxication, neoplasms, acute hemorrhage, splenectomy, acute appendicitis, pneumonia, intoxication by chemicals, or acute rheumatic fever. It may also occur as a normal protective response to physiologic stressors, such as strenuous exercise; emotional changes; temperature changes; anesthesia; surgery; pregnancy; and some drugs, toxins, and hormones.

leukopenia: A reduction of the number of leukocytes in the blood (below 5000/μL), which is caused by a variety of factors, such as anaphylactic shock and systemic lupus erythematosus, bone marrow failure associated with radiation therapy, dietary deficiencies, and in autoimmune diseases.

limbic lobe syndrome: Central nervous system disorder involving primary emotions (ie, those associated with pain, pleasure, anger, and fear).

lupus erythematosus: A chronic inflammatory disorder of connective tissues. It can result in several forms, including discoid lupus erythematosus (DLE), which affects only the skin, and systemic lupus erythematosus (SLE), which affects multiple organ systems, including the skin, and can be fatal (*see* discoid lupus erythematosus and systemic lupus erythematosus).

Lyme disease: An infectious multisystemic disorder caused by a spiral-shaped form of bacteria. It is carried by a deer tick. Initially, flu-like symptoms accompanied by a rash appear, followed by skin lesions that resemble a raised, red circle with a clear center, called *erythema migrans* or *bull's-eye rash*, often at the site of the tick bite. Within a few days the infection spreads, more lesions erupt, and a migratory, ring-like rash, conjunctivitis, or diffuse urticaria (hives) occur. Malaise and fatigue are constant and symptoms include headache, fever, chills, achiness, and regional lymphadenopathy. Lyme disease can progress to include neurologic abnormalities (meningoencephalitis with peripheral and cranial neuropathy, abnormal skin sensations, insomnia and sleep disorders, memory loss, difficulty concentrating, and hearing loss) and cardiac involvement (fluctuating atrioventricular heart block; irregular, rapid, or slowed heart beat; chest pain; fainting; dizziness; and shortness of breath). Ultimately, the end stage leads to joint changes characteristic of rheumatoid arthritis.

lymphedema: This is not a disease but a symptom of lymphatic transport malfunction that results in an accumulation of lymphatic and edema fluid. Primary lymphedema is defined as impaired lymphatic flow owing to congenital malformation of the lymphatic vessels. Secondary lymphedema is acquired and most common, resulting from surgical removal of the lymph nodes, fibrosis secondary to radiation, and traumatic injury to the lymphatic system.

malabsorption syndrome: This is a group of disorders (celiac disease, cystic fibrosis, Crohn's disease, chronic pancreatitis, pancreatic carcinoma, pernicious anemia) characterized by reduced intestinal absorption of dietary components and excessive loss of nutrients in the stool.

malignant melanoma: A neoplasm of the skin originating from melanocytes or cells that synthesize the pigment melanin. The melanomas occur most frequently in the skin but can also be found in the oral cavity, esophagus, anal canal, vagina, meninges, or within the eye.

Mallory-Weiss syndrome: A laceration of the lower end of the esophagus associated with bleeding. The most common cause is severe retching and vomiting as a result of alcohol abuse; eating disorders, such as bulimia; or in the case of a viral syndrome.

manic depressive disorder: Also called *bipolar disorder*, it is characterized by cyclical mood swings that often include intense outbursts of high energy and activity, elevated mood, a decreased need for sleep, and a flight of ideas (mania) followed by extreme depression. The cause is a biochemical dysfunction.

Marfan syndrome: A hereditary disorder characterized by abnormalities of the blood circulation and the eyes, abnormally long bones of the limbs, and very mobile joints.

Meniere's disease: A disorder of the labyrinth of the membranous inner ear function that can cause devastating hearing and vestibular symptoms. Deficits are related to volume and pressure changes within closed fluid systems. It leads to progressive loss of hearing, characterized by ringing in the ear, dizziness, nausea, and vomiting.

meningitis: Infection of the cerebrospinal fluid within the cranium and spinal cord; meninges of the brain and spinal cord become inflamed. Early features include fever and headache. The cardinal signs are a stiff and painful neck with pain in the lumbar areas and posterior aspects of the thigh. Meningitis may produce damage to the cerebral cortex, which may affect motor function, sensation, and perception, as well as other areas of the central nervous system. Meningitis is almost always a complication of another infection and can be caused by a wide variety of organisms.

meningocele: Hernial protrusion of the meninges through a defect in the vertebral column; a form of spina bifida consisting of a sac-like cyst of meninges filled with spinal fluid. External protrusion of the meninges due to failure of neural tube closure of the spine.

meningomyelocele: Hernial protrusion of a sac-like cyst of meninges, spinal fluid, and a portion of the spinal cord with its nerves through a defect in the vertebral column.

middle cerebral artery syndrome (MCA): A syndrome related to occlusion of the middle cerebral artery that results in contralateral hemiplegia and hemianesthesia, or loss of movement and sensation on one half of the body. If the dominant hemisphere is affected, global aphasia, or the loss of fluency, ability to name objects, comprehend auditory information, and repeat language, is the result.

migraine: A throbbing, episodic headache that is usually confined to one side of the head. The pain associated with migraine is associated with a change in the vasculature in the brain. The pain appears to come from a complex inflammatory process of the trigeminal and cervical dorsal nerve roots that innervate the cephalic arteries and venous sinuses.

mitral regurgitation (MR): There are many possible causes of MR, but mitral valve prolapse accounts for approximately half of all cases. Regurgitation occurs when the valve does not close properly, causing blood to flow back into the heart chamber.

mitral stenosis (MS): A narrowing or constriction of the mitral valve of the heart that prevents the valve from opening fully. It may be caused by scars or abnormal deposits on the leaflets. It causes obstruction to blood flow so the left atrium must work harder to sustain cardiac output. Because the mitral valve is thickened, it opens early during diastole with a "snap" that is audible on auscultation, then closes slowly with a resultant murmur.

mitral valve prolapse (MVP): Prolapse of the mitral valve occurs when enlarged leaflets bulge backward into the left atrium. It is also called *floppy valve syndrome*, *Barlow's syndrome*, and *click-murmur syndrome*. Mitral valve prolapse appears to be the result of connective tissue abnormalities in the valve leaflets.

mononeuropathy: Injury to a single nerve; commonly a result of trauma.

multiple myeloma: Also called *plasma cell myeloma*, it is a primary malignant neoplasm of plasma cells arising most often in bone marrow. Malignant plasma cells arise from B cells that produce abnormally large amounts of one class of immunoglobulin (usually IgG, occasionally IgA). The abnormal immunoglobulin produced by the malignant transformed plasma cell is called the *M-protein*. Bone pain is the most prominent symptom.

multiple organ dysfunction syndrome: Often the final complication of critical illness. It is the progressive failure of two or more organ systems after a serious illness or injury.

multiple sclerosis (MS): A virus-induced autoimmune disease mediated by lymphocytes and macrophages, which are the cells of the immune system that trigger the demyelination of the central nervous system. It is primarily the white matter that is damaged, but lesions of the gray matter have also been found. Characterized by local inflammation, edema, and demyelination, the disease causes a significant decrease in the conduction rate of the axon.

muscle tension headache: Tension headache associated with muscle contraction occurring in response to stress.

muscular dystrophy (MD): A group of inherited, progressive neuromuscular disorders with a genetic origin characterized by ongoing symmetrical muscle wasting without neural or sensory deficits but with increasing weakness, atrophy, deformity, and disability. Paradoxically, the wasted muscles tend to hypertrophy because of connective tissue and fat deposits. There are four types: Duchenne's (pseudohypertrophic), Becker's (benign pseudohypertrophic), facioscapulohumeral (Landouzy-Dejerine), and limb-girdle dystrophy.

myalgia: Tenderness or pain in the muscles; often called *muscular rheumatism*.

myasthenia gravis (MG): Chronic progressive autoimmune disorder of striated muscles that leads to weakness in the voluntary muscles, particularly those innervated by the bulbar nucleus. A disorder of neuromuscular transmission characterized by fluctuating weakness and fatigability of skeletal muscle. It is a fundamental defect of the neuromuscular junction in which the number of acetylcholine receptors are decreased and those that remain are flattened, which results in decreased efficiency of neuromuscular transmission.

myelodysplasia: A general term used to describe defective development of any part of the spinal cord but especially of the lower spinal cord levels.

myelomeningocele: Protrusion of the meninges and spinal cord due to failure of neural tube closure.

myocardial infarction (MI): Also known as a *heart attack* or *coronary*, it is the development of ischemia with resultant necrosis of myocardial tissue. Any prolonged obstruction depriving the heart muscle of oxygen can cause an MI.

myocarditis: A relatively uncommon inflammatory condition of the muscular walls of the heart most often the result of bacterial or viral infection.

myofascial pain dysfunction: A condition marked by the presence of tender myofascial trigger points. The trigger point is viewed as more of a clinical entity than a pathologic entity.

myopathy: Involvement of muscle typically reflected by proximal weakness, wasting, and hypotonia without sensory impairment.

myositis: A rare but potentially life-threatening entity characterized by severe pain and inflammation in the affected muscle. Inflammation is the result of a streptococcal infection and is often referred to as *streptococcal myositis*.

neurapraxia: Involves segmental demyelination, which slows or blocks conduction of the action potential at the point of demyelination on a myelinated nerve. Often occurs following nerve compression that induces mild ischemia in nerve fibers.

neuropathy: Any disease of the nerves (*see* peripheral neuropathies).

neurotmesis: The complete severance of nerve fiber and its supporting endoneurium, also producing axonal loss in which the connective tissue coverings are disrupted at the site of injury (eg, gunshot or stab wounds or avulsion injuries that disrupt a section of the nerve).

neutropenia: A condition associated with a reduction in circulating neutrophils (less than 2000/mL). This may occur in severe, prolonged infections when production of granulocytes cannot keep up with demand. Neutropenia may also occur in the presence of decreased bone marrow production, such as happens with radiation, chemotherapy, leukemia, and aplastic anemia.

non-insulin-dependent diabetes mellitus (NIDDM): Diabetes associated with obesity through a negative feedback mechanism in which excessive insulin levels decrease the number of insulin receptor sites on adipose cells. The decrease in insulin receptor sites decreases the amount of glucose that can enter cells. This promotes high blood glucose levels.

obesity: A medically defined weight greater than 20% of desirable weight for adults of a given sex, body structure, and height.

orchitis: Inflammation of the testis that can be acute or chronic and associated with epididymitis.

orthostatic hypotension: The term *orthostatic* (postural) *hypotension* signifies a decrease of 20 mmHg or greater in systolic blood pressure or a drop of 10 mmHg or more of both systolic and diastolic arterial blood pressure with a concomitant pulse increase of 15 beats/min or more on standing from a supine or sitting position.

Osgood-Schlatter disease: Also called *osteochondrosis*, it results from fibers of the patellar tendon pulling small bits of immature bone from the tibial tuberosity. Osgood-Schlatter disease is considered a form of tendonitis of the patellar tendon rather than a degenerative disease.

osteoarthritis (OA): A degenerative joint disease that is a slow, progressive degeneration of joint structures due to mechanical stresses, which results in loss of mobility, chronic pain, deformity, and loss of function. Joint degeneration results from periods of inflammation of the joints in response to wear and tear stresses.

osteoblastoma: A benign tumor of the bone similar to osteoid osteoma, only larger, with a tendency to expand.

osteochondroma: The most common primary benign neoplasm of bone.

osteogenesis imperfecta: Autosomal dominant disorder that occurs in one of 30,000 births. It is characterized by increased susceptibility to fractures. Normal intelligence and possible hearing loss are associated. Sometimes referred to as *brittle bones*, it is a rare congenital disorder of collagen synthesis affecting bones and connective tissue. Clinically, occasional fractures result from brittle bone with growth retardation and long bone deformities.

osteoid osteoma: A benign vascular osteoblastic lesion that is often found in the cortex of long bones, such as the femur, near the end of disphysis. Pathologic study shows areas of immature bone surrounded by prominent osteoblasts and osteoclasts. The lesion is vascular, but no cartilage is present. The tumor can lead to joint pain and dysfunction.

osteomalacia: Softening of bone without loss of bone matrix. It is a generalized bone condition in which insufficient mineralization (deficient bone calcification) of bone matrix results from calcium and/or phosphate deficiency. Sometimes referred to as the adult form of "rickets."

osteomyelitis: An inflammation of bone caused by an infectious organism. Acute osteomyelitis is a rapidly destructive pyogenic infection. Chronic osteomyelitis is a recognized complication of treatment of open fractures.

osteonecrosis: The term *osteonecrosis* refers to the death of bone and bone marrow cellular components in the absence of infection. Avascular necrosis and aseptic necrosis are synonyms for this condition. The femoral head is most commonly affected.

osteopenia: A condition that results in the loss of bone mass, usually in isolated areas. When this condition of demineralization progresses to include the entire skeletal system, it is termed *osteoporosis.*

osteoporosis: A reduction of bone mass per unit of bone volume. Reduction in bone mass associated with loss of bone mineral and matrix occurring when bone resorption is greater than formation; found in sedentary, postmenopausal women or following steroidal therapy.

osteosarcoma: Tumors, with malignant properties, that are usually destructive lesions with abundant sclerosis both from the tumor itself and from reactive bone formation. A characteristic of osteosarcoma is the production of osteoid by malignant, neoplastic cells.

Paget's disease: Paget's disease, or osteitis deformans, is a progressive disorder of abnormal bone remodeling. Initially, excessive bone resorption occurs followed by disorganized and excessive bone formation. The disease is characterized by a greatly accelerated remodeling process in which osteoclastic resorption is massive and osteoblastic bone formation is extensive. As a result, there is an irregular thickening and softening of the bones of the skull, pelvis, and extremities. It rarely occurs in those younger than 50 years of age.

pancreatitis: A potentially serious inflammation of the pancreas that may result in autodigestion of the pancreas by its own enzymes. Acute pancreatitis is thought to result from the "escape" of activated pancreatic enzymes from acinar cells into surrounding tissues. The pathogenesis is unknown, but it may include edema or obstruction of the ampulla of Vater with resultant reflux of bile into pancreatic ducts or direct injury to the acinar cells, which allows leakage of pancreatic enzymes into pancreatic tissue.

paraneoplastic syndromes: Neurologic complications in cancer caused by three phenomena: tumor metastases to the brain; endocrine, fluid, and electrolyte abnormalities; and paraneoplastic syndromes. When tumors produce signs and symptoms at a site distant from the tumor or its metastasized sites, these "remote effects" of malignancy are collectively referred to as *paraneoplastic syndromes.* Symptoms include anorexia, malaise, diarrhea, weight loss, and fever (non-specific symptoms); necrotizing vasculitis, Raynaud's disease, arthralgia, neurologic symptoms, nephrotic syndrome, palmar fasciitis and polyarthritis, scleroderma-like changes, enteric bacteria cultured from joints, bone pain, stress fractures, digital necrosis, and subcutaneous nodules.

Parkinson's disease: A chronic progressive disease of the motor component of the central nervous system characterized by rigidity, tremor, and bradykinesia. It is a degenerative disease of the substantia nigra in the basal ganglia. Abnormal functioning in the area of the basal ganglia in the brain is referred to as *parkinsonism*. Parkinson's disease usually affects the elderly population.

pediculosis: An infestation by *Pediculus humanus*, a very common parasite infecting the head, body, and genital area. More commonly referred to as lice.

peptic ulcer disease (PUD): A break in the protective mucosal lining exposing submucosal areas to gastric secretions. The word *peptic* refers to pepsin, a proteolytic enzyme, the principal digestive component of gastric juice, which acts as a catalyst in the chemical breakdown of protein.

pericarditis: Inflammation of the pericardium.

peripheral neuropathies: Trauma, inherited disorders, environmental toxins, and nutritional disorders may affect the myelin (myelinopathy), axon (axonopathy), or cell body of a peripheral nerve, leading to loss of sensation and subsequent loss of muscle function. Symptoms occur related to the affected nerves, or in many conditions, such as diabetic neuropathy, the pattern of loss is distal and in a sock-like or glove-like pattern.

peripheral vascular disease: Diseases affecting the peripheral blood vessels, including inflammatory diseases (eg, polyarteritis, arteritis, allergies, Kawasaki's disease, Buerger's disease), occlusive disorders (eg, arteriosclerosis, thromboangiitis obliterans, arterial thrombosis or embolism), venous disorders (eg, thrombophlebitis, varicose veins, chronic venous insufficiency), and vasomotor dysfunction (eg, Raynaud's disease, reflex sympathetic dystrophy).

peritonitis: Inflammation of the serous membrane lining the walls of the abdominal cavity caused by a number of situations that introduce microorganisms into the peritoneal cavity.

pervasive developmental disorder (PDD): Severe and pervasive impairment in the development of reciprocal social interaction or verbal and nonverbal communication skills, or when stereotyped behavior, interest, and activities are present, but the criteria do not allow to categorize features under autistic, Rett, childhood disintegrative, or Asperger's disorders.

phenylketonuria (PKU): Disorder in which a metabolic error occurs when an enzyme fails to convert phenylalanine to tyrosine, resulting in the accumulation of phenylalanine in the blood, causing mental retardation.

Pick's disease: A rare form of dementia involving the frontal and temporal regions of the cortex. Symptoms include prominent apathy, as well as memory disturbances, increased carelessness, poor personal hygiene, and decreased attention span. Often severe emotional displays of anxiety and agitation accompany this disease of the brain.

pickwickian syndrome: The complex of exogenous obesity, somnolence, hypoventilation, and erythrocytosis. Named after an obese character in a Dickens novel.

pleural effusion: The collection of fluid in the pleural space (between the membrane encasing the lung and the membrane lining the thoracic cavity) where there is normally only a small amount of fluid to prevent friction as the lung expands and deflates.

pleurisy: An inflammation of the pleura caused by infection, injury (eg, rib fracture), or tumor. It is often a complication of pneumonia but can also be secondary to tuberculosis, lung abscesses, influenza, systemic lupus erythematosus, rheumatoid arthritis, or pulmonary infarction.

pneumoconiosis: A group of lung diseases resulting from inhalation of particles of industrial substances, particularly inorganic dusts such as that of iron ore or coal with permanent deposition of substantial amount of such particles in the lung ("dusty lungs"). Common pneumoconiosis include coal worker's pneumoconiosis, silicosis, and asbestosis. Other types of pneumoconiosis include talc, beryllium lung disease, aluminum pneumoconiosis, cadmium's worker's disease, and siderosis (inhalation of iron or other metallic particles).

***Pneumocystis carinii* pneumonia:** A progressive, often fatal pneumonia that represents the most frequently occurring opportunistic infection in persons with AIDS.

pneumonia: An inflammation affecting the parenchyma of the lungs. It can be caused by bacterial, viral, or mycoplasmal infection; inhalation of toxic or caustic chemicals, smoke, dusts, or gases; or aspiration of food, fluids, or vomitus. It often follows influenza.

pneumothorax (Ptx): An accumulation of air or gas in the pleural cavity caused by a defect in the visceral pleura or chest walls. The result is the collapse of the lung on the affected side.

poliomyelitis: Inflammation of the gray matter of the spinal cord resulting in paralysis, atrophy of muscles, and deformities.

polyarteritis nodosa: Refers to a condition consisting of multiple sites of inflammatory and destructive lesions in the arterial system; the lesions are small masses of tissue in the form of nodes or projections (nodosum). The cause is unknown, although hepatitis B is present in 50% of cases, and polyarteritis occurs more commonly among intravenous drug abusers and other groups who have a high prevalence of hepatitis B.

polycythemia vera: Also known as *erythrocytosis*, it is a neoplastic disease of the bone marrow stem cell primarily affecting the erythroid cells, which produce erythrocytes, but causing overproduction of all three hematopoietic cell lines. It is characterized by an excessive number of erythrocytes, leading to an increased concentration of hemoglobin, increased hematocrit (measure of the volume of packed RBCs), and an increased hemoglobin level.

polymyalgia rheumatica: A disorder marked by diffuse pain and stiffness that primarily affects the shoulder and pelvic girdle musculature.

polymyositis: A diffuse, inflammatory myopathy that produces symmetrical weakness of striated muscle, primarily the proximal muscles of the shoulder and pelvic girdle, neck, and pharynx.

polyneuropathy: *See* peripheral neuropathies. Indicates involvement of several peripheral nerves.

polyp: A growth or mass protruding into the intestinal lumen from any area of mucous membrane.

polyradiculitis: Injury that affects several nerve roots and occurs when infections create an inflammatory response.

polyradiculoneuropathy: Inflammatory breakdown of myelin usually associated with motor and sensory deficits (*see* Guillain-Barré syndrome).

polyuria: A cardinal sign of diabetes, polyuria is excessive urination. The pathophysiologic basis is that water is not reabsorbed from renal tubules because of osmotic activity of glucose in the tubules.

portal hypertension: An abnormally high blood pressure in the portal venous system of the liver, occurring commonly in conditions such as cirrhosis, as a result of obstruction of portal blood flow.

posterior cerebral artery syndrome (PCA): When the proximal posterior cerebral artery is occluded, including penetrating branches, the area of the brain that is affected is the subthalamus, medial thalamus, and ipsilateral (same side) cerebral peduncle and midbrain. Signs include thalamic syndrome, including loss of pain and temperature (superficial sensation) and proprioception and touch (deep sensation). This may develop into intractable, searing pain, which can be incapacitating.

posterior cord syndrome: This is an extremely rare syndrome secondary to injury of the spinal cord. Motor function, pain, and light touch sensation are preserved. There is loss of proprioception below the level of the lesion, leading to a wide-based steppage gait.

posterior inferior cerebellar artery syndrome (PICA): Blood supply to the brainstem, medulla, and cerebellum is provided by the vertebral and posterior cerebellar arteries. When infarction occurs in the posterior inferior cerebellar artery, the lateral medulla and the posteroinferior cerebellum are affected, resulting in Wallenberg's syndrome, which is characterized by vertigo, nausea, hoarseness, and dysphagia (difficulty swallowing). Other symptoms include ipsilateral ataxia (ie, uncoordinated movement), ptosis (ie, eyelid droop), and impairment of sensation in the ipsilateral portion of the face and contralateral portion of the torso and limbs.

postpolio syndrome (PPS): Refers to new neuromuscular symptoms that occur decades after recovery from the acute paralytic episode (average postpolio interval is 25 years).

post-traumatic stress disorder (PTSD): Development of characteristic symptoms following exposure to an extreme traumatic stressor involving direct personal experience of an event that involves actual or threatened death or serious injury, or other threat to one's physical integrity; or witnessing an event that involves death, injury, or threat to someone else. Symptoms include intense fear, helplessness, or horror.

Pott's disease: Vertebral tuberculosis (TB).

Prader-Willi syndrome: Characterized by severe obesity; mental retardation; and small hands, feet, and genitalia. In infancy, problems with poor tone, feeding, and body temperature control are common. Over 50% of Prader-Willi children have a deletion of a chromosome.

pressure ulcer: A lesion caused by unrelieved pressure resulting in damage to the underlying tissue. Pressure ulcers usually occur over bony prominences and are graded or staged to classify the degree of tissue damage observed.

primary ciliary dyskinesia (PCD): PCD is an inherited, relatively rare condition associated with an abnormality of cilia, which may affect the lungs, sinuses, and ears. The mainstay of treatment is chest physical therapy. The condition involves recurrent infections of nose, ears, sinuses, and lungs. If untreated, it can lead to bronchiectasis, sinusitis, dextrocardia, and situs inversus.

prostatitis: Inflammation of the prostate gland, which can be acute or chronic and bacterial or nonbacterial.

pseudobulbar palsy: *See* amyotrophic lateral sclerosis (ALS).

psoriasis: A chronic, inherited recurrent inflammatory dermatosis characterized by well-defined erythematous plaques covered with a silvery scale.

psoriatic arthritis: A form of arthritis that differs from rheumatoid arthritis in that it more frequently involves the distal interphalangeal joints, asymmetrical distribution, and the presence of spondyloarthropathy. Joints are less tender, although pain and stiffness are increased by periods of immobility.

pulmonary edema: Also called *pulmonary congestion*, it is an excessive fluid build-up in the lungs, which may accumulate in the interstitial tissue, in the air spaces (alveoli), or in both. Pulmonary edema is a complication of many disease processes.

pulmonary embolism: The lodging of a blood clot in a pulmonary artery with subsequent obstruction of blood supply to the lung parenchyma.

pulmonary fibrosis: An excessive amount of fibrous or connective tissue in the lung, predominantly fibroblasts and small blood vessels, that progressively remove and replace normal tissue. Categorized as a restrictive lung disease.

pulmonary hypertension: High blood pressure in the pulmonary arteries defined as a rise in pulmonary artery pressure of 5 to 10 mmHg above normal (normal is 15 to 18 mmHg).

pyelonephritis: An infectious, inflammatory disease involving the kidney parenchyma and renal pelvis. Typically related to a bacterial infection.

pyloric stenosis: An obstruction at the pyloric sphincter (ie, the sphincter at the distal opening of the stomach into the duodenum).

pyoderma: Any purulent (containing or forming pus) skin disease.

rachischisis: Congenital fissure of the vertebral column; seen in spina bifida.

radiculoneuropathy: Indicates involvement of the nerve root as it emerges from the spinal cord.

Raynaud's disease/phenomenon: Intermittent episodes of small artery or arteriole constriction of the extremities causing temporary pallor and cyanosis of the digits and changes in skin temperature is called *Raynaud's phenomenon*. These episodes occur in response to cold temperature or strong emotions, such as anxiety or excitement. When this condition is a primary vasospastic disorder, it is called *Raynaud's disease*. If the disorder is secondary to another disease or underlying cause, the term *Raynaud's phenomenon* is used.

rectocele: Herniation of the rectum into the vagina.

reflex sympathetic dystrophy (RSD): Differentiation syndrome with autonomic nerve changes. Sympathetic dysfunction of the extremity following trauma, nerve injury, or central nervous system disorder; usually occurs secondary to a preexisting condition. For instance, adhesive capsulitis in the shoulder is often accompanied by vasomotor instability of the hand and known as *reflex sympathetic dystrophy* (formerly known as *shoulder-hand syndrome*). This condition is characterized by severe pain, swelling, and trophic skin changes of the hand (eg, thinning and shininess of the skin with loss of wrinkling, sometimes with increased hair growth). Skin and subcutaneous tissue atrophy and tendon flexion contractures develop.

Reiter's syndrome: One of the most common reactive arthritic conditions. Reactive arthritis is defined as a sterile inflammatory arthropathy distant in time and place from the initial inciting infectious process. Reiter's syndrome usually follows venereal disease or an episode of bacillary dysentery and is associated with typical extra-articular manifestations of arthritis.

renal calculi: Urinary stone disease is a common urinary tract disorder and can result from sex, age, geography, climate, diet, genetics, and environmental factors. Pathologically, there is an increased risk of stone formation due to the urine being super-saturated with calcium, salts, uric acid, magnesium ammonium phosphate, or cystine.

renal cystic disease: A renal cyst is a cavity filled with fluid or renal tubular elements making up a semisolid material. The presence of these cysts can lead to degeneration of renal tissue and obstruction of tubular flow.

renal failure: *See* chronic renal failure.

restrictive lung disease: A major category of pulmonary problems including any condition that limits lung expansion. Pulmonary function tests are characterized by a decrease in lung volume or total lung capacity.

Rett syndrome: Disorder characterized by the development of multiple specific deficits following a period of normal functioning at birth. There is a loss of previously acquired purposeful hand skills between ages 5 and 30 months, with the subsequent development of characteristic stereotyped hand movements resembling hand wringing or hand washing. Problems develop in the coordination of gait or trunk movements. There is also severe impairment in expressive and receptive language development, with severe psychomotor retardation.

Reye's syndrome: Illness that occurs following a viral infection. It is characterized by vomiting and brain dysfunction, such as disorientation, lethargy, and personality disorder, and may progress into coma. It usually affects children and teenagers.

rheumatic fever: One form of endocarditis (ie, infection of the heart) caused by streptococcal group A bacteria. It can be fatal or may lead to rheumatic heart disease, a chronic condition caused by scarring and deformity of the heart valves. It is called rheumatic fever because the two most common symptoms are fever and joint pain.

rheumatoid arthritis (RA): A chronic, systemic inflammatory disease of the joints. Chronic polyarthritis perpetuates a gradual destruction of joint tissues and can result in severe deformity and disability. Pathologically, the indicator of rheumatoid arthritis is a positive rheumatoid factor (antibodies that react with immunoglobulin antibodies found in the blood and in the synovium). Interaction between rheumatoid factor and the immunoglobulin triggers events that initiate an inflammatory reaction. It typically involves the joints of the fingers, hands, wrists, and ankles. Often the hips, knees, and shoulders are severely affected. As a systemic disease, it can affect the juncture at any articulation (eg, ribs to vertebrae, scapula to clavicle). The joints are affected symmetrically, and there is a considerable range of severity.

rickets: Condition affecting children characterized by soft and deformed bones resulting from inadequate calcium metabolism due to vitamin D deficiency.

right hemisphere syndrome: This syndrome, following a stroke, represents the inability to orient the body within external space and generate the appropriate motor responses. Hemineglect is a common feature of right hemisphere involvement. The individual does not respond to sensory stimuli on the left side.

sarcoidosis: A systemic disease of unknown origin involving any organ. Sarcoidosis is characterized by granulomatous inflammation present diffusely throughout the body. The lungs and lymph nodes are most commonly affected. Secondary sites include skin, eyes, liver, spleen, heart, and small bones in the hands and feet. Symptoms include dyspnea, cough, fever, malaise, weight loss, skin lesions, and erythema nodosum (multiple, tender, nonulcerating nodules).

sarcoma: Refers to a malignant tumor of mesenchymal origin.

Saturday night palsy: This is a radial nerve compression at the spiral groove of the humerus. Compression of the nerve causes segmental demyelination. Paralysis of upper extremity musculature and sensory loss is associated with the level of compression. It is also referred to as *crutch palsy*.

scabies: This is a skin eruption caused by a mite, *Sarcoptes scabiei*. The mite burrows into the skin and deposits eggs, which hatch, causing the skin eruption.

scapuloperoneal muscular dystrophy: This is a variation of facioscapulohumeral dystrophy (*see* muscular dystrophy) with involvement of the distal muscles of the lower extremities instead of the face and proximal muscles of the shoulder girdle.

Scheuermann's disease: *See* kyphoscoliosis.

sciatica: Radiculopathy in which the nerve root of the sciatic nerve is affected, most typically caused by compression. It results in low back pain with potential radiation down the back of the lower extremity consistent with the innervation of the sciatic nerve.

scleroderma: Systemic sclerosis (SS), or scleroderma, is an autoimmune disease of connective tissue characterized by excessive collagen deposition in the skin and internal organs.

scoliosis: An abnormal lateral curvature of the spine. The curvature of the spine may be to the right (more common in thoracic curves) or left (more common in lumbar curves). Rotation of the vertebral column around its axis occurs and may cause rib cage deformity. Scoliosis is often associated with kyphosis and lordosis.

septic arthritis: Osteomyelitis is one type of infection that is capable of extending into a joint and causing infection (ie, sepsis). Bacteria, viruses, and fungi can also affect the joints. Infection in the joint causes erosion of the joint capsule, leading to arthritic changes in the septic joint.

shoulder-hand syndrome: *See* reflex sympathetic dystrophy.

sickle cell anemia: A hereditary, chronic form of hemolytic anemia in which the rupture of erythrocytes (forming sickle cells) releases hemoglobin prematurely into the plasma, thereby reducing the delivery of oxygen to tissues.

sick sinus syndrome: Also called *brady-tachy syndrome*, it is a complex cardiac arrhythmia associated with coronary artery disease or drug therapy (eg, digitalis, calcium channel blockers, ß-blockers, antiarrhythmics). Sick sinus syndrome as a result of degeneration of conductive tissue necessary to maintain normal heart rhythm occurs most often among the elderly.

sleep apnea syndrome: Defined as episodes of cessation of breathing occurring at the transition from nonrapid eye movement (NREM) to rapid eye movement (REM) sleep, with repeated wakening and excessive daytime sleepiness.

somatoform disorder: The presence of physical symptoms that suggest a medical condition causing significant impairment in social, occupational, or other areas of functioning. The physical symptoms associated with somatoform disorders are not intentional or under voluntary control. It is a psychophysiologic disorder in which emotional problems or conflicts may develop physical symptoms as a means of coping.

spina bifida: Congenital malformation of the spine in which the walls of the spinal canal do not develop typically due to the lack of union between vertebrae; the degree of impairment depends on the location of the malformation. A term used to describe various forms of myelodysplasia. A defective closure of the bony encasement of the spinal cord (ie, the bony vertebral column is divided into two parts through which the spinal cord and meninges may or may not protrude). If the anomaly is not visible, the condition is called *spina bifida occulta*. If there is an external protrusion of the sac-like structure, it is called *spina bifida cystica*, which is further classified according to the extent of involvement (eg, meningocele, meningomyelocele, or myelomeningocele).

spinal cord injury (SCI): Injury to the spinal cord that results in temporary or permanent paralysis of the muscles of the limbs and the autonomic nervous system. SCI is categorized into traumatic and nontraumatic injuries. Traumatic injury is the most common and is due to a concussion, contusion, or laceration. The spinal cord is violently displaced or compressed. A concussion is an injury caused by a blow or violent shaking and results in temporary loss of function. Contusions are bruises with hemorrhage beneath the unbroken skin often associated with fractured bone segments striking the spinal cord. Laceration (ie, disruption of tissue) results from complete transection of the cord. Nontraumatic SCI is the result of tumors, infection, or bony changes in the spinal column.

spinal muscular atrophy: Also known as *Werdnig-Hoffmann disease*, it is a progressive infantile spinal muscular atrophy, and floppy infant syndrome. It is characterized by progressive weakness and wasting of muscles and is the second most common fatal autosomal recessive disorder after cystic fibrosis.

splenomegaly: The spleen's involvement in the lymphopoietic and mononuclear phagocyte systems predisposes it to multiple conditions, causing splenomegaly. The spleen becomes enlarged by an increase in the number of cellular elements, by the deposition of extracellular material, or in the presence of extracellular hemopoiesis that accompanies reactive bone marrow disorders and neoplasm.

spondylitis: *See* ankylosing spondylitis.

squamous cell carcinoma: The second most common skin cancer usually arising in sun-damaged skin, such as the rim of the ear, face, lips and mouth, and the dorsa of the hands.

staphylococcal infection: *Staphylococcus aureus* is one of the most common bacterial pathogens normally residing on the skin and easily inoculated into deeper tissues where it causes suppurative (pus formation) infections. "Staph" infections are associated with bacteremia, pneumonia, enterocolitis, osteomyelitis, food poisoning, and skin infections.

Still's disease: A form of juvenile rheumatoid arthritis characterized by systemic manifestations, including fever and rash. The rash typically appears on the trunk and extremities, leaving palms and soles unaffected. Inflammatory arthritis typically develops at some point.

streptococcal infection: *Streptococcus pyogenes* is one of the most frequent bacterial pathogens of humans and causes many diseases of diverse organ systems ranging from skin infections, to acute pharyngitis, to major-illnesses such as rheumatic fever, scarlet fever, pneumococcal pneumonia, otitis media, meningitis, and endocarditis.

stroke: Stroke, or cerebrovascular accident (CVA), is the result of thrombosis and/or embolic occlusion of a major artery in the brain, causing ischemia and death of brain tissue. An array of neurologic syndromes can result dependent on the artery occluded and the area of the brain affected (*see* middle cerebral artery syndrome, anterior cerebral artery syndrome, internal artery syndrome, posterior cerebral artery syndrome, vertebral and posterior inferior cerebellar artery syndrome, basilar artery syndrome, superior cerebellar artery syndrome, anterior inferior cerebellar artery syndrome, and lacunar syndrome). These syndromes reflect the dysfunction associated with disruption of blood flow in specific areas of the brain. The syndromes are named according to the arteries that feed the specific area.

substance abuse: Defined as the excessive use of mood-affecting chemicals that are a potential or real threat to either physical or mental health.

sudden infant death syndrome (SIDS): Rare form of death in infants ages 2 to 6 months in which the child dies mysteriously without cause.

superior cerebellar artery syndrome: Occlusion of the superior cerebellar artery results in severe ipsilateral cerebellar ataxia, nausea and vomiting, and dysarthria, which is a slurring of speech. Loss of pain and temperature in the contralateral extremities, torso, and face occurs. Dysmetria, characterized by the inability to place an extremity at a precise point in space, affects the ipsilateral upper extremity.

systemic lupus erythematosus (SLE): Sometimes referred to as *lupus*, it is a chronic inflammatory autoimmune disorder. The cause of SLE remains unknown, but evidence points to interrelated immunologic, environmental, hormonal, and genetic factors. The central immunologic disturbance is autoantibody production, which destroy the body's normal cells. Arthralgias and arthritis constitute the most common presenting manifestations.

systemic sclerosis: A diffuse connective tissue disease that causes fibrosis of the skin, joints, blood vessels, and internal organs. It is an autoimmune disorder (*see also* scleroderma).

Tay-Sachs disease: Genetic progressive disorder of the nervous system that causes profound mental retardation, deafness, blindness, paralysis, and seizures; life expectancy is 5 years.

temporal lobe syndrome: Temporal lobe syndrome involves the primary emotions (ie, those associated with pain, pleasure, anger, and fear). In this syndrome these emotions are amplified.

tendonitis: Inflammation of any tendon.

tenosynovitis: A rheumatologic condition found most often in diabetics. The is caused by accumulation of fibrous tissue in the tendon sheath and can cause aching, nodularity along the tendons, and contracture. It is most frequently associated with the flexor tendons.

thalassemia: A group of inherited chronic hemolytic anemias predominantly affecting people of Mediterranean or southern Chinese ancestry (thalassa means "sea," referring to early cases of sickle cell disease reported around the Mediterranean). Thalassemia is a sickle cell trait with clinical manifestations inclusive of defective synthesis of hemoglobin, structurally impaired RBCs, and shortened life span of erythrocytes.

thoracic outlet syndrome (TOS): A nerve entrapment syndrome caused by pressure from structures in the thoracic outlet on fibers of the brachial plexus; in addition, vascular symptoms can occur because of pressure on the subclavian artery. Chronic compression of nerves and arteries between the clavicle and first rib or impinging musculature results in edema and ischemia in the nerves. It initially creates a neurapraxia and segmental demyelination of the nerve.

thromboangiitis obliterans: *See* Buerger's disease.

thrombocytopenia: A decrease in the platelet count below 150,000/mm^3 of blood caused by inadequate platelet production from the bone marrow, increased platelet destruction outside the bone marrow, or splenic sequestration. Thrombocytopenia is a common complication of leukemia or metastatic cancer (bone marrow infiltration) and aggressive cancer chemotherapy (cytotoxic agents). Presenting symptoms are aplastic anemia and primary bleeding sites in the bone marrow and spleen and secondary bleeding occurring from small blood vessels in the skin, mucosa, and brain. Other symptoms include petechiae and/or purpura in the skin and mucosa, easy bruising, epistaxis, melena, hematuria, excessive menstrual bleeding, and gingival bleeding.

thrombocytosis: An increase in the number of circulating platelets greater than 400,000/mm^3. Overproduction of platelets is associated with conditions such as chronic nonlymphoblastic leukemia, polycythemia vera, and myelofibrosis (replacement of hematopoietic bone marrow with fibrous tissue). Blood viscosity is increased, leading to an increased risk of thrombosis or emboli.

thrombophlebitis: A partial or complete occlusion of a vein by a thrombus (clot) with secondary inflammatory reaction in the wall of the vein. It may affect the deep superficial veins.

torticollis: Torticollis means "twisted neck" and is a contracted state of the sternocleidomastoid muscle producing a bending of the head to the affected side with rotation of the chin to the opposite side.

traumatic brain injury (TBI): A closed head injury occurring when the soft tissue of the brain is forced into contact with the hard, bony, outer covering of the brain, the skull. The long-term effects associated with closed head injury vary, depending on the severity of the injury. A mild head injury occurs when there is no skull fracture or laceration of the brain. There is an altered state of consciousness though loss of consciousness does not always occur. Usually, neurologic examination is normal though postconcussive syndrome may develop, which severely limits an individual's ability to perform activities of daily living. Severe head injuries result from significant bruising and bleeding within the brain. Permanent disability cognitively and physically is often the consequence.

traumatic spinal cord injury: *See* spinal cord injury.

tricuspid atresia: A congenital heart disease in which there is a failure of the tricuspid valve to develop with a lack of communication from the right atrium to the right ventricle. Blood flows through an atrial septal defect or a patent ductus ovale to the left side of the heart and through a ventricular septal defect to the right ventricle and out to the lungs. There is complete mixing of unoxygenated and oxygenated blood in the left side of the heart, resulting in systemic desaturation and varying amounts of pulmonary obstruction.

tricuspid stenosis: Tricuspid stenosis occurs in people with severe mitral valve disease (usually rheumatic in origin) and is rare. A secondary complication is tricuspid regurgitation, which is associated with carcinoid syndrome, SLE, infective endocarditis, and in the presence of mitral valve disease. Surgical repair is more common than valvular replacement.

tuberculosis (TB): Respiratory disease caused by the tubercle bacilli. Formerly known as *consumption*, TB is an infectious, inflammatory systemic disease that affects the lungs and may disseminate to involve lymph nodes and other organs. It is caused by infection with *Mycobacterium tuberculosis* and is characterized by granulomas, caseous (resembling cheese) necrosis, and subsequent cavity formation.

Turner's syndrome: Absence of an X chromosome in females, resulting in lower amounts of estrogen and tendencies to be shorter in height, have fertility problems, and mild mental retardation or learning difficulties.

ulcerative colitis: An inflammatory intestinal tract disease with prominent erythema and ulceration affecting the colon and rectum. Inflammation and ulceration affect mucosal and submucosal layers. It is associated with mild to severe abdominal pain; chronic, severe diarrhea; bloody stools; mild to moderate anorexia; and mild to moderate joint pain.

urinary incontinence: The involuntary loss of urine that is sufficient to be a social and/or hygiene problem. There are five categories of urinary incontinence: stress incontinence is the loss of urine during activities that increase the intra-abdominal pressure, such as coughing, laughing, lifting; urge incontinence is the uncontrolled loss of urine that is preceded by an unexpected, strong urge to void; mixed or total incontinence is a combination of stress and urge incontinence; overflow incontinence is the uncontrolled loss of urine when intravesicular pressure exceeds outlet resistance, usually the result of a obstruction (eg, tumor) or neurologic symptoms; and functional incontinence, which is the functional inability to get to the bathroom or manage the clothing required to go to the bathroom.

urinary tract infection (UTI): An example of urinary tract infection affecting the lower urinary tract (ie, ureter, bladder, urethra) is cystitis. An example of urinary tract infection involving the upper urinary tract (ie, kidneys) is pyelonephritis (*see* pyelonephritis). Elderly individuals have a higher risk for this due to inactivity or immobility, which causes impaired bladder emptying; bladder ischemia resulting from urine retention; urinary overflow obstruction from renal calculi and prostatic hyperplasia; senile vaginitis; constipation; and diminished bactericidal activity of prostatic secretions. UTI is a bacterial infection with a bacteria count of greater than 100,000 organisms per mL of urine.

urticaria: An eruption of itching wheals (hives); a vascular reaction of the skin with the appearance of slightly elevated patches that are redder or paler than the surrounding skin.

uterine prolapse: The bulging of the uterus into the vagina.

varicose veins: Abnormal dilation of veins, usually the saphenous veins of the lower extremities, leading to tortuosity (twisting and turning) of the vessel, incompetence of the valves, and propensity to thrombosis.

vertebral cerebellar artery syndrome: Blood supply to the brainstem, medulla, and cerebellum is provided by the vertebral and posterior cerebellar arteries. An occlusion of the vertebral artery leading to a medial medullary infarction of the pyramid can result in contralateral hemiparesis of the arm and leg, sparing the face. If the medial lemniscus and the hypoglossal nerve fibers are involved, loss of joint position sense and ipsilateral tongue weakness can occur. The edema associated with cerebellar infarction can cause sudden respiratory arrest due to raised intracranial pressure in the posterior fossa. Gait unsteadiness, dizziness, nausea, and vomiting may be the only early symptoms.

vestibular dysfunction: Lesions of the vestibular system that cause dizziness, lightheadedness, disequilibrium, nystagmus (rhythmic eye movements), abnormalities of saccadic eye movements (fast eye movements), oscillopsia (illusion of environmental movement), and diminished vestibulospinal reflexes. Lesions of the vestibular system can be broadly categorized into five anatomic sites: the vestibular end organ and vestibular nerve terminals, the vestibular ganglia and nerve within the internal auditory canal, the cerebellopontine angle, the brainstem and cerebellum, and the vestibular projections to the cerebral cortex. The causes are varied and include bacterial infection, viral infection, vascular disease, neoplasia, trauma, metabolic disorders, and toxic drugs.

Vogt's disease: *See* athetoid cerebral palsy.

von Recklinghausen's disease: Multiple neurofibromata of nerve sheaths that occur along peripheral nerves and on spinal and cranial nerve roots. The area over the tumor may be hyperpigmented. Symptoms may be completely absent or may be those of pain due to pressure on spinal cord and nerves.

Wallenberg's syndrome: *See* posterior inferior cerebellar artery syndrome.

wallerian degeneration: Anterograde (distal) degeneration of the axon (unlike segmental demyelination which leaves the axon intact as myelin breaks down).

Weber's syndrome: When a third cranial nerve palsy occurs with contralateral hemiplegia. Paralysis of oculomotor nerve on one side with contralateral spastic hemiplegia is referred to as *Weber's paralysis*.

Wernicke's aphasia: Infarct to a specific area of the brain that severely affects the person's level of comprehension. The person is able to visualize but is frequently nonfunctional. Usually involves a vitamin deficiency of vitamin B_1 and vitamin B_{12}.

Williams syndrome: Syndrome caused by a genetic defect, characterized by cardiovascular problems, high blood calcium levels, mental retardation, developmental delays, and a "little pixie face" with puffy eyes and a turned-up nose.

Wilms' tumor: Wilms' tumor is a nephroblastoma and is the most common malignant neoplasm in children. The tumor appears to be fleshy but may have areas of necrosis that lead to cavity formation. The most common presenting feature is a large abdominal mass and abdominal pain. Hematuria may occur, as well as hypertension, anorexia, nausea, and vomiting.

Wilson's disease: Also known as *hepatolenticular degeneration*, it is a progressive disease inherited as an autosomal recessive trait that produces a defect in the metabolism of copper, with accumulation of copper in the liver, brain, kidney, cornea, and other tissues. The disease is characterized by the presence of Kayser-Fleischer rings around the iris of the eye (from copper deposition), cirrhosis of the liver, and degenerative changes in the brain, particularly the basal ganglia.

xeroderma: A mild form of ichthyosis; excessive dryness of the skin.

BIBLIOGRAPHY

American Physical Therapy Association. Guide to physical therapy practice. *J Am Phys Assoc*. 1997;77(11).

Bottomley JM, Lewis CB. *Geriatric Rehabilitation: A Clinical Approach*. 2nd ed. Upper Saddle River, NJ: Prentice Hall Publishers; 2003.

Goodman CC, Boissonnault WG. *Pathology: Implications for the Physical Therapist*. Philadelphia, Pa: WB Saunders; 1998.

International Classification of Diseases: Clinical Modification. 9th rev. New York, NY: World Health Organization; 1997.

Tan JC. *Physical Medicine and Rehabilitation: Diagnostics, Therapeutics, and Basic Problems*. St. Louis, Mo: Mosby-Year Book; 1998.

Thomas CL. *Taber's Cyclopedic Medical Dictionary*. 18th ed. Philadelphia, Pa: FA Davis; 1997.

Physical Therapy Tests and Measures

TESTS AND MEASURES

- Muscle Strength
- Joint Range of Motion
- Cardiovascular and Pulmonary Function
- Pain Assessment
- Neuromuscular System
- Neurophysiologic Assessment
- Motor Control
- Sensory Testing
- Balance Assessment
- Gait Assessment
- Measures of Intelligence
- Levels of Consciousness
- Mental Status/Cognitive Disability Measures
- Depression
- Developmental and Neonatal Assessment
- Pediatric Assessment of Function
- Self-Perception Examinations
- Functional Assessment
- Elders and Caregivers Assessment
- Work Assessment
- Environmental Evaluation
- Orthopedic Examination (by Body Part)

MUSCLE STRENGTH

dynamic tests: Isokinetic testing uses an electromechanical device that prevents a moving body segment from exceeding a preset angular speed. The axis of the device is aligned with the anatomic axis of the joint that is being tested, and the lever arm is attached to the subject's limb (eg, Cybex, Lido, Kinetron). Isokinetic tests measure torque, work, and power.

hand-held dynamometer (HHD): A hand-held device that incorporates spring scales or strain gauges to measure applied force in kilograms or pounds. For hand strength testing, two devices are in common clinical use: grip strength (eg, Jamar dynamometer, Nicholas dynamometer) and pinch meters (eg, TEC).

manual muscle test (MMT): Standard positions that attempt to isolate muscle function are employed while resistance to motion is applied throughout the range or at a specific point in the range (break test). The muscle is graded numerically, descriptively, or by percentage grades.

modified sphygmomanometer (SM): Instrumented muscle test used to quantify the resistance used during a manually resisted isometric contraction (eg, blood pressure cuff).

trunk testing: Trunk testing devices include measurement of isometric and dynamic trunk strength. Similar to the electro-mechanical devices used for dynamic tests, trunk testing is helpful in functional strength tests of trunk musculature (eg, Cybex, Lido, Kin-Com, B-200, etc).

Bibliography

Andersson GBJ. Methods and application of functional muscle testing. In: Weinstein JL, ed. *Clinical Efficacy and Outcome in the Diagnosis and Treatment of Low Back Pain*. New York, NY: Raven Press; 1992:93-99.

Daniels L, Worthingham C. *Muscle Testing: Technique of Manual Examination*. 5th ed. Philadelphia, Pa: WB Saunders; 1986.

Hislop HJ, Perrine JJ. The isokinetic concept of exercise. *Phys Ther*. 1967;47(2):114-117.

Kendall FP, McCreary EK, Provance PG. *Muscle Testing and Function*. 4th ed. Baltimore, Md: Williams and Wilkins; 1993.

JOINT RANGE OF MOTION

attraction methods: Procedure using a tape measure to record a decrease in distance between two points marked on the skin over the spine as it extends.

distraction methods: Procedure using a tape measure to record an increase in distance between two points marked on the skin as the spine flexes.

goniometer: A device with an axis, which is aligned with the axis of the joint being measured, and two long arms, which are aligned with standard landmarks along the moving segments of the extremity.

gravity protractor: A fluid-filled disk or a disk-shaped weighted needle indicator that measures the plane and range of motion based on the fluid or needle movement. A device commonly used in carpentry.

modified Schöber technique: Skin distraction-attraction method using a midline point 5 cm below the lumbosacral junction and a point 10 cm above it.

pelvic inclinometer: A device, designed with calipers with a mounted gravity protractor, able to measure the change in position of two separate points by the placement of either end of the calipers over an identifiable area used as a landmark.

pendulum goniometer: Goniometer usually made of metal with two movement arms. One arm is allowed to move freely in accordance with the line of gravity and is used as a vertical reference.

spinal inclinometer: A circular, fluid-filled disk with a weighted needle indicator, which is maintained in the vertical, that is placed over the spine and used to measure range of motion in degrees as the spine moves.

3-Space Isotrak: An electromagnetic device for measurement of three-dimensional movements.

Bibliography

American Academy of Orthopedic Surgeons. *Joint Motion Method of Measuring and Recording*. Chicago, Ill: Authors; 1965.

Batti'e M, Bigos S, Sheely A, Wortley M. Spinal flexibility and factors that influence it. *Phys Ther*. 1987;69(12):1025-1033.

Boone DC, Azen SP, Lin C, Spence C, Baron C, Lee L. Reliability of goniometric measurements. *Phys Ther*. 1978;58(11):1355-1360.

Cave ER, Roberts SM. A method for measuring and recording joint function. *J Bone Joint Surg*. 1936;18:455-465.

Gajdosik RL, Bohannon RW. Clinical measurement of range of motion review of goniometry emphasizing reliability and validity. *Phys Ther*. 1987;67(12):1867-1872.

Miller PJ. Assessment of joint motion. In: Rothstein JM, ed. *Measurement in Physical Therapy*. New York, NY: Churchill Livingstone; 1985:103-136.

Miller SA, Mayer T, Cox R, Gatchel RJ. Reliability problems associated with the modified Schöber technique for true lumbar flexion measurement. *Spine*. 1992;17:345-348.

Moore ML. The measurement of joint motion: Part I—introductory review of the literature. *Physical Therapy Review*. 1949;29:195-205.

Moore ML. The measurement of joint motion: Part II—the technique of goniometry. *Physical Therapy Review*. 1949;29:256-264.

Petherick M, Rheault W, Kimble S, Lechner C, Senear V. Concurrent validity and intertester reliability of universal and fluid-based goniometers for active elbow range of motion. *Phys Ther*. 1988;68:966-969.

CARDIOVASCULAR AND PULMONARY FUNCTION

Balke protocol: A treadmill test in which there is a constant speed of 3.0 mph with the grade starting at 0% and increased by 3.5% every 2 minutes. Used for individuals with impaired pulmonary or cardiovascular function.

bicycle test: A test using a bicycle ergometer set at a specific workload (ie, watts or kg/min). Workload is gradually increased based on patient/client response.

blood pressure: Resting and exercise measurements of blood pressure measure the cardiovascular response to activity.

Bruce protocol: A treadmill test with the speed initially at 1.7% and the grade at 10%, gradually increasing in seven stages every 3 minutes. Used for relatively fit individuals to test all systems' response to exercise.

Buerger-Allen test: Measures the time it takes for blood to fill the lower extremity vessels when legs go from a horizontal to dependent position and the time it takes for blood to drain from the legs when they are elevated. A measure used in rating peripheral vascular involvement.

chair step test: A progressive test with four levels or stages conducted sitting by placing feet on increasingly higher levels in a stepping fashion. Reciprocal arm movements may be added with the stepping. Vital signs are monitored.

dyspnea scale: A scale that has the individual subjectively rate the sensation of difficulty breathing during exercise.

functional exercise test: The measurement of vital signs during activities of daily living.

graded exercise test: Physical performance of measured, incremental workloads with measurement of physiologic response. Used to assess physiologic response to exercise stress for determination of cardiac and respiratory status.

heart rate: The easiest way to monitor cardiovascular responses to activity. There is a linear relationship between heart rate, the intensity of aerobic exercise, and the oxygen consumption.

Korotkoff's method (test, sounds): The auscultatory method for determining blood pressure in the presence of an aneurysm. The sounds heard during auscultation of blood pressure are produced by a sudden distention of the artery (aneurysm), the walls of which were previously relaxed because of the surrounding pneumatic cuff. In aneurysm, if the blood pressure in the peripheral circulation remains fairly high while the artery above the aneurysm is compressed, the collateral circulation is good.

maximal exercise test: Maximal ability to perform exercise with large muscle groups (eg, on bike, treadmill, etc). The individual reaches his or her maximal capabilities and is not able to continue the exercise and reaches several other criteria indicating maximum exercise.

perceived exertion: A rating scale used by the exercising individual that reflects his or her perception of exercise intensity from very, very light to very, very hard.

pulmonary function tests: Measures of air flow and air flow resistance, lung volumes, and gas exchange.

pulse oximeter: Noninvasive measure of oxyhemoglobin saturation, which is the oxygen saturation of hemoglobin in arterial blood (resting normal value is generally 95% or more).

pulses: Palpation of pulses to determine their intensity from 0 (no pulse) to 1+ (diminished pulse) to 2+ (normal) to 3+ (bounding and usually visible without palpation).

respiratory rate: Counting the number of breaths per minute. Resting rate is usually 12 to 16 breaths in adults and can increase in frequency to 36 to 46 breaths per minute during maximal exercise.

submaximal exercise test: A test that ends at a predetermined endpoint, such as a heart rate of 150 beats per minute or the appearance of significant symptoms.

tidal volume and minute ventilation: Tidal volume is the volume of air breathed in one inhalation and exhalation. Minute ventilation is the product of the tidal volume times the breathing frequency.

walk test: An indirect means to measure cardiovascular endurance in the clinical setting by noting the distance walked in a fixed period of time, such as 3, 6, or 12 minutes, with the individual walking as far and as fast as possible.

Bibliography

Altug Z, Hoffman JL, Martin JL. *Manual of Clinical Exercise Testing, Prescription, and Rehabilitation*. Norwalk, Conn: Appleton & Lange; 1993.

American College of Sports Medicine. *ACSM's Guidelines for Exercise Testing and Prescription*. 5th ed. Baltimore, Md: Williams and Wilkins; 1995.

Borg G. Psychophysical bases of perceived exertion. *Med Sci Sports Exer*. 1982;14:377-387.

Bruce RA, Kusami F, Hosmer D. Maximal oxygen intake and nomographic assessment of functional aerobic impairment in cardiovascular disease. *Am Heart J*. 1973;85:546-562.

Ellestad NH. *Stress Testing: Principles and Practice*. Philadelphia, Pa: FA Davis; 1979.

Englehard C, Protas EJ, Stanley R. Diurnal variations in blood pressure and walking distance in elderly nursing home residents. *Phys Ther*. 1993;73:S60.

Froelicher VF. *Manual of Exercise Testing*. 2nd ed. St. Louis, Mo: Mosby-Year Book; 1994.

McGavin CR, Cupta SP, McHardy GJR. Twelve-minute walking test for assessing disability in chronic bronchitis. *Br Med J*. 1976;1:822-826.

Mengelkock LJ, Marin D, Lawler J. A review of the principles of pulse oximetry and accuracy of pulse oximeter estimates during exercise. *Phys Ther*. 1994;74:40-49.

Montoye HJ, Kemper HCG, Saris WHM, Washburn RA. *Measuring Physical Activity and Energy Expenditure*. Champaign, Ill: Human Kinetics; 1996.

Protas EJ. Pulmonary function testing. In: Rothstein JM, ed. *Measurement in Physical Therapy*. New York, NY: Churchill-Livingstone; 1985:229-254.

Sinacore DR, Ehsani AA. Measurement of cardiovascular function. In: Rothstein JM, ed. *Measurement in Physical Therapy*. New York, NY: Churchill-Livingstone; 1985:255-280.

Smith EL, Gilligan C. Physical activity prescription for this older adult. *Physician and Sports Medicine*. 1983;11:91-101.

Ward A, Ebbeling CB, Ahlquist LE. Indirect methods for estimation of aerobic power. In: Maud PJ, Foster C, eds. *Physiological Assessment of Human Fitness*. Champaign, Ill: Human Kinetics; 1995:47-56.

PAIN ASSESSMENT

descriptor differential scale: Twelve descriptor items are presented, each centered over 21 horizontal dashes. At the extreme left dash is a minus sign, and at the extreme right dash is a plus sign. Individuals are asked to rate the magnitude of their pain in terms of each descriptor.

McGill pain questionnaire: The most widely used and thoroughly researched assessment tool for pain. The individual is asked to identify the area of pain on an anterior/posterior drawing of the body. The next part categorizes 102 words that describe different aspects of pain into 20 subclasses. The subclasses consist of words that describe sensory qualities of pain (eg, time, space, pressure, heat, etc) and affective qualities of pain (eg, tension, fear, autonomic properties, etc). The next part assesses how the pain changes over time, and the last part rates the evaluative qualities of pain (eg, intensity of the pain experience).

numerical rating scale: A scale that has the individual rate his or her perceived level of pain intensity on a numerical scale from 0 to 10 (an 11-point scale where 0 is no pain and 10 is extreme pain).

Oswestry low back pain disability questionnaire: A self-rating scale that illustrates the degree of functional impairment the individual is experiencing. It consists of 10 questions regarding pain intensity, personal care, lifting, walking, sitting, standing, sleeping, sex life, social life, and traveling.

pain discomfort scale: A scale that rates discomfort for 10 statements based on the level of agreement from 0 = "This is very untrue for me" to 4 = "This is very true for me."

pain location, body diagrams, and mapping: A front-to-back drawing of the body in which the individual is asked to color or shade areas on the drawing that correspond to areas of his or her pain.

verbal rating scale: A list of adjectives that describe different levels of pain intensity, ranging from no pain to extreme pain.

visual analogue scale: Another measure used to assess pain intensity and typically consisting of a 10- to 15-cm line, with each end anchored by one extreme of perceived pain intensity from "no pain" to "pain as bad as it could be."

Bibliography

Fairbanks J, Couper J, Davies J, O'Brien J. The Oswestry low back pain disability questionnaire. *Physiotherapy*. 1980;66(8):271-273.

Gracely RH, Kwilosz DM. The descriptor differential scale: applying psychophysical principles to clinical pain assessment. *Pain*. 1988;35:279-288.

Jensen MP, Karoly P. Self-report scales and procedures for assessing pain in adults. In: Turk DC, Melzack R, eds. *Handbook of Pain Assessment*. New York, NY: Guilford Press; 1992:131-151.

Jensen MP, Karoly P, Braver S. The measurement of clinical pain intensity: a comparison of six methods. *Pain*. 1986;27:117-126.

Jensen MP, Karoly P, Harris P. Assessing the affective component of chronic pain: development of the pain discomfort scale. *J Psychosom Res*. 1991;35(2/3):149-154.

Margolis RB, Chibnall JT, Tait RC. Test-retest reliability of the pain drawing instrument. *Pain*. 1988;3:49-51.

Melzack R. The McGill pain questionnaire: major properties and scoring methods. *Pain*. 1975;1:277-299.

Turk DC, Melzack R. The measurement of pain and the assessment of people experiencing pain. In: Turk DC, Melzack R, eds. *Handbook of Pain Assessment*. New York, NY: Guilford Press; 1992:3-12.

Neuromuscular System

electromyography: Recording of electrical activity of muscles through the use of needles or surface electrodes.

Bibliography

Hammond EJ. Electrodiagnosis of the neuromuscular system. In: Van Deusen J, Brunt D, eds. *Assessment in Occupational Therapy and Physical Therapy*. Philadelphia, Pa: WB Saunders; 1997:175-197.

Neurophysiologic Assessment

modified Ashworth scale: An objective means to assess the severity of spasticity. Involves manually moving a limb through the range to stretch specific muscle groups. The resistance encountered during the passive muscle stretch is graded on a 5-point ordinal scale from 0 to 4, with 0 representing normal tone and 4 depicting severe spasticity.

pendulum test: A test for spasticity. The subject's lower limb is extended to full extension at the knee in a sitting position. The examiner then releases the extremity and allows it to fall free. The leg swings like a pendulum before the motion is damped by the viscoelastic properties of the limb. Hypertonicity is assessed by taking the angular difference between maximum knee flexion and the angle of flexion at which the knee first reversed direction toward extension in the swing.

tendon reflexes: Slight stretching of a muscle activates the neuromuscular spindle, which sends an electrical message to the spinal cord via the large muscle spindle afferent, exciting the motor neurons and resulting in the contraction of the stretched muscle.

Bibliography

Bohannon RW, Smith MB. Interrater reliability of a modified Ashworth scale of muscle spasticity. *Phys Ther.* 1987;67(2):206-207.

Greenberg DA, Aminoff MJ, Simon RP. *Clinical Neurology.* 2nd ed. Norwalk, Conn: Appleton & Lange; 1993.

Milanov IG. Flexor reflex for assessment of common interneuron activity in spasticity. *Electromyogr Clin Neurophysiol.* 1992;32:621-629.

Motor Control

action research arm test: Used for assessing upper extremity function in individuals following a stroke, it is a hierarchically arranged evaluation of grasp, grip, pinch, and gross arm movement.

arm function test: An upper extremity assessment that includes assessment of arm and trunk movement through evaluation of performance in turning a cranked wheel. Hand function is assessed through eight functional tasks, and passive movement, muscle tone, and pain are evaluated.

Ashburn's physical assessment for stroke patients: Provides an ordinal scale, divided into three major sections: lower limb, upper limb, and balance and movement activities.

Carr and Shepherd's motor assessment scale (MAS): This scale measures motor function following stroke in eight tasks: supine to side lying onto intact side, supine to sitting over side of bed, balanced sitting, sit to stand, walking, upper arm function, hand movements, and advanced hand activities. The assumptions are that recovery is characterized by stereotyped movements in synergies and recovery proceeds in a proximal to distal sequence. Each item is scored on a 7-point scale from 0 to 6.

Fugl-Meyer assessment (FMA): An assessment scale using Brunnström's sequence of recovery as a framework in developing an ordinal scale for assessing motor performance in individuals after a stroke. This tool has five components: joint motion and pain, sensation, balance, upper extremity motor function, and lower extremity motor function.

functional test for the hemiparetic upper extremity: Assesses integrated arm and hand function through the performance of 17 standardized tasks, ordered hierarchically and graded on a pass-fail basis. Most activities are timed.

Halsted-Reitan neuropsychological battery: Battery that tests perceptual, intellectual, and motor skills and performance.

Montreal evaluation: Based on the Bobath approach to hemiplegia, this tool measures six parameters of function, each scored on a 4-point scale ranging from 0 for most severe impairment to 3 for normal performance. The functional parameters measured are mental clarity, muscle tone, reflex activity, voluntary movement, automatic reactions, and pain.

Rivermead motor assessment protocol: A motor function test that requires individuals to complete a series of functional movements in three categories: gross function, leg and trunk function, and arm function. This tool uses Guttman scaling (ie, cumulative scales that present a set of items that reflect increasing intensities of the characteristics being measured).

Bibliography

Ashburn A. A physical assessment for stroke patients. *Physiotherapy*. 1982;68:109-113.

Corriveau H, Guarna F, Dutil E, et al. An evaluation of the hemiplegic subject based on the Bobath approach. Part II: the evaluation protocol. *Scand J Rehabil Med*. 1988;20:5-11.

DeSouza LH, Langton Hewer RL, Miller S. Assessment of recovery of arm control in hemiplegic stroke patients. Arm function tests. *International Rehabil Med*. 1980;2:3-9.

Duncan PW, Badke MB. *Stroke Rehabilitation: The Recovery of Motor Control*. St. Louis, Mo: Mosby-Year Book; 1987.

Fugl-Meyer AR. Post-stroke hemiplegia: assessment of physical properties. *Scand J Rehabil Med*. 1980;7(suppl):83-93.

Guarna F, Corriveau H, Chamberland J, et al. An evaluation of the hemiplegic subject based on the Bobath approach. Part I: the model. *Scand J Rehabil Med*. 1988;20:1-4.

Lyle RC. A performance test for assessment of upper limb function in physical rehabilitation treatment and research. *Int J Rehabil Res*. 1981;4:483-492.

Wilson DJ, Baker LL, Craddock JA. Functional test for the hemiparetic upper extremity. *Am J Occup Ther*. 1984;38:159-164.

SENSORY TESTING

Bender visual motor gestalt test: Perceptual motor test developed by Bender that consists of geometric shapes.

confrontational visual testing: Evaluation for visual field deficits, such as homonymous hemianopsia or depth perception. The individual focuses on a targeted area, and a stimulus target is moved in an arc from the periphery. The individual indicates when the target stimulus comes into view. For depth perception, the individual identifies which object of the two is closer.

Disk-Criminator: A common clinical method of assessment of tactile sensibility through reports of two-point discrimination. Disk-Criminator has a set of two points placed around a disk; each set of points is a different distance apart.

pain: Assessed by randomly applying the blunt or sharp ends of a pin to the individual's skin for appropriate identification.

proprioception: Clinical testing for position sense is done by identifying the position that an extremity is placed in verbally, or repeating the position has been placed in and then taken out of, or reproducing the position of one side on the other side.

Semmes-Weinstein monofilament aesthesiometer test: Nylon filaments on rods, graded as to thickness of the filament, determine an objective level of touch-pressure sensation. The ability to feel the 4.17 filament indicates normal sensation. The ability to feel the 5.07 filament indicates the presence of protective sensation, and the inability to feel the 6.0 filament indicates a loss of sensation. Fine gradations of the filaments range between 4.17 to 6.0, so an absolute level of sensation can be determined.

temperature: Assessed by test tubes of hot and cold water applied randomly to the individual's skin.

vibration test: Traditionally, a procedure in which a tuning fork, randomly applied to bony prominences, is graded based on the report of the subject's sensitivity to the vibration of the tuning fork. The examiner starts the fork vibration, applies it to the subject, and asks the individual to indicate when the vibration stops. If vibration continues to be felt by the examiner's fingertips, but the individual reports its sensation, the vibratory sense is recorded as diminished. If vibration by the subject is not felt, it is graded absent. If both the examiner and subject report cessation of vibration at the same time (assuming the examiner's vibratory sensation is intact), it is graded as normal.

weighted touch-pressure tool: A metal capsule into which graded weights are inserted (0.5, 1.0, and 2.0 oz) to determine touch-pressure sensitivity. (Note: not as sensitive as the Semmes-Weinstein monofilaments.)

Bibliography

Bell-Krotoski J, Weinstein S, Weinstein C. Testing sensibility, including touch-pressure, two-point discrimination, point localization, and vibration. *J Hand Ther*. 1993;6:114-123.

Benton A, Sivan A, des Hamsher K, Varney N, Spreen O. *Contributions of Neuropsychological Assessment*. 2nd ed. New York, NY: Oxford University Press; 1994.

Dellon AL. A numerical grading scale for peripheral nerve function. *J Hand Ther*. 1993;6:152-160.

Van Deusen J, Jackson Foss J. Sensory deficits. In: Van Deusen J, Brunt D, eds. *Assessment in Occupational Therapy and Physical Therapy*. Philadelphia, Pa: WB Saunders; 1997:295-301.

BALANCE ASSESSMENT

Berg balance scale: A scale that measures balance and mobility during 14 functional activities. Useful in a frailer population. Graded according to ability to do independently without assistance to unable to do on a point scale.

functional reach test: With a ruler taped to a wall, the patient/client stands at the end of the ruler and reaches as far as he or she can before having to take a step to catch him- or herself. The distance along the ruler that is reached is recorded.

get-up and go: This is a test that measures balance, gait, and overall mobility. In this test, the patient/client is asked to stand up from a chair, stand still, then walk toward a wall, and before reaching the wall, turn without touching and return to the chair. Observation is made of steadiness, difficulty in getting into or out of the chair, gait, ability to turn, and strategies for accommodating for balance loss.

postural stress test: This test requires the patient/client to stand quietly and progresses to a final stage of maintaining balance while arms are extended with a weight around the wrist and then suddenly dropped.

Rhomberg: *See* sharpened Rhomberg. This test is just the standing eyes open, eyes closed portion of the subsequent test.

sharpened Rhomberg: A test of static balance with progressively difficult postures to maintain. First with the feet together, eyes open, then closed; then with feet in semi-tandem, eyes open, then closed; then in a full tandem position, eyes open, eyes closed. Both sides are tested, so it is a six-part test. Significant postural sway, a loss of balance, or the inability to stand with the eyes closed is indicative of a cerebral injury.

sternal nudge: In standing, the patient/client is pushed gently in all directions and balance strategies are observed.

Tinetti assessment tool: This tool combines assessment of balance and gait. There is a cumulative score for balance that is rated against a possible 16 total points indicative of no balance problems and is reported as a fraction (eg, 10/16). Likewise, the gait score has a high score of 12 and is reported as a fraction (eg, 8/12). A total score for balance and gait uses a fraction of N/28.

Bibliography

Bannister R, ed. *Brain's Clinical Neurology.* 6th ed. New York, NY: Oxford University Press; 1985.

Berg K, Wood-Dauphinee S, Williams J, et al. Measuring balance in the elderly: preliminary development of an instrument. *Physiother Can.* 1989;42:304-311.

Duncan PW, Weiner DK, Chandler J, et al. Functional reach: a new clinical measure of balance. *J Gerontol.* 1990;45:M192-M197.

Mathias S, Nayak USL, Isaacs B. Balance in elderly patients: the get-up and go test. *Arch Phys Med Rehabil.* 1986;67:385-389.

Tinetti ME. Performance-oriented assessment of mobility problems in elderly patients. *J Am Geriatr Soc.* 1986;34:119-126.

Wolfson L, Whipple R, Amernan P, et al. Stressing the postural response: a quantitative method for teaching balance performance. *J Am Geriatr Soc.* 1986;34:845-850.

GAIT ASSESSMENT

ambulation profiles: Clinical tests of locomotion skill or quantitative methods of assessing ambulatory function, which include standing balance, ability to negotiate turns, ability to rise from a chair, and in some profiles, cardiorespiratory or muscular endurance, along with standard gait parameters.

functional ambulation profile: A tool that is particularly useful for patients/clients who have suffered from a stroke. It measures bilateral and unilateral stance time (eyes open and eyes closed), weight transfer from one foot to the other, and ambulation efficiency.

gait abnormality rating scale (GARS): This tool was developed to detect fallers and to quantify aspects of gait patterns.

observational gait analysis (OGA): Analysis of the parameters of gait by actual in-time observation or frame-by-frame assessment using videotaped observation.

Bibliography

Criak RL, Oatis CA. *Gait Analysis: Theory and Application*. St. Louis, Mo: Mosby-Year Book; 1995.

Nelson AJ. Function ambulation profile. *Phys The*r. 1974;54:1059-1065.

Observational Gait Analysis. Downey, Calif: Los Amigos Research and Education Institute, The Pathokinesiology Service and the Physical Therapy Department, Rancho Los Amigos Medical Center; 1993.

Perry J. *Gait Analysis: Normal and Pathological Function*. Thorofare, NJ: SLACK Incorporated; 1992.

Wolfson L, Whipple R, Amerman P. Gait assessment in the elderly. A gait abnormality rating scale and its relation to falls. *J Gerontology*. 1990;45(1):M14.

MEASURES OF INTELLIGENCE

Wechsler Adult Intelligence Scale-Revised (WAIS-R): Test of general intelligence.

Wechsler Preschool and Primary Scale of Intelligence (WPPSI): Individual intelligence test of children aged 4 to 6½.

LEVELS OF CONSCIOUSNESS

Glasgow coma scale (GCS): A tool used to assess the level of consciousness following traumatic brain injury. Using this scale, three aspects of coma are observed independently: eye opening, best motor response, and verbal response. A score of 8 or less indicates coma.

levels of cognitive function scale (LCFS): Eight stages of cognitive function and recovery following a traumatic brain injury developed at Rancho Los Amigos Hospital in 1972.

Luria Nebraska neuropsychological battery: General neuropsychological assessment of brain injury based on the work of Luria.

Bibliography

Jennett B, Teasdale G. *Management of Head Injuries*. Philadelphia, Pa: FA Davis; 1981.

MENTAL STATUS/COGNITIVE DISABILITY MEASURES

Allen cognitive level test (ACL): Test that screens and assesses individual cognitive levels through performance of set tasks. Designed to provide a quick assessment of a person's ability to function based on simple to complex activities and rating of 1 to 6, where 1 is the lowest level and 6 the highest.

cognitive performance test (CPT): Assesses the functional level of a patient/client with Alzheimer's disease and is in a standardized activity of daily living format.

dementia rating scale (DRS): Measures the differences between demented individuals and normals in the areas of neurologic, behavioral, and cognitive functions. It includes 36 tasks with five subscales for attention, initiation and perseveration, construction, conceptualization, and memory.

Galveston orientation and amnesia test (GOAT): Assesses general orientation to person, place, and time and estimation of time after injury. This test has been standardized on patients/clients with closed head injury.

low cognitive level (LCL): A test designed to assess the performance of patients/clients functioning at a low level of cognition (eg, individuals with Alzheimer's or other dementia).

mental status questionnaire (MSQ): Composed of 10 questions and is easy to administer. It is used frequently in research due to its convenience.

Mini-Mental State Exam (MMSE): A mental status assessment that assesses orientation, the ability to follow verbal and written directions, attention, recall, language, reading, writing, and copying.

Myers-Briggs test: Based on Karl Jung's profile of psychological types, this test describes 16 trait combinations and their associated patterns of action.

Ranchos Los Amigos levels: Rancho Los Amigos Hospital described eight progressive levels of cognitive functioning and behavioral response, which are widely observed and referred to as no response/coma; generalized response; localized response; confused and agitated; confused, inappropriate, and nonagitated; confused and appropriate; automatic and appropriate; and purposeful and appropriate.

Bibliography

Allen CK, Allen R. Cognitive disabilities: measuring the social consequences of mental disorders. *J Clin Psychiatry.* 1987;48(5):185-190.

Folstein MF, Folstein SE, McHugh PR. Mini-Mental State: a practical method for grading the cognitive state of patients for the clinician. *J Psychiatr Res.* 1975;12:189-198.

Kahn RL, Goldfarb AL, Pollack M, et al. Brief objective measures for the determination of mental status in the aged. *Am J Psychiatry.* 1960;117:326.

Levin H, O'Donnell V, Grossman R. The Galveston Orientation and Amnesia Test: a practical scale to assess cognition after head injury. *J Nerv Ment Dis*. 1979;11:675-684.

Mattis S. *Dementia Rating Scale, Professional Manual*. Odessa, Fla: Psychological Assessment Resources Inc; 1973.

DEPRESSION

Beck depression inventory: Twenty sets of statements with a scoring mechanism from 0 to 3, which rates from no depression at 0 to progressive levels of depression to 3. A cutoff score of 13 (summing the entire set of 21) is indicative of depression.

geriatric depression scale: A 30-item, yes-or-no questionnaire in which one point for each response that matches the yes or no answer after the question is tallied. A score of 5 on this form may indicate depression.

Popoff index of depression: A good test for community-dwelling elders. There is a covert, overt, and healthy response to each of 15 statements. If an individual selects all overt answers, he or she is considered severely depressed. If the covert response is chosen most often, the individual is also considered depressed, but somatizising his or her depression in physical complaints. Healthy responses indicate the absence of depression.

Zung self-rating scale: Composed of 10 negative and 10 positive statements, with the respondent giving an answer that correlates with a 1 to 4 rating. Eighty is the highest score and most indicative of severe depression.

Bibliography

Brink T, Yesavage J, Lum D, et al. Screening tests for geriatric depression. *Clin Gerontologist*. 1982;1:37-42.

Gallagher D. The Beck depression inventory and older adults review of its development and utility. In: Brink T, ed. *Clinical Gerontology: A Guide to Assessment and Intervention*. New York, NY: Haworth Press; 1986:149-163.

Popoff S. A simple method for diagnosis of depression in geriatric medical patients. *Clin Med*. 1969;76:24-29.

Zung W, Richard D, Shrot M. Self-rating depression scale in an outpatient clinic. *Archive Geriatric Psychiat*. 1965;13:508-515.

Developmental and Neonatal Assessment

Apgar score: Evaluation of the infant's condition in terms of heart rate, respiratory effort, muscle tone, reflex irritability, and skin color at 1 and 5 minutes after birth.

assessment of premature infant behavior (APIB): Provides a comprehensive neurobehavioral assessment of premature infants. It is a standardized assessment of subsystem stability before, during, and after administration of 27 items and 19 reflexes arranged according to amount of stimulation provided. Scoring and interpretation are complex and require in-depth training.

Battelle developmental inventory: A tool developed to identify developmental strengths and weaknesses of both children with disabilities and nondisabled children between the ages of 0 to 8 years. The domain of measurement includes personal-social, adaptive, motor, communication, and cognition skills.

Bayley scales of infant development II (BSID-II): Assesses current developmental function, diagnoses-based developmental delay, and plan intervention strategies in infants 1 to 42 months of age. It is a standardized test that measures the subscales of motor, mental, and behavioral rating scales.

Brazleton neonatal behavioral assessment scale: Scale that assesses the neurological condition of neonates, including reflexes, muscle tone, responsiveness to objects and people, motor capacities, and ability to control behavior and attention.

Denver II: Criteria-referenced screening instrument that tests personal/social, communication, self-help, and gross and fine motor skills. Provides an initial screen of well children, between the ages of 0 to 6 years, suspected of having or being at risk for developmental delay. It is a norm-referenced test that measures the domains of personal-social, fine motor adaptive, language, and gross motor functions.

early intervention developmental profile (EIDP): A comprehensive developmental assessment and systematic intervention system for young children and newborn to 6 year olds. It is a general overview of developmental milestones based on age-specific skills for children with all types of disabilities. The domains measured include perceptual/fine motor, cognition, language, social/emotional, self-care, and gross motor functioning.

Hawaii early learning profile (HELP): Criteria-referenced test for children ages 0 to 36 months that assesses personal, social, communication, cognition, self-help, gross motor, fine motor, and visual-motor integration.

Milani-Comparetti: Motor development screening test for infants and young children. Standardized screening tool for neurodevelopmental disorders.

Miller assessment for preschoolers (MAP): Assists in the identification of preschoolers, between the ages of 2 years, 9 months and 5 years, 8 months, with mild to severe developmental delays. It is a norm-referenced test that measures sensory and motor abilities, cognitive functioning, and combined abilities of these areas.

movement assessment of infants screening test (MAI-ST): An assessment tool developed to identify movement patterns that interfere with normal development for infants 2 to 18 months of age. The domains that it measures include muscle tone, primitive reflexes, and volitional movement.

neonatal behavioral assessment scale (NBAS): Assesses the infant's current behavior capabilities in response to environmental stimuli and handling providing a "snapshot" of the infant. This is used in premature neonates aged 37 to 44 weeks gestational age. Designed to show parents their infant's capabilities with emphasis on eliciting the best response in 37 items scored on a 9-point scale and 19 reflexes scored on a 3-point scale. This assessment is also called the *Brazleton neonatal scale*.

neonatal neurobehavioral examination (NNE): A standardized battery of tests for neonates 32 to 42 weeks of gestational age. The purpose is to describe neurobehavioral characteristics at specific conceptual ages in quantitative terms. The domains of measurement include tone and motor patterns, primitive reflexes, and behavioral responses.

Bibliography

Als H, Duffy FH, McAnulty GB. Behavioral differences between preterm and full-term newborns as measured with the APIB system scores: I. *Infant Behavior and Development*. 1988;11:305-318.

Als H, Duffy FH, McAnulty GB. The APIB, an assessment of functional competence in preterm and full-term newborns regardless of gestational age at birth: II. *Infant Behavior and Development*. 1988;11:319-331.

Bayley N. *Bayley Scales of Infant Development*. 2nd ed. San Antonio, Texas: The Psychological Corp; 1993.

Brazelton TB. *Neonatal Behavioral Assessment Scale*. 2nd ed. Philadelphia, Pa: JB Lippincott; 1984.

Brown SL, D'Eugenio DB, Drews JE, et al. Preschool assessment and application. In: D'Eugenio DB, Moersch M, eds. *Developmental Programming for Infants and Young Children*. Vol 4. Ann Arbor, Mich: University of Michigan Press; 1981.

Chandler LS. Screening for movement dysfunction in infancy. *Physical and Occupational Therapy in Pediatrics*. 1986;6(3-4):171-190.

Chandler LS, Andrews MS, Swanson M, Larson AH. *Chandler Movement Assessment of Infants—Screening Test*. Unpublished manuscript (available from primary author). 1988.

Frankenberg WK, Dodds J, Archer P, et al. *Denver II: Screening Manual*. Denver, Colo: Denver Developmental Materials Inc; 1990.

Miller LJ. *Miller Assessment for Preschoolers Manual*. Rev ed. San Antonio, Texas: The Psychological Corp; 1988.

Miller LJ, Schouten PG. Age related effects on the predictive validity of the Miller Assessment for Preschoolers. *Journal of Psychoeducational Assessment*. 1988;6:99-106.

Morgan AE, Koch V, Lee V, Aldag J. Neonatal Neurobehavioral Examination: a new instrument for quantitative analysis of neonatal neurological status. *Phys Ther*. 1988;68:1352-1356.

Newborg J, Stock JR, Wnek L, et al. *Battelle Developmental Inventory: Examiner's Manual*. Chicago, Ill: Riverside; 1988.

Rogers RJ, D'Eugenio DB. Assessment and application. In: D'Eugenio DB, Moersch M, eds. *Developmental Programming for Infants and Young Children*. Vol 4. Ann Arbor, Mich: University of Michigan Press; 1977.

PEDIATRIC ASSESSMENT OF FUNCTION

Alberta infant motor scale (AIMS): An assessment for 0- to 18-month-old children that measures gross motor maturation and monitors motor behaviors essential to evaluation of development of at-risk infants over time. It is a norm-referenced tool that contains 58 items observing the child in four positions: prone, supine, sitting, and standing. The score sheet has drawings with key descriptions of postures or movement components that must be present to receive credit. Positional and total scores are obtained and graphed, and percentiles are estimated.

Bruininks-Oseretsky motor development scale (BOTMP): An assessment for 4.5- to 14.5-year-old children that tests developmental components of gross and fine motor skills. It is a norm-referenced test that measures the domains of four fine motor subtests and five gross motor subtests.

DeGangi-Berk test of sensory integration (TSI): An assessment for 3- to 5-year-old children that detects sensory integrative dysfunction. There are 36 items on three subtests: postural control, bilateral motor integration, and reflex integration. Scores are interpreted as normal, at-risk, or deficient.

Erhardt developmental prehension assessment (EDPA): An assessment for children from birth to 6 years of age that measures qualitative change in the development of hand function in children with developmental delays. It is a criterion-based test comparing quality and level of performance to developmental progression of hand function. Provides a sequential description of fine motor skills, measures voluntary and involuntary arm-hand patterns from the prenatal period to 15 months, and measures pencil grasp/prewriting skills from ages 1 to 6 years.

Gesell preschool test: Norm-referenced test for children 2.5 to 6 years that assesses personal, social, communication, and gross motor and fine motor skills.

gross motor function measure (GMFM): An assessment for children with cerebral palsy that measures changes in gross motor function over time. It is a criterion-based observation that evaluates five dimensions: lying and rolling; sitting; crawling and kneeling; standing; and walking, running, and jumping. Items are scored on a 4-point scale.

infant neurological international battery (INFANIB): A tool used to assess 1- to 15-month-old children for neurologic integrity from neonatal intensive care unit through follow-up. It is a standardized assessment with 20 items.

motor-fine visual perceptual test (MVPT): Norm-referenced test for children 4 to 8 years that assesses visual perception.

movement assessment of infants (MAI): An assessment in the first year of life (from 0 to 12 months) that is a systematic assessment of motor behaviors and identifies motor dysfunction and monitors the effects of intervention. It is a standardized, criterion-referenced assessment that evaluates muscle tone, primitive reflexes, automatic reactions, and volitional movement.

Peabody developmental motor scales (PDMS): Assesses a child's gross and fine motor skills in relation to adaptive capacities in 0- to 83-month old children. The PDMS identifies areas of strengths and weaknesses that facilitate programming, including reflexes, balance, nonlocomotor and locomotor function, and receipt and propulsion of objects. The fine motor scale includes grasping, hand use, eye-hand coordination, and manual dexterity.

pediatric assessment of self-care activities: Assessment that determines the child's degree of independence according to defined developmental sequences of feeding, toileting, hygiene, and dressing, including the use of fasteners.

posture and fine motor skills assessment of infant (PFMAI): Assesses the developmental age of 2 to 6 months and identifies quality of motor function and major motor problems typically not identified until the child is older. The child's postural control and proximal stability are observed in prone and supine. Then, fine motor and distal control are observed.

quick neurology screening test: Informal screening for children aged 5 to 18 years that tests gross motor, praxis, fine motor, visual-motor integration, visual perception, tactile, and vestibular.

sensorimotor performance analysis (SPA): A screening tool for 5- to 21-year-olds that analyzes the underlying sensorimotor components of performance during fine and gross motor tasks. It is a criterion-referenced, observational assessment of postural mechanisms, sensory processing, developmental lags, postural tone, and bilateral integration.

sensory assessment: A standardized sensory assessment that evaluates pressure sensitivity, moving two-point discrimination, stereognosis, proprioception, and directionality.

Sensory Integration and Praxis Test (SIPT): Evaluates children, ages 4 to 8 years, 11 months, in the areas of form and space, somatosensory and vestibular processing, bilateral integration and sequencing, and praxis. The test consists of 17 subtests that require integration of bilateral function in either gross, fine, or oral motor movements, as well as tactile perception.

sensory rating scale: An assessment for 0- to 3-year-old children that identifies and quantifies sensory responses. The domains of measurement include touch, movement and gravity, hearing, vision, taste and smell, temperature, and general sensitivity.

test of visual perceptive skills (nonmotor) (TVPS): Norm-referenced test for children 4 to 12 years that assesses visual perception.

toddler and infant motor evaluation (TIME): A comprehensive, diagnostic assessment of 4-month to 3.5-year-old children with suspected motor delays that assists with appropriate program planning. It is a standardized test that measures mobility, stability, motor organization, functional performance, and social/emotional abilities.

Bibliography

Berk RA, DeGangi G. *DeGangi-Berk Test of Sensory Integration.* Los Angeles, Calif: Western Psychological Services; 1987.

Bruininks RH. *Bruininks-Oseretsky Test of Motor Proficiency: Examiner's Manual.* Circle Pines, Minn: American Guidance Service; 1978.

Case-Smith J. Postural and fine motor control in preterm infants in the first six months. *Phys Occup Ther Pediatr*. 1993;13(1):1-17.

Chandler LS, Andrews MS, Swanson MW. *Movement Assessment of Infants: A Manual*. Rolling Bay, Wash: Movement Assessment of Infants; 1980.

Cooper J, Majnerner A, Rosenblatt B, Birnbaum R. A standardized sensory assessment for children of school-age. *Phys Occup Ther Pediatr*. 1993;13(1):61-80.

Ellison PH. Scoring sheet for the Infant Neurological International Battery (INFANIB). *Phys Ther*. 1986;66:548-550.

Erhardt RP. *Developmental Hand Function: Theory, Assessment, Treatment*. Laurel, Md: Ramsco Publishing Company; 1982.

Folio MR, Fewell RR. *Peabody Developmental Motor Scales and Activity Card*. Chicago, Ill: Riverside; 1983.

Miller LJ, Roid GH. *The T.I.M.E. Toddler and Infant Motor Evaluation: A Standardized Assessment*. Tucson, Ariz: Therapy Skill Builders; 1994.

Piper MC, Darrah J. *Motor Assessment of the Developing Infant*. Philadelphia, Pa: WB Saunders; 1994.

Provost B, Oetter P. The Sensory Rating Scale for Infants and Young Children: development and reliability. *Phys Occup Ther Pediatr*. 1993;13(4):15-35.

Richter EW, Montgomery PC. *The Sensorimotor Performance Analysis*. Hugo, Minn: PDP Press; 1989.

Russell DJ, Rosenbaum PL, Gowland C, et al. *Manual for the Gross Motor Function Measure: A Measure of Gross Motor Function in Cerebral Palsy*. Ontario, Canada: McMaster University; 1990.

SELF-PERCEPTION EXAMINATIONS

additive activities profile test (ADAPT): Self-administered test that relates activities of daily living to physical fitness.

Borg perceived exertion: A cardiac patient's/client's assessment of his or her own level of exertion on stress tests.

Canadian Occupational Performance Measure (COPM): An individualized measure of a patient's/client's perception of performance and satisfaction in areas of self-care, productivity, and leisure.

SF-36: A set of 36 questions directed at the patient's/client's assessment of his or her functional capacity vs. actual observation of performance. The questions are in the area of activities of daily living as well as items that reflect depression and quality of life.

Bibliography

Law M, Baptiste S, Carswell A, et al. *Canadian Occupational Performance Measure*. 2nd ed. Toronto, Canada: CAOT Publications; 1994.

Functional Assessment

assessment of older people's self-maintenance and instrumental activities of daily living: Assessment containing a physical self-maintenance scale and an instrumental activities of daily living scale. Used with older adults to gather information.

Barthel index: One of the oldest self-care measures. It was initially developed to measure changes in functional status for patients/clients undergoing inpatient rehabilitation. It includes 10 activities rated using a 2-point or 3-point ordinal scale. It is a moderately sensitive screening assessment used mainly in geriatrics.

functional independence measure (FIM): An assessment used to describe the degree of disability experienced by an adult rehabilitation patient/client and to evaluate changes in groups of patients/clients over time. The FIM uses a seven-point scale to evaluate 18 items in areas of self-care, sphincter control, mobility, locomotion, communication, and social cognition.

functional life scale: Measures the effects of a person's impairments on his or her ability to participate in daily activities at home rather than in a rehabilitation setting. It uses 44 items, each rated on a five-point scale.

functional status index (FSI): A self-report tool in which patients/clients are asked to rate their performance as well as the degree of pain and difficulty in accomplishing tasks. It includes 18 items in the areas of gross mobility, hand activities, personal care, home chores, and social activities.

geriatric functional rating scale: Assessment used to assist in making independent living decisions.

Karnofsky performance status scale: A functional performance scale used in oncology to indicate the patient's/client's activity level in the hospital, home, or community.

Katz index of activities of daily living: The Katz index is a short ADL index designed to classify individuals in rehabilitation who have self-care problems and to predict need for later attendant requirements. It includes six items: bathing, dressing, toileting, transfers, continence, and feeding. Each item is scored on a nominal scale of independence or dependence.

Kenny self-care evaluation: Assessment of self-care abilities that evaluates changes in self-care over time in adults. Seventeen items are rated from 0 to 4, with 0 indicating dependent and 4 indicating independent. Items include bed activities, transfers, locomotion, dressing, personal hygiene, and feeding.

Klein-Bell activities of daily living scale: Evaluates change in self-care abilities over time for adults and children. This scale documents basic ADL in the areas of dressing, elimination, mobility, bathing, hygiene, eating, and emergency telephone communication. Each area is broken down into component tasks and scored as achieved or not achieved.

Kurtzke expanded disability status scale (EDSS): A scale used with patients/clients with multiple sclerosis used to monitor changes in disability levels; it has value in determining prognosis.

Minimum Data Set (MDS): Comprehensive screening tool reflecting quality of life concerns, includes activities of daily living, self-performance, disease diagnosis, and activity pursuits (requirement for nursing homes using third-party payers).

OARS multidimensional functional assessment questionnaire: The Older American Resources and Services (OARS) was one of the first formal approaches developed to assess the function of elders in multiple domains. It is composed of an instrument to assess functional activities (the Multidimensional Functional Assessment Questionnaire [MFAQ]) and a questionnaire to identify the resources that an elder uses.

Philadelphia geriatric center multilevel assessment instrument (MAI): Based on Lawton's conceptual model of adult behavior, which is hierarchically organized by the complexity of behavior. It measures five behavioral domains: physical health cognition, self-care, and instrumental ADLs; time use (employment, hobbies, recreation); social interaction; personal adjustment (morale, psychiatric symptoms); and perceived environment (housing, neighborhood, personal security).

PULSES profile: Designed to provide a descriptive measure of severity of disability and to evaluate change over time in adults with physical impairments. Scores are assigned using a 4-point scale for items in areas of physical condition (P), upper extremity function (U), lower extremity function (L), sensory components (S), excretory function (E), and support factors (S).

resident assessment instrument: Nationwide tool used to periodically measure the functional performance of each nursing home resident and identify problem areas that may be open to intervention.

safety and functional ADL evaluation (SAFE): Evaluates the independence and degree of required supervision in bathing, dressing, feeding, bowel and bladder control, transfers, and mobility.

structured assessment of independent living skills (SAILS): Assesses everyday activities in patients/clients with dementia to determine problems and potential safety issues. It is a criterion-based measure that includes items in the areas of fine motor skills, gross motor skills, dressing skills, eating skills, cognitive tasks, receptive language, expressive language, time and orientation, money-related skills, instrumental activities, and social interaction.

Bibliography

Baird SB, McCorkle R, Grant M. *Cancer Nursing: A Comprehensive Textbook.* Philadelphia, Pa: WB Saunders; 1991.

Fillenbaum GG, Smyer MA. The development, validity, and reliability of the OARS Multidimensional Functional Assessment Questionnaire. *J Gerontol.* 1981;36:428-434.

George LK, Fillenbaum GG. OARS methodology: a decade of experience in geriatric assessment. *J Am Geriatr Soc.* 1985;33:607-615.

Granger CV, Albrecht GL, Hamilton BB. Outcome of comprehensive medical rehabilitation measurement by Pulses Profile and the Barthel index. *Arch Phys Med Rehabil.* 1979;60:145-154.

Iversen IA, Silberberg NE, Stever RC, Schoening HA. *The Revised Kenny Self-Care Evaluation: A Numerical Measure of Independence in Activities of Daily Living.* Minneapolis, Minn: Sister Kenny Institute; 1973.

Jette AM. Functional Status Index: reliability of the chronic disease evaluation instrument. *Arch Phys Med Rehabil.* 1980;61:395-401.

Jette AM. The Functional Status Index: reliability and validity of the self-report functional disability measure. *J Rheumatol.* 1987;14:15-19.

Katz S, Downs RD, Cash HR, Grotz RC. Progress in the development of ADL. *Gerontologist.* 1970;10:20-30.

Klein RM, Bell B. Self-care skills: behavioral measurement with the Klein-Bell ADL scale. *Arch Phys Med Rehabil.* 1982;63:335-338.

Kurtzke J. Rating neurological impairment in multiple sclerosis: an expanded disability status scale (EDSS). *Neurology.* 1983;33:1444.

Law M, Usher P. Validation of the Klein-Bell ADL scale for pediatric occupational therapy. *Can J Occup Ther.* 1987;55:63-68.

Leon J, Lair T. *Functional Status of the Non-Institutionalized Elderly: Estimates of ADL and IADL Difficulties.* Rockville, Md: National Medical Expenditure Survey Research Findings 4. Agency for Health Care Policy Research. Public Health Service, DHHS Publication No (PHS) 90-3462; 1990.

Long WB, Sacco WJ, Coombes SS, et al. Determining normative standards for Functional Independence Measure: transitions in rehabilitation. *Arch Phys Med Rehabil.* 1994;75:144-148.

Mahoney FI, Barthel DW. Functional evaluation: the Barthel Index. *Maryland State Medical Journal*. 1965;14:61-65.

Mahurin RK, DeBettignies BH, Pirozzolo FJ. Structured Assessment of Independent Living Skills: preliminary report of performance measure of functional abilities in dementia. *J Gerontol*. 1991;46:58-66.

Oczkowski WJ, Barreca S. The Functional Independence Measure: its use to identify rehabilitation needs in stroke survivors. *Arch Phys Med Rehabil*. 1993;74:1291-1294.

Settle C, Holm MB. Program planning: the clinical utility of three activities of daily living assessment tools. *Am J Occup Ther*. 1993;487:911-918.

ELDERS AND CAREGIVERS ASSESSMENT

assessment of living skills and resources (ALSAR): A multidimensional assessment of the elderly that includes information on balance of functional ability (eg, ability to stay in a community setting vs. being institutionalized) and available resources.

Kohlman evaluation of living skills (KELS): Standardized test combining interview and task performance, used to evaluate an individual's ability to function safely and independently in the community.

Bibliography

Williams JH, Drinka TJ, Greenberg JR, et al. Development and testing of the assessment of living skills and resources (ALSAR) in elderly community-dwelling veterans. *Gerontologist*. 1991;31(1):84-91.

WORK ASSESSMENT

Baltimore therapeutic equipment (BTE) work simulator: A computerized treatment and evaluation device that has a variety of attachments intended to reproduce all motions needed to simulate almost any job, activity, or activity of daily living function.

blankenship system: A computerized system for evaluating the effect that any pathology has on an injured worker's ability to work.

EPIC lift capacity (ELC) test: An outgrowth of the WEST II (see following page), which is a progressive isoinertial test composed of six subjects and used to evaluate lift capacity across a broad spectrum of disability groups.

functional capacity evaluations (FCEs): Return-to-work functional capacity evaluations that evaluate low back problems, upper extremity and hand injuries, cervical injuries, and lower extremity injuries. The physical demand levels are rated as sedentary, light, medium, and heavy work. Computerized testing is generally used, looking at isometric, isoinertional, and isokinetic abilities.

hand tool dexterity test: A measure of efficiency using regular mechanics tools. This test measures manipulative skill independence in performing manual tasks.

key method: A whole-body assessment that is a standardized, computerized, objective evaluation used for return-to-work decisions. Over 27 functional tests measure weight lifting, pushing and pulling, carrying, work day tolerance, sitting, standing, upper extremity function, walking tolerance, and posture within four levels of increasing work intensity.

Purdue pegboard: Measures dexterity for two types of activity: one involving gross movements of the hands, fingers, and arms and the other, primarily fingertip dexterity.

testing, orientation, and work evaluation in rehabilitation (TOWER): First work sampling system, developed in 1936 for individuals with physical disabilities. It is now used for all types of people, including those with emotional disabilities.

VALPAR component work samples: A defined work activity involving tasks, materials, and tools that are similar to those in an actual job or occupation. They are criterion-referenced instruments designed to determine whether an individual can perform certain tasks.

Work Evaluations Systems Technologies II (WEST II): Equipment that simulates work tasks and is used in preplacement or pre-employment screening, work evaluation, work hardening, and performance of FCEs.

Bibliography

Bennett GK. *Hand Tool Dexterity Test: Manual.* San Diego, Calif: The Psychological Corp; 1981.

Blankenship KL. *The Blankenship System: Functional Capacity Evaluation. The Procedure Manual.* Macon, Ga: Blankenship Corp, Panaprint, Inc; 1994.

Christopherson BB, Hayes PD. *VALPAR Component Work Samples: Uses in Allied Health.* Tucson, Ariz: VALPAR International Corp; 1992.

Field JE, Field TF. The classification of jobs according to worker trait factors. In: *Dictionary of Occupational Titles*. 4th ed. Athens, Ga: Elliot and Fitzpatrick; 1988.

Isernhagen SJ. *Work Injury: Management and Prevention*. Gaithersburg, Md: Aspen Publishers; 1988.

Mayer TG, Gatchel RJ. *Functional Restoration for Spinal Disorders: The Sports Medicine Approach*. Philadelphia, Pa: Lea & Febiger; 1988.

Tiffin J. *Purdue Pegboard Examiner's Manual*. Bloomington, Ind: Serence Research Associates; 1987.

ENVIRONMENTAL EVALUATION

Functional Home Assessment Profile: A tool developed to allow performance-based environmental risk assessment. Performance during routine activities is graded and scored for 0 = no risk, 1 = low risk, and 2 = moderate to high risk. The frequency of the activity on a weekly basis is also recorded.

Home Assessment Checklist for Fall Hazards: A tool used to evaluate the safety of an individual's home.

Institutional Environmental Evaluation: A tool used to evaluate the safety of a hospital, nursing home, or other public facility.

Multiphasic Environmental Assessment Procedure (MEAP): Collection of checklists and questionnaires designed to evaluate the quality of living in a given sheltered care facility. The assessment focuses on the structural components of the facility, the social atmosphere, programs offered, and the attributes of the resident and staff.

Post-Occupancy Evaluation (POE): Generic, comprehensive, and systematic approach to assessing any physical environment that is currently in use.

Bibliography

Chandler JM, Duncan PW, Prescott BL, et al. *The Functional Home Assessment Profile: Reliability of a New Instrument*. In review.

Council on Aging. *The Sixth Sense*. Washington, DC: The National Council on Aging; 1997.

Tideiksaar R. Fall prevention in the home. *Topics in Geriatric Rehabilitation*. 1987;3(1):59.

ORTHOPEDIC EXAMINATION (BY BODY PART)

Temporomandibular

Chvostek Test: The examiner taps over the masseter and the parotid gland. Twitching of the facial muscles, especially the masseter, is indicative of positive findings for facial nerve pathology.

Loading Test: The examiner places a cotton roll between the molars on the uninvolved side and instructs the subject to bite down forcefully. The reporting of pain by the subject indicates a positive finding, which may be reflective of an anteriorly dislocated disc at the TMJ.

Palpation Test: The examiner places his or her fingers in the subject's ears. The subject is instructed to repeatedly open and close the mouth while the examiner applies pressure in an anterior direction. A report of pain or discomfort during the opening and closing of the mouth indicates a positive test. This may result from an inflammation of the synovium of the joint.

Cervical Spine

Foraminal Compression Test (Spurling): The examiner applies a downward pressure while the subject laterally flexes the head. The test is repeated on both sides. A reporting of pain into the upper extremity toward the same side that the head is flexed is positive, indicating pressure on a nerve root. This level of involvement may be correlated by the dermatomal distribution of pain.

Foraminal Distraction Test: The examiner distracts the subject's head from the trunk. The finding is positive for nerve root compression when existing complaints of pain decrease or disappear.

Swallowing Test: Ask the subject to swallow. Increased pain or difficulty swallowing (dysphagia) is a positive sign of anterior cervical spine obstructions, such as vertebral subluxations, osteophyte protrusion, soft tissue swelling, or tumors in the anterior cervical spine.

Valsalva's maneuver: The examiner asks the subject to take a deep breath and hold while bearing down as if having a bowel movement. Increased pain due to increased intrathecal pressure, which may be secondary to a space-occupying lesion, herniated disk, tumor, or osteophyte in the cervical canal, is positive.

Vertebral Artery Test: With the subject lying in supine with his or her head free of support (supported by examiner), the examiner extends, rotates, and laterally flexes the cervical spine to each side. Dizziness, blurred vision, nystagmus, slurred speech, or loss of consciousness are indicative of partial or complete occlusion of the vertebral artery. (Note: If trying to determine vestibular versus orthopedic involvement, start with rotation before extending and laterally flexing).

Shoulder

acromioclavicular (AC) joint compression test: With the subject seated and the arm relaxed at the side, the examiner places one hand on the clavicle and the other on the spine of the scapula. The examiner gently squeezes the hands together, noting any movement at the AC joint. Pain and/or movement of the clavicle is positive, indicating an AC and/or coracoclavicular ligament sprain.

acromioclavicular (AC) joint distraction test: With the subject sitting and hands in his or her lap, the examiner applies gentle downward pressure on the arm, noting any movement at the AC joint. Pain and/or movement of the scapula inferior to the clavicle is positive, indicating AC and coracoclavicular ligament sprains.

Adson's maneuver: Examiner places his or her fingers over the radial artery (distally). Externally rotate and extend the subject's arm and then tell the subject to extend and rotate the neck toward the test arm and take a deep breath. A diminished or absent radial pulse is indicative of thoracic outlet syndrome, secondary to compression of the subclavian artery by the scalene muscles.

Allen's test: Subject with the shoulder in 90 degrees of abduction and external rotation and the elbow flexed at 90 degrees. The examiner palpates the radial pulse. A diminished pulse is indicative of thoracic outlet syndrome.

Apley's scratch test: Part I: The subject is instructed to take one hand and touch the opposite shoulder. Repeat to the other side. Asymmetrical results from side-to-side are positive. Inability to touch the opposite shoulder is indicative of limited gleno-humeral adduction, internal rotation, and horizontal flexion. Limits in scapular protraction may also produce asymmetrical results. Part II: Next, the subject is instructed to bring his or her arm overhead and reach behind the neck, as if scratching the upper back. This is repeated on both sides. Asymmetrical results are positive, indicating limited glenohumeral abduction and external rotation, and scapular upward rotation and elevation. Part III: The subject is instructed to place the hand behind the back and reach upwards (as in hooking a bra). This is repeated on the opposite side. Asymmetrical results are positive and indicate limited glenohumeral adduction and internal rotation, and scapular retraction and downward rotation.

apprehension test (anterior): With the subject supine and the shoulder in 90 degrees of abduction, the examiner slowly, externally rotates the shoulder. This test is interpreted as positive when the subject either looks apprehensive or expresses apprehension. This test mimics anterior dislocation of the glenohumeral joint.

apprehension test (posterior): With the subject supine, the examiner places the shoulder in a position of 90 degrees of flexion and internal rotation, while applying a posterior force through the long axis of the humerus. This test is positive when the subject either looks apprehensive or expresses apprehension. This test mimics posterior dislocation of the glenohumeral joint.

brachial plexus stretch test: With the subject seated, the examiner laterally flexes the subject's head while applying gentle pressure on the shoulder. Pain radiating down the arm on that side is a positive finding for brachial plexus involvement.

cross-over impingement test: With the subject's trunk stabilized and his or her shoulder at 90 degrees flexion, maximally resist adduction across the chest. Superior shoulder pain is indicative of acromioclavicular joint pathology. Anterior pain is indicative of subscapularis, supraspinatus, and/or biceps long head pathology. Posterior shoulder pain is indicative of infraspinatus, teres minor, and/or posterior capsule pathology.

drop arm test: The examiner passively abducts the subject's arm to 90 degrees and then instructs the subject to slowly lower the arm to the side. If the subject is unable to slowly return the arm to the side and/or has significant pain, this test is indicative of rotator cuff pathology.

empty can (supraspinatus) test: With subject's arms abducted to 90 degrees, horizontally adducted 30 degrees, and internally rotated so the thumbs face down, the examiner resists the subject's attempts to actively abduct both shoulders. Involvement of the supraspinatus muscle and/or tendon is suspected with noted weakness and/or a report of pain.

grind test: The subject lies supine with the shoulder abducted to 90 degrees and the elbow flexed to 90 degrees. The examiner applies compression at the proximal humerus while attempting to rotate the humeral head 360 degrees around the surface of the glenoid fossa. A positive test results in a grinding or clucking sensation possibly indicative of a glenoid labrum tear.

Neer impingement test: The examiner places one hand on the scapula and the other at the elbow. With the scapula stabilized, maximally forward flex the shoulder. Shoulder pain and apprehension are indicative of impingement of the supraspinatus and/or biceps long head tendons.

O'Brien test: The subject places the shoulder in 90 degrees of forward flexion, 30 to 45 degrees of horizontal adduction, and maximal internal rotation. The subject horizontally adducts and flexes against the examiner's manual resistance. Pain and/or popping are indicative of a superior labrum anterior-posterior (SLAP) lesion.

piano key sign: The examiner applies pressure to the subject's distal clavicle in an inferior direction. The examiner is able to depress the clavicle into its normal resting position and subsequently watch the clavicle elevate again once pressure is removed. This is indicative of instability of the AC joint.

Roos test: The subject places both shoulders in 90 degrees of abduction and external rotation, and the elbows in 90 degrees of flexion and then rapidly opens and closes both hands for 3 minutes. The inability to maintain the test position, diminished motor function of the hands, and/or loss of sensation in the upper extremities are indicative of thoracic outlet syndrome, secondary to neurovascular compromise.

Speed's test: With the subject's shoulder flexed to 90 degrees, the elbow fully extended, and the forearm supinated, the examiner resists the subject's attempt to actively forward flex the arm. Tenderness and/or pain in the bicipital groove is a positive finding that may indicate bicipital tendinitis.

sternoclavicular (SC) joint stress test: The examiner applies gentle downward and inward pressure on the clavicle, noting any movement at the SC joint. Pain and/or movement of the clavicle indicates a sternoclavicular ligament sprain, possibly involving the costoclavicular ligament.

sulcus sign: With the subject seated and his or her hands in the lap, the examiner stabilizes the scapula and applies an inferior (distraction) force at the elbow. Excessive inferior humeral translation with a visible and/or palpable "sulcus" deformity ("step-off") immediately inferior to the acromion (laterally) is indicative of multidirectional instability.

Yergason test: With the subject seated, the elbow flexed to 90 degrees (stabilized against the thorax), and the forearm pronated, the examiner places one hand along the forearm and the other hand on the upper portion of the humerus (near the bicipital groove). The examiner resists the attempt to supinate the forearm and externally rotate the humerus. Pain that is reported in the area of the bicipital groove is a positive finding that may indicate bicipital tendinitis.

Elbow

elbow flexion test: The subject is instructed to maximally flex the elbow and hold this position for 3 to 5 minutes. Radiating pain into the median nerve distribution is a positive finding for cubital fossa syndrome.

hyperextension test: With the subject's elbow fully extended and the forearm supinated, the examiner grasps the distal humerus at the epicondyle region with one hand, while the other hand grasps the distal forearm. The examiner passively extends the elbow to its limit. Elbow extension beyond 0 degrees is considered hyperextension. A positive finding may be attributed to a torn or stretched anterior capsule of the elbow.

passive tennis elbow test: The subject fully extends his or her elbow and the examiner passively pronates the forearm and flexes the wrist. A reporting of pain along the lateral epicondyle region may indicate lateral epicondylitis.

pinch grip test: The subject is instructed to pinch the tips of the thumb and index finger together. Inability to do this is a positive finding. This is indicative of pathology of the anterior interosseous nerve.

resistive tennis elbow test (Cozen's test): With the subject seated, the examiner stabilizes the elbow while palpating along the lateral epicondyle. With a closed fist, the subject pronates and radially deviates the forearm and extends the wrist against the examiner's resistance. A report of pain along the lateral epicondyle region or objective muscle weakness indicates lateral epicondylitis.

Tinel's sign: With the subject seated and elbow in slight flexion, the examiner grasps the wrist (laterally). He or she stabilizes the wrist, tapping the ulnar nerve in the ulnar notch (between the olecranon process and medial epicondyle—commonly called the "crazy bone") with the index finger. Tingling along the ulnar distribution of the forearm, hand, and fingers is indicative of ulnar nerve compromise.

valgus stress test: The subject is seated with his or her elbow flexed to 20 to 30 degrees. The examiner places one hand around the subject's wrist (medially) and the other over the elbow (laterally). With the wrist stabilized, the examiner applies valgus stress to the elbow. Medial elbow pain and/or increased valgus movement indicate ulnar or medial collateral ligament damage.

varus stress test: The subject is seated with his or her elbow flexed to 20 to 30 degrees. The examiner places one hand around the subject's wrist (laterally) and the other over the elbow (medially). With the wrist stabilized, the examiner applies varus stress to the elbow. Lateral elbow pain and/or increased varus movement indicate radial or lateral collateral ligament damage.

Wrist and Hand

Bunnel Littner test: With the subject's metacarpophalangeal joint in slight extension, the examiner passively flexes the proximal interphalangeal joint of the same ray and assesses the amount of flexion at the PIP. The examiner then passively and slightly flexes the MCP and again assesses the amount of flexion at the PIP. A positive finding is that the PIP does not flex while the MCP is extended. If the PIP does flex fully once the MCP is slightly flexed, this is indicative of intrinsic muscle tightness. If flexion of the PIP remains limited once the MCP is slightly flexed, capsular tightness can be assumed.

compression test: With the subject's affected finger extended, the examiner holds the distal phalanx and applies compression along the long axis of the bone. Pain at the site of injury is indicative of a fracture.

digital Allen's test: The subject is instructed to make a fist several times in order to "pump" the blood out of the hand and fingers. The subject is then instructed to maintain a fist while the examiner compresses the radial artery with the thumb and the ulnar artery with the fingers. As the subject relaxes the hand, the examiner releases pressure from one artery at a time and observes the color of the hand. A delay in or absence of flushing of the radial or ulnar half of the hand and fingers is indicative of partial or complete occlusion of the radial or ulnar arteries.

Finkelstein test: The subject forms a fist around the thumb. The examiner grasps the forearm with one hand and the fist with the other, with the subject's thumb in the examiner's thenar eminence. While stabilizing the forearm, the examiner ulnarly deviates the wrist. Pain over the abductor pollicis longus and extensor pollicis brevis tendons distally is indicative of tenosynovitis in these tendons.

Froment's paper sign: The subject is instructed to hold a piece of paper between the thumb and index finger. The examiner tries to pull the paper. Flexion of the distal interphalangeal joint of the thumb is indicative of adductor pollicis muscle paralysis due to ulnar nerve damage.

long finger flexor test: The examiner isolates the proximal or distal interphalangeal joint by stabilizing the metacarpophalangeal or metacarpophalangeal and proximal interphalangeal joint of the finger being tested. The subject is instructed to flex the proximal or distal interphalangeal joint. Inability to flex the proximal interphalangeal joint indicates compromise of the flexor digitorum superficialis muscle. Inability to flex the distal interphalangeal joint indicates compromise of the flexor digitorum profundus muscle.

Murphy's sign: The subject is instructed to make a fist. The examiner notes the position of the third metacarpal. If the subject's third metacarpal is level with the second and fourth, a dislocated lunate is indicated.

Phalen test: The subject is sitting with the dorsal aspects of both hands in full contact, such that both wrists are maximally flexed. A steady compression force is applied through the forearms by the examiner for 1 minute. Numbness and tingling in the median nerve distribution are indicative of carpal tunnel syndrome, secondary to median nerve compression.

tap or percussion test: With the subject's finger extended, the examiner applies a firm tap to the end of the finger being tested (a percussion hammer can also be used). Pain at the site of injury is indicative of a fracture.

Tinel's sign: The examiner taps the volar aspect of the subject's wrist over the area of the carpal tunnel. Complaints of tingling, paresthesia, or pain by the subject in the area of the thumb, index finger, middle finger, and radial one-half of the ring finger is indicative of a compression of the median nerve in the carpal tunnel (carpal tunnel syndrome).

Watson test: The examiner stabilizes the distal forearm at the distal radial-ulnar joint, while grasping the scaphoid bone. The examiner mobilizes the scaphoid bone anteriorly and posteriorly while ulnarly and radially deviating the subject's wrist. Positive findings include a palpable subluxation and reduction of the scaphoid and may be an indication of a carpal ligament tear.

wrinkle test (shrivel test): The subject's fingers are placed in warm water for ~10 minutes. Upon removal, the examiner assesses the skin around the pulp area for any wrinkling. A positive test is seen when the involved finger shows no signs of wrinkling, indicating denervated tissue.

Thoracic Spine

anterior/posterior rib compression test: With the subject supine, the examiner places his or her hands anteriorly and posteriorly, compresses the rib cage anterior to posterior, and quickly releases. Pain with compression or release of pressure indicates the possibility of a rib fracture, rib contusion, or costochondral separation.

inspiration/expiration breathing test: The subject is instructed to breath normally and then take a deep breath followed by rapid expiration. Normal breathing that is rapid and shallow is indicative of a rib fracture. Pain with inspiration may suggest a rib fracture, rib contusion, costochondral separation, or external intercostal muscle strain. Pain with forced expiration may indicate costochondral separation or internal intercostal muscle sprain.

Kernig/Brudzinski test: With the subject in supine and the hands cupped behind the head, the subject is instructed to flex the cervical spine by lifting the head. Each hip and then knee is unilaterally flexed to 90 degrees by the subject, while the opposite leg remains on the table. The test is confirmed by increased pain, localized or radiating into the lower extremity, with neck and hip flexed. The pain is relieved when the knee is flexed. The pain is indicative of meningeal irritation, nerve root impingement, or dural irritation that is exaggerated by elongating the spinal cord.

lateral rib compression test: With the subject supine, the examiner compresses the lateral aspect of the rib cage bilaterally and then quickly releases. Pain with compression or release indicates the possibility of a rib fracture, rib contusion, or costochondral separation.

Lumbar Spine

bilateral straight leg raise test: With the subject in supine, raise both legs simultaneously until pain or tightness is noted. Low back pain occurring at hip flexion of less than 70 degrees is indicative of sacroiliac joint involvement. Low back pain occurring at hip flexion of more than 70 degrees is indicative of lumbar spine involvement.

bowstring test (cram test): With the subject supine, the examiner performs a passive straight leg raise (SLR). If the subject reports radiating pain with the SLR, the examiner flexes the knee to ~20 degrees and then applies pressure to the popliteal area in an attempt to reproduce the radicular pain. Painful reproduction of the pain indicates tension on the sciatic nerve.

Hoover test: In supine, the subject is asked to perform a unilateral straight leg raise. The inability to lift the leg may reflect a neuromuscular weakness.

Kernig/Brudzinski test: With the subject in supine and the hands cupped behind the head, the subject is instructed to flex the cervical spine by lifting the head. Each hip and then knee is unilaterally flexed to 90 degrees by the subject, while the opposite leg remains on the table. The test is confirmed by increased pain, localized or radiating into the lower extremity, with neck and hip flexed. The pain is relieved when the knee is flexed. The pain is indicative of meningeal irritation, nerve root impingement, or dural irritation that is exaggerated by elongating the spinal cord.

90-90 straight leg raise test: With the subject lying supine, stabilizing both hips at 90 degrees of flexion with both hands, and the knees bent in a relaxed position, the subject is instructed to actively extend one knee at a time as much as possible. If the knee is flexed greater than 20 degrees, the hamstrings are considered tight.

piriformis test: With the subject side lying, the top leg in 60 degrees of hip flexion, and the knee in relaxed flexion, the examiner stabilizes the pelvis and applies an adduction (downward) force on the knee. Tightness or pain in the hip and buttock areas is indicative of piriformis tightness. Pain in the buttock and posterior thigh is indicative of sciatic nerve impingement secondary to piriformis tightness.

sitting root test: The subject sits with his or her hip flexed to 90 degrees and the cervical spine in flexion. The subject actively extends the knee. If the subject arches backward and/or complains of pain in the regions of the buttock, posterior thigh, and calf during knee extension, this is indicative of possible sciatic nerve pain.

spring test: With the subject lying prone, the examiner applies a downward "springing" force through the spinous process of each vertebra to assess anterior-posterior motion. This process should be repeated for each transverse process to assess rotary motion. Increases or decreases in motion at one vertebra compared to another are indicative of hypermobility or hypomobility, respectively.

stoop test: The subject is asked to walk briskly for a period of 1 minute. The examiner assesses the onset of pain in the buttock and lower limb areas. If present, the subject forward flexes the trunk. Pain in the buttock and lower limb areas brought on by brisk walking that is relieved with forward flexion indicates that there is a relationship between the neurogenic intermittent claudication, posture, and walking.

Thomas test: With the subject in supine and legs extended over the end of a table at the knees, have the subject flex both knees toward the chest. The examiner places one hand under the lumbar spine to monitor lumbar lordosis or pelvic tilt. The subject slowly lowers the test leg until the leg is fully relaxed or until either anterior pelvic tilt or an increase in lumbar lordosis occurs. A lack of hip extension with knee flexion more than 45 degrees is indicative of iliopsoas muscle tightness. Full hip extension with knee flexion less than 45 degrees is indicative of rectus femoris muscle tightness. A lack of hip extension with knee flexion less than 45 degrees is indicative of iliopsoas and rectus femoris muscle tightness. Hip external rotation is indicative of iliotibial band (particularly the tensor fascia latae) tightness.

Trendelenburg's test: The subject stands on one lower extremity and remains in this position for ~10 seconds and then switches legs. A positive finding is seen when the pelvis on the unsupported side drops lower than the pelvis on the supported side. This indicates a weakness of the gluteus medius on the supported side.

unilateral straight leg raise (Lasegue) test: With the subject lying in supine with both hips and knees extended, the examiner slowly raises the leg until pain or tightness is noted. Slowly lower the leg until pain or tightness resolves, at which point dorsiflex the ankle and have the subject flex the neck. Leg and/or low back pain occurring with dorsiflexion and/or neck flexion is indicative of dural involvement. A lack of pain reproduction is indicative of either hamstring tightness or possibly lumbar spine or sacroiliac joint involvement. If the latter is determined, proceed to the bilateral straight leg raise test to differentiate between lumbar spine and sacroiliac joint involvement.

Valsalva's maneuver: The examiner asks the subject to take a deep breath and hold while bearing down. The test is positive if there is increased pain due to increased intrathecal pressure, which may be secondary to a space-occupying lesion, herniated disk, tumor, or osteophyte in the lumbar canal.

Sacral Spine

long-sitting test: With the subject supine and both hips and knees extended, the examiner places his or her thumbs on the medial malleoli, passively flexes both knees and hips and then fully extends and compares the position of the malleoli relative to each other. The subject then assumes a long-sitting position, and malleoli position is reassessed. A leg that appears longer in supine but shorter in long-sitting is indicative of an ipsilateral anteriorly rotated ilium. Conversely, a leg that appears shorter in supine but longer in long-sitting is indicative of an ipsilateral posteriorly rotated ilium.

Patrick's or FABER test: With the subject supine, the examiner passively flexes, abducts, and externally rotates the hip; flexes the knee; and places the foot on top of the opposite knee (frog position). The examiner slowly abducts the extremity being tested toward the table. A positive test results when the involved extremity does not abduct below the level of the noninvolved extremity. This indicates iliopsoas, sacroiliac, or even hip joint problems.

sacroiliac (SI) joint fixation test: With the subject standing, the examiner places the thumbs over the posterior superior iliac spines (PSIS) and notes whether they are level. If they are asymmetrical, it is indicative of fixation on one side or the other. The examiner then places one thumb over the PSIS on the right or left side, and the other thumb over the S2 spinous process. The subject is then instructed to actively flex each hip (one at a time) with the knee flexed to 90 degrees. The thumb over the PSIS should drop relative to the spinous process. If there is no change or the thumb moves superiorly, hypomobility is indicated. (Repeat on the other side). The examiner then leaves one thumb over the PSIS and places the other on the ischial tuberosity. The subject is instructed again to actively flex the hip to 90 degrees. The thumb over the ischial tuberosity should move inferiorly. If the thumb moves superiorly, hypomobility is indicated. (Repeat on the other side).

sacroiliac (SI) joint stress test: There are four positions in this test: With the subject lying supine the examiner applies an outward and downward pressure on the anterior pelvis with the heel of the hand (arms crossed). Unilateral pain at the SI or in the gluteal or leg region indicates anterior SI ligament sprain; With the subject side lying, the examiner applies downward pressure on the pelvis. Increased pain or pressure is indicative of SI joint pathology, possibly involving the posterior SI ligaments; With the subject lying supine and the examiner's hands on the lateral aspect of the iliac crests, the examiner applies inward and downward pressure. Increased pain or pressure is indicative of SI joint pathology, possibly involving the posterior SI ligaments; With the subject prone, the examiner places one hand on top of the other over the sacrum and applies downward pressure. Pain at the SI joint is indicative of SI joint pathology.

Hip

Craig's test: With the subject prone and the testing leg's knee flexed to 90 degrees, the examiner palpates the greater trochanter, then passively internally and externally rotates the femur until the greater trochanter is parallel to the table. The subject is asked to hold this position, and the examiner measures the angle between the long axis of the lower leg and the perpendicular axis to the table using a goniometer. If the angle is greater than 15 degrees, femoral anteversion is indicated. If the angle is less than 8 degrees, femoral retroversion is indicated. In gait, an anteverted femur will result in toeing-in and retroversion will be observed as toeing-out. Both lead to malalignment problems.

Ely's test: In prone, the examiner passively flexes the subject's knee and notes the reaction at the hip. When the knee is flexed, if the hip also flexes, a tight rectus femoris is indicated.

hip scouring or quadrant test: With the subject supine, the examiner passively flexes and adducts the hip (the knee is also in full flexion), and applies downward pressure along the shaft of the femur while simultaneously adducting and externally rotating the hip. Next, the hip is adducted and internally rotated, maintaining the downward pressure. The examiner notes any unusual movement (eg, catching, grinding) or subject apprehension. Pain or apprehension is indicative of hip joint pathology, such as arthritis, osteochondral defects, avascular necrosis, or acetabular labrum defects.

leg length discrepancy test: With the subject supine and legs extended, a tape measure is used to measure the distance between the anterior superior iliac spine (ASIS) and the medial malleolus. A difference of more than 1 cm is indicative of discrepancies in either length of the femur or tibia or the angle of femoral neck inclination (ie, coxa vara or valga).

Nélaton's line: With the subject supine and legs extended, the examiner puts a finger on the anterior superior iliac spine and one on the ischial tuberosity and imagines a line between those points. The position of the greater trochanter is palpated in relation to the line. If the greater trochanter is above the line, coxa vara or a decreased angle of inclination is present. Coxa vara presents as a valgus knee position (knock-kneed) and represents malalignment of the lower extremity.

90-90 straight leg raise test: With the subject lying supine, both hips at 90 degrees of flexion and stabilized with both hands, and the knees bent in a relaxed position, the subject is instructed to actively extend one knee at a time as much as possible. If the knee is flexed greater than 20 degrees, the hamstrings are considered tight.

Ober's test: With the subject side lying with both legs out straight, the examiner stabilizes the pelvis to prevent rolling and abducts and extends the top hip in order to position the iliotibial band (ITB) behind the greater trochanter. The subject slowly adducts the leg. A positive finding is the inability to adduct and touch the table. This indicates a tight tensor fascia latae and iliotibial band. The leg will remain abducted in mid-air. The tensor fascia latae can be isolated from the iliotibial band by bending the knee to 90 degrees.

Patrick's or FABER test: With the subject supine, the examiner passively flexes, abducts, and externally rotates the hip, flexes the knee, and places the foot on top of the opposite knee (frog position). The examiner slowly abducts the extremity being tested toward the table. A positive test results when the involved extremity does not abduct below the level of the noninvolved extremity. This indicates iliopsoas, sacroiliac, or even hip joint problems.

piriformis test: With the subject side lying, the top leg in 60 degrees of hip flexion, and the knee in relaxed flexion, the examiner stabilizes the pelvis and applies an adduction (downward) force on the knee. Tightness or pain in the hip and buttock areas is indicative of piriformis tightness. Pain in the buttock and posterior thigh is indicative of sciatic nerve impingement secondary to piriformis tightness.

Thomas test: With the subject in supine and the legs extended over the end of a table at the knees, have the subject flex both knees toward the chest. The examiner places one hand under the lumbar spine to monitor lumbar lordosis or pelvic tilt. The subject slowly lowers the test leg until the leg is fully relaxed or until either anterior pelvic tilt or an increase in lumbar lordosis occurs. A lack of hip extension with knee flexion more than 45 degrees is indicative of iliopsoas muscle tightness. Full hip extension with knee flexion less than 45 degrees is indicative of rectus femoris muscle tightness. A lack of hip extension with knee flexion more than 45 degrees is indicative of iliopsoas and rectus femoris muscle tightness. Hip external rotation is indicative of iliotibial band (particularly the tensor fascia latae) tightness.

Trendelenburg's test: The subject stands on one lower extremity and remains in this position for ~10 seconds and then switches legs. A positive finding is seen when the pelvis on the unsupported side drops lower than the pelvis on the supported side. This indicates a weakness of the gluteus medius on the supported side.

Knee

anterior drawer test: With the subject supine, the hip flexed to 45 degrees, and the knee flexed to 90 degrees, the examiner applies an anterior force to the proximal tibia. (Note: Make sure the hamstrings stay relaxed.) Increased anterior tibial displacement is indicative of a partial or complete tear of the anterior cruciate ligament.

anterior Lachman's test: With the subject supine and the knee flexed to 20 to 30 degrees, the examiner applies an anterior force to the tibia while stabilizing the femur. Excessive anterior translation of the tibia with a diminished or absent endpoint is indicative of a partial or complete tear of the anterior cruciate ligament.

Apley compression test: With the subject in prone and the knee flexed to 90 degrees, the examiner medially and laterally rotates the tibia while applying a downward force through the heel. Pain, clicking, and/or restriction is indicative of either a medial or lateral meniscus tear, depending on the location of symptoms.

ballotable patella or patella tap test: With the subject in supine, the examiner compresses the suprapatellar pouch with one hand and compresses the patella into the femur with two fingers of the thumb of the other hand. Downward movement of the patella followed by a rebound will give the appearance of a floating or ballotable patella and is indicative of moderate to severe joint effusion.

bounce home test: With the subject in supine, the examiner passively flexes the knee and then allows the knee to fall passively into extension. A rubbery end-feel or springy block is indicative of a meniscal tear.

external rotation recurvatum test: With the subject supine, the examiner grasps a great toe in each hand and lifts both legs off the table. An increase in hyperextension and external tibial rotation is indicative of posterolateral rotary instability, secondary to damage of the posterior cruciate ligament, lateral collateral ligament, posterolateral capsule, and arcuate complex.

Godfrey 90/90: With the subject supine and both hip and knee supported in 90 degrees of flexion, the examiner passively stabilizes the hip and knee while assessing the location of the tibia along the longitudinal axis. If one tibia is resting more inferior than the other side, it may indicate a posterior sag or instability. This may be related to posterior cruciate ligament laxity or avulsion.

gravity drawer sign (posterior sag test): With the subject supine, the knee flexed to 90 degrees, and the hip in 45 degrees of flexion, the examiner observes the position of the tibia relative to the femur in the sagittal plane. The subject is then instructed to actively contract the quadriceps while maintaining the position. Posterior displacement of the tibia upon the femur is an indicator of posterior instability. This could be the result of injury to the posterior cruciate ligament, arcuate ligament complex, and posterior oblique ligament.

Hughston plica test: With the subject supine, the examiner passively flexes and extends the knee while internally rotating the tibia and simultaneously pushing the patella medially. Pain and/or popping over the medial aspect of the knee is indicative of an abnormal plica.

Hughston posterolateral drawer test: With the subject supine, the hip flexed to 45 degrees, the knee flexed to 90 degrees, and the tibia externally rotated 20 to 30 degrees, the examiner applies a posterior force to the proximal tibia. Increased posterior tibial displacement is indicative of posterolateral rotary instability, secondary to damage of the posterior cruciate ligament, posterolateral capsule, lateral collateral ligament, and arcuate complex.

Hughston posteromedial drawer test: With the subject supine, the hip flexed to 45 degrees, the knee flexed to 90 degrees, and the tibia internally rotated 20 to 30 degrees, the examiner applies a posterior force to the proximal tibia. Increased posterior tibial displacement is indicative of posteromedial rotary instability, secondary to damage of the posterior cruciate ligament, posteromedial capsule, medial collateral ligament, and posterior oblique ligament.

jerk test: The subject is supine with the hip flexed to 45 degrees. The examiner passively flexes the knee to 90 degrees, then extends the knee while applying a valgus force and internally rotating the tibia. If a shift or "clunk" is felt at 30 degrees of knee flexion during extension, this is indicative of anterolateral rotary instability. If shift occurs, it will reduce upon further passive extension of the knee.

McMurray test: With subject in supine, knee fully flexed, and tibia externally rotated, the examiner introduces a valgus force and extends the knee (medial meniscus). Repeat with tibia externally rotated with the application of a varus force (lateral meniscus). A "click" along the medial joint line is indicative of a medial meniscus tear. A "click" along the lateral joint line is indicative of a lateral meniscus tear.

medial-lateral grind test: With the subject supine, the examiner passively flexes the hip and knee maximally and applies a circular motion with the tibia, rotating the tibia clockwise and counter-clockwise. Pain, grinding, or clicking is indicative of a meniscus tear.

noble test: With the subject in supine and the knee flexed to 90 degrees, the examiner passively extends and flexes the knee, maintaining pressure over the lateral epicondyle. If pain is present under the examiner's thumb in 30 degrees, iliotibial band friction syndrome is indicated.

patella apprehension test: With the subject supine and the knees extended, the examiner gently pushes the patella laterally using both thumbs on the medial border of the patella. If the subject is apprehensive or the quadriceps contract to protect against subluxation, the test is indicative of patellar subluxation or dislocation due to laxity of the medial retinaculum.

patella tendon/patella ligament length test: With the subject lying supine, the examiner measures the distance between the superior pole of the patella and the inferior pole of the patella. Next, the distance between the inferior pole and the tibial tuberosity is measured. A ratio is taken of the first and second measurements. A ratio greater than 1 indicates patella baja, while a ratio of less than 1 indicates patella alta. If the ratio is 1, it is normal.

patellar grind test: With the subject supine and the knees extended, the subject is asked to contract the quadriceps while the examiner applies downward and inferior pressure on the patella. Pain with movement of the patella or an inability to complete the test is indicative of chondromalacia patella.

pivot shift test: With the subject in supine and the knee in full extension, the examiner internally rotates the tibia while applying a valgus force and slowly flexing the knee. A palpable "clunk" or shift at ~20 to 30 degrees of flexion is indicative of anterolateral rotary instability, secondary to tearing of the anterior cruciate ligament and posterolateral capsule.

posterior drawer test: With the subject supine, the hip flexed to 45 degrees, and the knee flexed to 90 degrees, the examiner applies a posterior force to the proximal tibia. Increased posterior displacement indicates partial or complete tear of the posterior cruciate ligament.

posterior Lachman's test: With the subject supine and the knee flexed to 20 to 30 degrees, the examiner applies a posterior force to the tibia while stabilizing the femur. Excessive posterior translation of the tibia with a diminished or absent endpoint is indicative of a partial or complete tear of the posterior cruciate ligament.

quadriceps or Q-angle test: With the subject supine and the legs extended, place the axis of a goniometer over the midpoint of the patella and align the arms of the goniometer with the ASIS (proximally) and the tibial tubercle (distally). The result is the Q-angle. Normal is 13 degrees for males and 18 degrees for females. Angles greater or less than these norms are indicative of patellofemoral pathology.

Renne test: While the subject stands, the examiner places a thumb over the lateral epicondyle and instructs the subject to support the body weight on that leg and knee and actively flex as if performing a squat. The examiner applies pressure with the thumb over the lateral epicondyle. If pain is present when the knee is positioned in 30 degrees of flexion, iliotibial band friction syndrome is indicated.

reverse pivot shift (Jakob) test: With the subject supine and the knee in 40 to 50 degrees of flexion, the examiner externally rotates the tibia with one hand and applies a valgus force with the other while slowly extending the knee. The examiner observes if the lateral tibial plateau subluxes posteriorly in the flexed position. With extension, this subluxation is reduced at ~20 degrees and a palpable "clunk" or shift is indicative of posterolateral rotary instability secondary to involvement of the posterior cruciate ligament, lateral collateral ligament, posterolateral capsule, and arcuate complex.

Slocum test with external tibial rotation: With the subject supine, the hip flexed to 45 degrees, the knee flexed to 90 degrees, and the tibia externally rotated 15 to 20 degrees, the examiner applies an anterior force to the proximal tibia. Increased anterior tibial displacement is indicative of anterolateral rotary instability, secondary to a partial or complete tear of the anterior cruciate ligament, medial collateral ligament, and posteromedial capsule.

Slocum test with internal tibial rotation: With the subject supine, the hip flexed to 45 degrees, the knee flexed to 90 degrees, and the tibia internally rotated 15 to 20 degrees, the examiner applies an anterior force to the proximal tibia. Increased anterior tibial displacement is indicative of anterolateral rotary instability, secondary to a partial or complete tear of the anterior cruciate ligament and posterolateral capsule.

valgus stress test: With the subject supine with the knee in full extension, the examiner places one hand on the medial ankle and the other on the lateral knee. Stabilizing the ankle, a valgus force is applied. Medial knee pain and/or increased valgus movement with diminished or absent endpoint is indicative of damage to the medial collateral ligament, posterior cruciate ligament, and posteromedial capsule. If the test is repeated with the knee flexed 20 to 30 degrees, this isolates damage to the medial collateral ligament.

varus stress test: The subject is supine with knee in full extension. The examiner places one hand on the lateral ankle and the other on the medial knee. Stabilizing the ankle, a varus force is applied. Lateral knee pain and/or increased varus movement with diminished or absent endpoint is indicative of damage to the lateral collateral ligament, posterior cruciate ligament, and arcuate complex. If the test is repeated with the knee flexed 20 to 30 degrees, this isolates damage to the lateral collateral ligament.

Ankle and Foot

anterior drawer test: The subject is seated with his or her knee flexed to 90 degrees and foot relaxed (slight plantarflexion). While stabilizing the distal tibia and fibula, the examiner applies an anterior force to the calcaneus and talus. Anterior translation of the talus away from the ankle mortise is indicative of anterior talofibular ligament sprain.

compression test: The subject lies in supine with his or her foot off the examining table. The examiner squeezes the tibia and fibula together at some point away from the painful area. Pain at the site of injury may be indicative of a fracture. Pain will be exaggerated at the fracture site by compression.

Feiss' line: The subject is seated on the examining table with the leg extended. The examiner places a mark on the tip of the medial malleolus and at the base of the first metatarsophalangeal joint. A line is drawn between the two points, and the position of the navicular is noted. The subject then stands with his or her feet 3 to 6 inches apart. Observe the position of the navicular tuberosity in relation to the line. The navicular should be in line with the other two points. If the tuberosity of the navicular is below the line when seated, the subject has congenital pes planus. If the tuberosity is in line with the other two points while seated and then falls below the line upon standing, functional pes planus is indicated.

Homans' sign: With the subject in supine and the knee fully extended, the examiner passively dorsiflexes the foot. A production of pain in the calf due to the passive stretch is positive for thrombophlebitis. Pain may also be elicited with palpation of the calf in conjunction with the passive stretch.

interdigital neuroma test: The subject is seated on the exam table with his or her leg extended. The examiner squeezes the metatarsal heads together and holds them for 1 minute. Pain, tingling, or numbness in the foot, toes, or ankle is indicative of an interdigital neuroma. Pain is usually relieved when pressure is released.

long bone compression test: The subject is seated with his or her leg extended and foot just off the end of the exam table. The examiner applies compression along the long axis of the bone of the toe or metatarsal being tested. Pain at the site of injury is indicative of a fracture.

talar tilt test: The subject is side lying on the opposite side of testing with the foot hanging off the examining table. The examiner first places the foot in the anatomical position (neutral dorsi- and plantarflexion), then tilts the talus into an adducted position. Excessive range indicates a tear of the calcaneofibular ligament (compare to the other ankle).

tap or percussion test: The subject is supine with the foot just off the examining table. The examiner positions the ankle in maximal dorsiflexion and applies a firm tap to the bottom of the heel. Pain at the site of injury indicates a fracture. The vibration of tapping along the long axis of the bones will exaggerate pain at the fracture site.

Thomas test: The subject is in the prone position with his or her foot hanging off the table and the gastrocnemius-soleus complex relaxed. The examiner squeezes the belly of these muscles. A normal response would be to see the foot plantar flex. Absence of plantarflexion indicates a possible rupture of the Achilles' tendon.

Bibliography

Goldstein TS. *Geriatric Orthopaedics: Rehabilitative Management of Common Problems.* 2nd ed. Gaithersburg, Md: Aspen Publishers Inc; 1999.

Hoppenfeld S. *Physical Examination of the Spine and Extremities.* Norwalk, Conn: Appleton-Century-Crofts; 1976.

Konin JG, Wiksten DL, Isear JA. *Special Tests for Orthopedic Examination.* Thorofare, NJ: SLACK Incorporated; 1997.

Lewis CB, Knortz KA. *Orthopedic Assessment and Treatment of the Geriatric Patient*. St. Louis, Mo: Mosby-Year Book; 1993.

Magee DJ. *Orthopedic Physical Assessment*. 2nd ed. Philadelphia, Pa: WB Saunders; 1992.

GENERAL REFERENCES

Bohannon RW. Simple clinical measures. *Phys Ther*. 1997;67(12):1845-1850.

Delitto A. Subjective measures and clinical decision making. *Phys Ther*. 1989;69(7):585-589.

Jette AM. Measuring subjective clinical outcomes. *Phys Ther*. 1989;69(7):580-584.

Michels E. Evaluation and research in physical therapy. *Phys Ther*. 1982;62:828-834.

Rothstein JM. On defining subjective and objective measurements. *Phys Ther*. 1989;69(7):577-579.

Rothstein JM, Echternach JL. *Primer on Measurement: An Introductory Guide to Measurement Issues*. Alexandria, Va: American Physical Therapy Association; 1993:59-69.

Task Force on Standards for Measurement of Physical Therapy. Standards for tests and measurements in physical therapy practice. *Phys Ther*. 1991;71:589-622.

Van Deusen J, Brunt D. *Assessment in Occupational Therapy and Physical Therapy*. Philadelphia, Pa: WB Saunders; 1991.

Physical Therapy Interventions

Specific Therapeutic Interventions Defined

aerobic exercise: The use of ergometers, treadmills, steppers, aquatics, pulleys, weights, hydraulics, elastic resistance bands, robotics, and mechanical or electromechanical devices to improve fitness (a general term indicating a level of cardiovascular functioning, flexibility, and strength for optimum performance and well-being), endurance (the ability to work for prolonged periods without fatigue), maximum oxygen consumption (efficient intake and utilization of oxygen indicating physiological efficiency), conditioning (an augmentation of energy capacity), adaptation (ability of cardiovascular system to meet energy requirements at increasing levels of activity), and prevention of deconditioning (resulting from bedrest or sedentary lifestyle habits); submaximal, rhythmic, repetitive exercise requiring an increase in oxygen uptake.

aquatic exercise: A comprehensive therapeutic approach of exercise in water designed to aid in gaining strength, flexibility, and endurance; improve circulation; and promote relaxation. Aquatic therapy is a very helpful modality in treating balance problems. The resistance provided by movement through water has been shown to improve strength of muscle and of bone, as well as have a cardiovascular conditioning effect.

balance and coordination exercise: The use of functional activities and "motor practice" to assist the patient/client to learn strategies to prevent falls and coordination problems. Any of the evaluative techniques described in Appendix 19 (but not limited to) can also be employed as therapeutic tools for enhancing balance. Specialized programs that focus on systemic adaptation to position changes are also used for vestibular dysfunction.

biofeedback: The use of biofeedback enables an individual to use visual and auditory representations of physiological events, which are normally not perceived. Visual or auditory signals are indications of electromyographic activity and, through adequate training, an individual can learn to initiate and control appropriate muscle responses.

Bobath method: A neurodevelopmental approach, used primarily with cerebral palsy patients/clients but also applicable to dealing with stroke, using involuntary responses to movement of the head and body (eg, postural reflexes and equilibrium reactions) for purposes of modifying muscle tone or eliciting desired movements. The utilization of associated reactions is avoided; such movements are hypothesized to hamper progress beyond the stage in which reflexes and reactions dominate toward performance of normal, discrete voluntary movements. Supplemental proprioceptive stimuli (muscle stretch and "tapping") are used to facilitate and direct the individual's emerging responses to the head, neck, and body movement stimuli, which elicit equilibrium reactions.

body mechanics and ergonomics training: The instruction in proper alignment of body parts for activities at work, home, recreation, and sport to prevent injury.

Brunnström technique: A treatment approach based on the use of limb synergies and other available movement patterns in activities classified in six stages of recovery from hemiplegia. A method of "central facilitation" of the neuromuscular system that emphasizes the use of homolateral and bilateral associated reactions to recruit contraction of weak muscles through irradiation or overflow of activity from residually functional musculature during maximally resisted voluntary movement. Incorporates discrete proprioceptive and cutaneous stimuli as adjuncts for facilitation of individual muscles. Brunnström recognizes the importance of "shaping" or progressively refining the patient's/client's recovering motor skills, advocating the initial use of synergies and reflex patterns to begin the recovery process and then continuing to modify these patterns into more complex functional movements. Useful in the treatment of stroke and other pathologies in which tone is present.

Buerger-Allen exercise: An exercise protocol for peripheral vascular disease in which the positional change of the extremity, coupled with active muscle contraction (pumping of the feet, etc), uses gravity to enhance the filling and emptying of blood from the extremity. The positions include horizontal positioning of the extremity, elevation of the extremity above the level of the heart (emptying of the extremity), and a dependent position (filling of the extremity).

chest physical therapy: A multifaceted area of professional practice that deals with the evaluation and treatment of patients/clients with acute or chronic lung disorders. Goals of chest physical therapy are to prevent airway obstruction and accumulation of secretions that interfere with normal respiration, improve airway clearance and ventilation through mobilization and drainage of secretions, improve endurance and general exercise tolerance, reduce energy costs during respiration through breathing retraining, prevent or correct postural deformities, promote relaxation, maintain or improve chest mobility, and improve cough effectiveness. This is accomplished through breathing exercises (eg, diaphragmatic breathing, segmental expansion, inspiratory resistance exercises, etc), vibration, shaking, percussion, postural drainage, suctioning, coughing, instruction in energy conservation techniques, and conditioning exercises.

Codman exercise: The use of gravity to facilitate relaxation and movement of the shoulder joint. With the trunk flexed at the waist and the arm hanging straight down and relaxed, pendulum-type movements in all planes are performed.

compression therapies: Any therapy using compression to reduce or prevent edema and promote healing. Compression therapies include vasopneumatic compression pumps, compression bandaging and garments, taping, and total contact casting.

connective tissue massage: Deep massage of the connective tissues (ie, fascia) aimed at breaking adhesions, reducing friction between the muscles and connective tissues to improve mobility and flexibility, and enhancing circulation to promote healing. Used as a manual therapy to reduce restrictions of soft tissues that create muscle imbalances and lead to dysfunctional motor patterns.

contrast baths: Alternating hot and cold baths to promote vasodilatation and vasoconstriction of the local blood vessels. They are used to decrease joint stiffness and pain and improve peripheral blood flow.

cryotherapy (cold): The use of cold as a therapeutic agent. It is used for posttraumatic edema and inflammation. It has been found to alter the conduction velocity and synaptic activity of peripheral nerves, decreasing sensory and motor conduction velocities for management of pain and muscle spasms. The use of cryotherapy is based on the physiologic responses to a decrease in tissue temperature. Cold decreases blood flow and tissue metabolism, thus decreasing bleeding and acute inflammation. Spasticity and muscle guarding spasms can be diminished, allowing for a greater ease of motion. Pain threshold is elevated, thus allowing exercises to be carried out with increased comfort. Application of cryotherapy can include ice packs, ice massage, ice towels, cold baths, vapocoolant sprays, or controlled cold-compression units.

electrical stimulation: The use of direct current (DC) or alternating current (AC) therapeutically in many clinical conditions. Continuous DC will not elicit muscle contraction as the body accommodates to continuous flow of current (muscles respond best to "make and break" of the flow or a change in direction, polarity). Continuous DC is primarily used for iontophoresis (*see* iontophoresis). As electricity flows naturally from positive to negative, the negative pole produces the greater stimulation and is recommended as the stimulating electrode. Interrupted DC of sufficiently long duration is helpful in producing muscle contraction in denervated musculature. Continuous AC may be utilized to tetanize musculature to obtain relaxation of spasm. Surged AC is used to stimulate slow-twitch fibers because peak intensities are reached over a brief period of delay, whereas pulsed or interrupted AC is more effective in stimulating fast-twitch fibers because peak intensities are reached instantaneously. An optimum frequency for general stimulation is between 80 and 100 Hz as the net frequency (*see* also high-voltage [high-galvanic] pulsed current electrical stimulation [HVPC]).

fluidotherapy: A dry heat agent that transfers energy by forced convection providing heat. Warm air is circulated through a container holding fine cellulose particles. The solid particles become suspended when air is forced through them, thus the properties of fluidotherapy are similar to those of liquids. The viscosity of the air-fluidized system is low, permitting exercise with relative ease. Patients/clients with rheumatoid arthritis, osteoarthritis, Silastic joint replacements, wounds, sprains and strains, and amputations benefit from this exercise/heat modality. It has been used to promote relaxation, increase blood flow to an area, and decrease pain.

Frenkel exercises: They were developed principally for locomotor ataxia in which ataxia is due to loss of proprioception. They are useful in cerebellar ataxia. Frenkel exercises are begun from one of four positions: lying, sitting, standing, or walking. Concentration of attention on each movement is mandatory and each movement is done slowly and with repetition. The physiological basis for these exercises is the attempt to regain coordination by utilization of other senses (eg, visual in locomotor ataxia and proprioceptive-visual in cerebellar dysfunction), by voluntary relearning of functions lost by repetition of neurological deficiencies, and by retraining of functional patterns.

functional training and retraining: The use of functional activities as a therapeutic intervention to improve mobility, flexibility, strength, and endurance, while assimilating activities required to perform basic ADLs and IADLs.

gait training and retraining: The use of ambulation with special attention to muscle imbalances, stance and swing phases of gait, and biomechanical components of walking (eg, heel strike, push off, etc), where the individual focuses on locomotor or neurological deficits to correct deficient patterns. It may include the use of assistive devices.

Guthrie-Smith exercises: The use of a sling suspension frame in which springs or pulleys provide resistance or assistance to the movement of an extremity.

Helbrandt exercises: The use of reflexes to facilitate muscle contraction and functional movement in which a crossed reflex is used to exercise one muscle and strengthen its contralateral mate.

high-voltage (high-galvanic) pulsed current electrical stimulation (HVPC): A "twin-peak monophasic" wave form of electrical current used for wound healing, edema reduction, modulation of pain, neuromuscular stimulation, and enhancement of the vascular system. High-voltage galvanic stimulation utilizes the deeper penetration of higher-frequency (shorter-wave length) currents in the low microseconds range to eliminate discomfort by bypassing the superficial sensory nerve endings in the skin.

hot packs: Hot packs provide a superficial, moist heat. They are used for muscle pain, stiffness, and spasm; to increase circulation; and to prepare soft tissues for other therapeutic interventions.

hydrotherapy: The broad category of treatment using any water modality as a therapeutic intervention. It can include aquatic therapy, whirlpool therapy, contrast baths, or pulsatile lavage.

industrial rehabilitation: Functional capacity testing and conditioning for job-related skills. Training in skills required to function in a given employment position. Instruction in biomechanics, body mechanics, physical conditioning, and ergonomic modification to reduce the potential for job-related injury and prepare an individual for entry or re-entry to his or her job or career.

infrared: A form of electromagnetic radiation beyond the red end (lower, invisible wavelength range) of the visible band of colors. Radiation in this range is absorbed by the body as heat. Infrared therapy heats tissues, increases circulation, produces vasodilation, produces mild analgesia, increases phagocytosis, increases metabolic processes, and increases permeability of tissue membranes.

interferential electrical stimulation: A form of electrical stimulation with the physical phenomenon of wave interference when two more sinusoidal waves originate exactly in phase from separate currents and are coherent with respect to frequency and amplitude. Interferential current stimulation utilizes medium-frequency currents (4000 Hz to 4100 Hz), which are crossed subcutaneously. The resulting interferential pattern cancels out the difference in frequencies and leaves the balance in the range of 80 Hz to 100 Hz. This characteristic allows frequencies to penetrate to a tissue level considerably deeper than if administered with surface electrodes using the same range with low-volt apparatus. Interferential electrical stimulation has been found to be useful in the treatment of neuritis, musculoskeletal conditions (excellent mode for breaking up calcifications and adhesions), vascular conditions (Raynaud's disease), urogenital dysfunction (pelvic floor), and pain. Interferential current can be used as a substitute for traditional TENS to produce analgesia in conditions with acute, superficial, deep aching, and chronic pain.

iontophoresis: A electrotherapeutic modality that creates ion transfer. It is the introduction of topically applied, physiologically active ions into the epidermis and mucous membranes of the body by the use of continuous direct current. The electrical principle of iontophoresis is that an electrically charged electrode will repel a similarly charged ion. This modality is used to "drive in" local anesthetics, anti-inflammatory agents, and edema reduction agents and is used to treat a variety of skin conditions. It has been found to be helpful in the treatment of calcium deposits, softening scars and adhesions, fungus infections, musculoskeletal inflammation conditions, edema reduction, muscle relaxant and vasodilatation, hyperhidrosis, bursitis, neuritis, and slow healing wounds and ulcers.

isokinetic exercise: The control of the speed of muscle under water, or with the use of springs, in order to provide continuously uniform stress through the full range of motion of most joints.

isometric exercise: A form of resistance exercise in which there is no movement, so muscles are strengthened in a "static" position using manual or fixed-arm apparatus resistance.

Jacobson's relaxation exercise: Progressive isometric contraction of each muscle of the body leading to relaxation and awareness of the area. A form of biofeedback used to decrease overall stress.

joint manipulation techniques: A passive movement, using physiologic or accessory motions, that may be applied with a thrust (a sudden, high-velocity, short-amplitude motion) or when the patient/client is under anesthesia.

joint mobilization techniques: A passive movement performed by the therapist using oscillatory motion or a sustained stretch intended to decrease pain or increase mobility of a joint. The techniques may use physiologic movements (movements that the patient/client can do voluntarily) or accessory movements (movements within the joint and surrounding tissues that are necessary for normal range of motion but that cannot be performed by the patient/client). Component motions are those motions that accompany active motion but are not under voluntary control; the term is often used synonymously with accessory movement (eg, upward rotation of the scapula and clavicle, which occur with shoulder flexion). Joint play describes the motions that occur in the joint and describes the distensibility or "give" in the joint capsule, which allows the bones to move. The term arthrokinematics is used when these motions of the bone surfaces within the joint are described.

Kegel exercises: Contraction of the pelvic floor muscles in the treatment of urinary incontinence. The purpose of the exercises is to strengthen the hypotonic pelvic floor muscles to prevent leakage of urine from the bladder by repositioning the bladder into its normal position.

Kenny method: A muscle reeducation technique developed for lower motor neuron diseases. Sister Kenny used heat treatments and exercise based on the normal processes of learning starting with reflex activity in an attempt to stimulate proprioceptive pathways by passive movement of the extremity.

lymphatic drainage: The increase in hydrostatic pressure by manual massage techniques or mechanical compression to assist in reducing lymphedema and prevent further edema secondary to obstruction of the lymphatic system from trauma, infection, radiation, or surgery.

massage: Massage is a "hands-on" kneading, stroking, or frictional circular rubbing of the muscles to relieve spasm and pain, promote circulation, increase extensibility of the muscle, and provide sensory input to neurologically impaired muscles. Massage is an effective manual therapy for edema management in acute and chronic conditions and in pathologies of the lymphatic system (*see* lymphatic drainage). Massage techniques consist of three generally used strokes: effleurage or stroking, pétrissage or kneading, and friction. The techniques are performed either over the muscle belly or over a portion of the muscle that is involved.

muscle energy techniques: Physical therapy manual exercises that bring about controlled movement of joints and muscle through skilled application and direction of energy created within the muscle by concentrated efforts of the patient.

muscle reeducation: Techniques employed to reeducate the afferent side of the motor pattern. If sensation is normal, the techniques developed by Sister Kenny are effective; if sensation is not intact, biofeedback techniques may be necessary to facilitate normal muscle function.

myofascial release techniques: The use of deep friction and stroking of the fascia of the body to improve the ability of the fascia to deform and move within the body. This manual therapy is used to reduce or eliminate pain, speed the healing process, diminish structural imbalances, and improve the patient's/client's general functional abilities.

neurodevelopmental treatment (NDT): The reflexive inhibitory patterns used in Bobath's NDT approach using natural inhibitory mechanisms to gain new range and movement. Intervention approach developed to address abnormal tonicity in a muscle, and elimination of unwanted muscle activity and retraining of normal, functional patterns of movement in individuals with acquired brain dysfunction due to stroke, etc (*see* Bobath method).

neuromuscular electrical stimulation (NMES): The use of electrical current to strengthen or maintain muscle mass, maintain or gain range of motion, facilitate voluntary motor control, temporarily reduce the effects of spasticity, and temporarily provide for orthotic substitution.

orthotic training: Instruction by the physical therapist in the proper application and use of an orthotic device, including donning, precautions and skin management, gait training, functional training, and orthotic evaluation for wear and tear.

paraffin bath: The use of melted paraffin and mineral oil as a form of heat treatment for painful joints and muscles.

pendulum exercises: *See* Codman exercises.

phonophoresis: Similar to iontophoresis in concept, but differing in the physical chemistry involved, phonophoresis provides the introduction of molecules into the tissues by means of the energy of the sound wave front. In contrast to the ions introduced with direct current, phonophoresis requires that the body break down the molecules into the appropriate ions and radicals for use. Ultrasound is used to drive anti-inflammatory drugs and local analgesics through the skin to underlying tissues. It is hypothesized that phonophoresis is able to penetrate deeper than iontophoresis, thereby providing medications to deeper tissues.

progressive resistance exercises (PRE): The original method of PRE was developed by DeLorme using weights on the distal end of the extremity and contracting the muscles against the force of gravity to strengthen the muscle. The number of repetitions and the amount of weight is gradually increased. DeLorme also incorporated the use of counterbalancing the weight of the extremity with a cable or pulley arrangement for muscles of less than fair strength and thus giving load-assisting exercise to muscle groups that cannot perform antigravity motions. This method is used in many free-weight and machine resistive systems (eg, Cybex, Polaris, etc).

proprioceptive neuromuscular facilitation (PNF): A therapeutic approach developed by Knott and Voss in which the therapist attempts to facilitate the contraction of muscle groups in particular synergistic patterns (diagonal-spiral movements), which begin with placing the muscles to be facilitated under maximal stretch and end with the muscles at the maximally shortened end of their range. Graded resistance is applied to maintain facilitatory stretch afferent input during shortening and to recruit activity in the weak muscles through overflow from strong muscles during maximal effort.

prosthetic training: Instruction by the physical therapist in the proper application and use of a prosthetic limb, including donning, precautions and skin management, compression and edema control techniques, gait training, functional training, and prosthetic evaluation for wear and tear.

range of motion (ROM): Passive ROM is movement within the unrestricted range for a segment that is produced by an external force with no voluntary muscle contraction. Active ROM is movement within the unrestricted range for a segment that is produced by an active muscle contraction of the muscles crossing the joint. Active assistive ROM is a type of active range in which assistance is provided by an outside force, either manually or mechanically, to assist the prime mover muscles through the available range for the segment. Functional excursion is the distance that a muscle is capable of shortening after it has been elongated to its maximum.

resistance exercise: A form of active exercise in which a dynamic or static muscular contraction is resisted manually or mechanically to increase strength, endurance, and power of muscle contraction.

Rood approach: The application of cutaneous stimuli to discrete areas of the skin in order to modify tone and promote the contraction of underlying muscles. Rood developed the use of stimulus applications, such as "brushing," vibration, and "icing" using stroking techniques. The mechanical and thermal stimulation of the skin overlying a particular muscle leads to activation of the efferents innervating stretch receptors in the muscle. This, in turn, brings about increased sensitivity of stretch receptors in the muscle by virtue of which tone (ie, baseline tension in the absence of deliberate movement) as well as its contractile response to stretch is enhanced.

short-wave diathermy: Electrotherapeutic modality that generates high-frequency currents, producing heat deep within the tissues by induction. Condenser-type electrode or induction drums are used to apply the current. Short-wave diathermy uses high-frequency alternating currents that oscillate at frequencies between 10 and 50 MHz. Application of diathermy involves transmission and absorption of electromagnetic energy by the body, with subsequent conversion of the nonionizing radiation into therapeutic heat by resisting tissues. The utilization of diathermy in physical therapy includes functional restoration and analgesia and facilitation of healing of recently injured soft tissue. Medically, diathermy is used to create hyperthermia for tumor eradication.

stretching techniques: Stretching of soft tissues to elongate contractile or noncontractile tissues can be done through passive stretching or active inhibition of the muscles. Manual passive stretching is done by the therapist applying an external manual force, controlling direction, speed, intensity, and duration of the stretch and elongating contracted or restricted tissues beyond their resting length. Prolonged mechanical passive stretching is a low-intensity external force applied to shortened tissues over a prolonged period of time with mechanical equipment. Cyclic mechanical stretching is passive stretching using a mechanical device that ranges the extremity in a cyclic mode. Active inhibition refers to techniques in which the patient/client reflexively relaxes the muscle to be elongated prior to the stretching maneuver. Contract-relax (hold-relax) is when the patient/client performs an isometric contraction of the tight muscle before it is passively lengthened. This inhibition technique was originally associated with PNF, and the term *muscle energy* is also used by manual therapists to describe inhibition techniques used to elongate muscles and improve joint mobility in the spine or extremities. Contract-relax-contract (hold-relax-contract), a variation of the contract-relax technique, is contraction of the tight muscle and relaxation of the tight muscle followed by a concentric contraction of the muscle opposite the tight muscle. As the muscle opposite the tight muscle shortens, the tight muscle lengthens, combining autogenic inhibition and reciprocal inhibition to lengthen a tight muscle. Agonist contraction is when the patient/client dynamically contracts the muscle opposite the tight muscle against resistance causing reciprocal inhibition and lengthening of the tight muscle.

traction techniques: A steady (continuous) or intermittent (alternately applied and released in a rhythmic pattern) force is applied mechanically, manually, or positionally to separate the surfaces of bone at a joint.

transcutaneous electrical nerve stimulation (TENS): TENS is an electrotherapeutic modality specifically oriented to the stimulation of nerve fibers known to be involved with transmitting signals to the brain that are interpreted by the thalamus as pain. The waveforms used with TENS equipment are targeted to be received by large-diameter, myelinated A fibers, which are reserved for proprioceptive transmission. Generally, TENS is administered just below the stimulation of muscle contraction. It is useful for management of pain postsurgically as well as in pain associated with labor.

ultrasound: Though grouped amidst "electrotherapy" modalities, ultrasound generates sound waves, rather than electrical waves, which penetrate 1 cm to 3 cm into the tissues and produce mechanical oscillation within a frequency high enough to produce warmth, soften scar tissue by breaking molecular bonds, and increase metabolism, thereby improving nutrition, at the cellular level. Ultrasound is frequently used for joint contractures, scar tissues, reduction of pain and muscle spasm, bursitis and tendinitis, breaking up calcium deposits, phonophoresis, plantar warts, and wound healing.

ultraviolet therapy: A form of electromagnetic radiation beyond the violet end (higher, invisible wavelength range) of the visible band of colors. Ultraviolet has a profound physiological effect that is therapeutically valuable. Steroid metabolism is stimulated by ultraviolet radiation; vasomotor responses are enhanced; bactericidal qualities are enhanced, and ultraviolet has been found to have an anti-rachitic (ie, preventing rickets) effect.

whirlpool therapy: The hydrotherapy technique of placing an involved part or the whole body in circulating warm or cold water to increase circulation; increase connective tissue extensibility; modulate pain; reduce or eliminate soft tissue swelling, inflammation, or restriction; increase the rate of healing; and promote relaxation.

wound debridement: The cutting away of dead or contaminated tissue or foreign material to clean a wound and promote healthy tissue healing. Nonselective techniques can include enzymatic debridement; wet, wet-to-dry, or wet-to-moist dressings; total contact casts; whirlpool, supplemental oxygen, or electrotherapeutic modalities. Selective techniques include enzymatic debridement; sharp debridement; autolysis; topical agents; topical oxygen; or electrotherapeutic modalities.

BIBLIOGRAPHY

Basmajian JV. *Therapeutic Exercise*. 4th ed. Baltimore, Md: Williams and Wilkins; 1984.

Kisner C, Colby LA. *Therapeutic Exercise: Foundations and Techniques*. 2nd ed. Philadelphia, Pa: FA Davis; 1990.

Michlovitz SL. *Thermal Agents in Rehabilitation*. Philadelphia, Pa: FA Davis; 1986.

Nelson RM, Currier DP. *Clinical Electrotherapy*. 2nd ed. Norwalk, Conn: Appleton & Lange; 1991.

O'Sullivan SB, Schmitz TJ. *Physical Rehabilitation: Assessment and Treatment*. 2nd ed. Philadelphia, Pa: FA Davis; 1988.

Scully RM, Barnes MR. *Physical Therapy*. Philadelphia, Pa: JB Lippincott; 1989.

Sullivan PE, Markos PD, Minor MAD. *An Integrated Approach to Therapeutic Exercise: Theory & Clinical Application*. Reston, Va: Prentice-Hall; 1982.

Normal Measures for Range of Motion of the Joints

SPINE RANGE OF MOTION

	Cervical	*Lumbar*
Forward Flexion	0 to 45 degrees	0 to 95 degrees
Extension	0 to 50 degrees	0 to 35 degrees
Lateral Flexion	0 to 45 degrees	0 to 40 degrees
Rotation	0 to 60 degrees	0 to 35 degrees

UPPER EXTREMITY RANGE OF MOTION

Shoulder

Flexion	0 to 180 degrees
Extension	0 to 60 degrees
Abduction	0 to 180 degrees
Adduction	0 to 75 degrees
Horizontal Abduction	0 to 90 degrees
Horizontal Adduction	0 to 45 degrees
Internal Rotation	0 to 70 to 90 degrees
External Rotation	0 to 90 degrees

Elbow and Forearm

Extension to Flexion	0 to 150 degrees
Supination	0 to 80 to 90 degrees
Pronation	0 to 80 to 90 degrees

Wrist

Flexion	0 to 80 to 90 degrees
Extension	0 to 70 degrees
Ulnar Deviation	0 to 30 to 35 degrees
Radial Deviation	0 to 20 degrees

Thumb (first digit)

CM Flexion	0 to 15 degrees
CM Extension	0 to 20 degrees
MCP Flexion	0 to 50 to 90 degrees
MCP Extension	0 to 10 degrees

IP Flexion	0 to 80 to 110 degrees
IP Extension	0 to 10 degrees
Abduction	0 to 70 degrees
Opposition	0 (cm)

Fingers (second through fifth digits)

MCP Flexion	0 to 90 degrees
PIP Flexion	0 to 100 to 110 degrees
PIP Extension	0 to 10 degrees
DIP Flexion	0 to 90 to 110 degrees
DIP Extension	0 to 10 degrees
Abduction	No norm
Adduction	No norm

LOWER EXTREMITY RANGE OF MOTION

Hip

Flexion	0 to 120 degrees
Extension	0 to 10 degrees
Abduction	0 to 45 degrees
Adduction	0 to 30 degrees
Medial Rotation	0 to 45 degrees
Lateral Rotation	0 to 45 degrees

Knee

| Extension to Flexion | 0 to 135 to 145 degrees |

Ankle to Foot

Dorsiflexion	0 to 20 degrees
Plantarflexion	0 to 45 degrees
Inversion	0 to 30 degrees
Eversion	0 to 20 degrees

Great Toe (first digit)

MTP Flexion	0 to 45 degrees
MTP Extension	0 to 90 degrees
IP Flexion	0 to 90 degrees
IP Extension	0 to 70 degrees

Lesser Toes (second through fifth digit)

MTP Flexion	0 to 40 degrees
MTP Extension	0 to 45 degrees
PIP Flexion	0 to 45 degrees
DIP Flexion	0 to 70 degrees

MTP = metatarsalphalangeal
DIP = distal interphalangeal
IP = interphalangeal
MCP = metacarpophalangeal
PIP = proximal interphalangeal

Normal Ranges for Laboratory Values

NORMAL VALUES: HEMATOLOGY

Lab Test	Normal Value	Clinical Significance
Bleeding time	30 sec to 6 min	Prolonged in pupura hemorrhagia, where platelets are reduced, and in chloroform and phosphorus poisoning
Clotting time	5 to 10 min	Prolonged in hemorrhagic disease and in various coagulation factor deficiencies
Factor V assay	75% to 125%	Pro-accelerin factor
Factor VIII assay (antihemophiliac factor)	50% to 200%	Deficient in classical hemophilia
Factor IX assay (plasma thromboplastin component)	75% to 125%	Deficient in pseudohemophilia (Christmas disease)
Factor X	75% to 125%	Stuart clotting defect
Fibrinogen	0.2 to 0.4 g/100 mL	Increased in pregnancy, pneumonia, infections accompanied by leukocytosis, and nephrosis; decreased in acute yellow atrophy of liver, cirrhosis, typhoid fever, chloroform poisoning, and abruptio placentae

Lab Test	Normal Value	Clinical Significance
Fibrinolysins (whole blood clot lysis time)	No lysis in 24 hours	Increased activity associated with massive hemorrhage, extensive surgery, and transfusion reactions
Partial thromboplastin time	35 to 45 sec	Prolonged in factor VIII, IX, and X deficiency
Prothrombin consumption	Over 25 sec	Impaired in factor VIII, IX, and X deficiency
Prothrombin time	70% to 100% of control	Prolonged in factor X deficiency, and other hemorrhagic diseases, and in cirrhosis, hepatitis, and acute toxic necrosis of the liver
Erythrocyte count	Male: 4,200,000 to 6,000,000/mm^3 Female: 4,200,000 to 5,400,000/mm^3	Increased in severe diarrhea and dehydration, polycythemia rubra vera, secondary polycythemia, acute poisoning, pulmonary fibrosis, and Ayerza's disease; decreased in all anemias, leukemia, and after hemorrhage, when blood volume has been restored
Erythrocyte sedimentation rate	Male: 0 to 9 mm/hr Female: 0 to 20 mm/hr	Increased in tissue destruction, whether inflammatory or degenerative, and during menstruation, pregnancy, and in acute febrile diseases
Hematocrit	Male: 42% to 50% Female: 40% to 48%	Decreased in severe anemias, anemia of pregnancy, acute massive blood loss; increased in erythrocytosis of any cause and in dehydration or hemoconcentration associated with shock
Hemoglobin	Male: 13 to 16 g/ 100 mL Female: 12 to 14 g/ 100 mL	Decreased in various anemias, pregnancy, severe or prolonged hemorrhage, and with excessive fluid intake; increased in polycythemia, chronic obstructive pulmonary diseases, failure of oxygenation because of congestive heart failure, and normally, in people living at high altitudes

Lab Test	Normal Value	Clinical Significance
Leukocyte count	Total: 5000 to 10,000 cu mm	Elevated in acute infectious diseases—predominately in neutrophilic fraction with bacterial diseases, and in lymphocytic and monocytic fractions in viral diseases. Eosinophils elevated in collagen diseases, allergy, and intestinal parasitosis. Elevated in acute leukemia, following menstruation, and following surgery or trauma. Depressed in aplastic anemia, agranulocytosis, and by toxic agents, such as chemotherapeutic agents used in treating malignancy
Neutrophils	60% to 70%	
Eosinophils	1% to 4%	
Basophils	0% to 0.5%	
Lymphocytes	20% to 30%	
Monocytes	2% to 6%	
Erythrocyte indices		
Mean corpuscular volume (MCV)	80 to 94 cu μ	Increased in macrocytic anemias, decreased in microcytic anemia
Mean corpuscular hemoglobin (MCH)	27 to 32 μμg per cell	Increased in macrocytic anemias, decreased in microcytic anemia
Mean corpuscular hemoglobin concentration (MCHC)	33% to 38%	Decreased in severe hypochromic anemia
Reticulocytes	0.5% to 1.5% of red cells	Increased with any condition stimulating increased bone marrow activity (ie, infection, blood loss [acute or chronic], following iron therapy in iron deficiency anemia, polycythemia rubra vera); decreased with any condition depressing bone marrow activity, acute leukemia, late stage of severe anemias

Lab Test	Normal Value	Clinical Significance
Leukocyte alkaline phosphatase	Score of 40 to 100	Decreased in chronic myelocytic leukemia and chronic lymphocytic leukemia; increased in nonleukemic leukocytosis and myeloproliferative diseases
Osmotic fragility of red cells	Increase if hemolysis occurs in over 0.5% NaCl Decrease if hemolysis is incomplete in 0.3% NaCl	Increased in congenital spherocytosis, idiopathic acquired hemolytic anemia, isoimmune hemolytic disease, ABO hemolytic disease of newborn; decreased in sickle cell anemia, thalassemia
Platelet count	200,000 to 350,000 per cu mm	Increased with chronic leukemia, hemoconcentration; decreased in thrombocytopenic purpura, acute leukemia, aplastic anemia, and during cancer chemotherapy

NORMAL BLOOD OR SERUM VALUES: CHEMISTRY

Lab Test	Normal Value	Clinical Significance	
		(Increased)	(Decreased)
Acetoacetate and acetone	0.3 to 2.0 mg/100 mL	Diabetic acidosis Fasting Toxemia of pregnancy Carbohydrate-free diet	

Lab Test	Normal Value	Clinical Significance	
		(Increased)	*(Decreased)*
Aldolase	3 to 8 units/mL	High-fat diet Hepatic necrosis Granulocytic leukemia Myocardial infarction Skeletal muscle disease	
Alpha amino nitrogen	3.0 to 5.5 mg/100 mL	Phosphorus, arsenic, chloroform, carbon tetrachloride poisoning Infectious hepatitis Eclampsia	Pneumococcal pneumonia Administration of anterior pituitary extracts Administration of insulin
Ammonia	50 to 170 µg/100 mL*	Severe liver disease Hepatic decompensation	
Amylase	80 to 150 units/mL	Acute pancreatitis Mumps Duodenal ulcer Carcinoma of head of pancreas Prolonged elevation with pseudocyst of pancreas	Chronic pancreatitis Pancreatic fibrosis and atrophy Cirrhosis of liver Acute alcoholism Toxemia of pregnancy Rheumatic fever Collagen diseases
Ascorbic acid	0.4 to 1.5 mg/100 mL		Deficient vitamin C intake Renal and hepatic disease Congestive heart failure

*Whole blood

Lab Test	Normal Value	Clinical Significance	
		(Increased)	*(Decreased)*
Bilirubin	Total: 0.1 to 1.0 mg/100 mL Direct: 0.1 to 0.2 mg/100 mL Indirect: 0.1 to 0.8 mg/100 mL	Hemolytic anemia (indirect) Biliary obstruction Hepatocellular damage Pernicious anemia Hemolytic disease of newborn Eclampsia	
Bromsulphalein (BSP)	Less than 5% retention in 45 min	Acute hepatic diseases	
Calcium	9 to 11 mg/100 mL	Tumor or hyperplasia of parathyroid Hyperparathyroidism Hypervitaminosis D Multiple myeloma Nephritis with uremia	Hypoparathyroidism Diarrhea Celiac disease Rickets Osteomalacia Malnutrition Nephrosis After parathyroidectomy
CO_2 content	Adults: 24 to 32 mEq/L Infants: 20 to 26 mEq/L	Tetany Respiratory diseases Intestinal obstruction Vomiting	Acidosis Nephritis Eclampsia Diarrhea Anesthesia

Lab Test	Normal Value	Clinical Significance	
		(Increased)	(Decreased)
Carotene, Beta	100 to 300 μg/100 mL	Carotenemia	Malabsorption syndromes
		Hypothyroidism	Hepatic disease
		Diabetes	Dietary deficiencies
		Hyperlipemia	
Cephalin flocculation	Negative to 1+	Severe liver disease	
		Atypical viral pneumonia	
		Malaria	
		Lues	
		Infectious mononucleosis	
		Congestive heart failure	
Ceruloplasmin	27 to 43 mg/dL	Pregnancy	Wilson's disease (hepato-lenticular degeneration)
		Myocardial infarction	
		Hepatic cirrhosis	
Chloride	95 to 105 mEq/L	Nephritis	Diabetes
		Urinary obstruction	Diarrhea
		Cardiac decomposition	Vomiting
		Anemia	Pneumonia
		Ether anesthesia	Heavy metal poisoning
			Cushing's syndrome
			Burns
			Intestinal obstruction
			Febrile conditions

Lab Test	Normal Value	Clinical Significance	
		(Increased)	(Decreased)
Cholesterol	150 to 270 mg/100 mL	Lipemia Obstructive jaundice Diabetes Hypothyroidism	Pernicious anemia Hemolytic jaundice Hyperthyroidism Severe infection Terminal states of disease
Cholesterol esters	65% to 70% of total liver disease		The esterified fraction decreases in liver disease
Cholinesterase	Plasma: 1.15 to 1.65 units Red cells: 0.65 to 1.0 units	Nephrosis Exercise	Nerve gas intoxication (greater effect on red cell activity) Insecticides, organic phosphates (greater effect on plasma activity)
Congo red	60% to 100% remains in bloodstream		Deposits in amyloid tissue absorb congo red. In amyloid disease, less than 40% of the dye will remain in the plasma In severe cases, less than 10% is retained

Lab Test	Normal Value	Clinical Significance	
		(Increased)	(Decreased)
Copper	Males: 97 to 130 µg/100 mL Females: 105 to 140 µg/100 mL	Cirrhosis of the liver Pregnancy	Wilson's disease
Creatine	3 to 7 mg/100 mL	Biliary obstruction Pregnancy Nephritis Renal destruction Trauma to muscle Pseudohypertrophic muscular dystrophy	
Creatine phosphokinase (CPK)	Males: 0 to 20 I.U./L Females: 0 to 14 I.U./L	Myocardial infarction Skeletal muscle diseases Nephritis	
Creatinine	1 to 2 mg/100 mL	Chronic renal disease	
Cryoglobulin	Zero	Multiple myeloma Chronic lymphocytic leukemia Lymphosarcoma Systemic lupus erythematosus Rheumatoid arthritis Subacute bacterial endocarditis Some malignancies	

Lab Test	Normal Value	Clinical Significance (Increased)	(Decreased)
Fatty acids	Total: 250 to 390 mg/100 mL	Diabetes Anemia Nephrosis Hypothyroidism Nephritis	Hyperthyroidism
Fibrinogen**	0.1 to 0.4 g/100 mL	Pneumonia Acute infections Pregnancy Nephrosis Carcinoma	Cirrhosis Acute toxic necrosis of liver Anemia Typhoid fever Chloroform or phosphorus poisoning Abruptio placentae
Glucose	65 to 110 mg/100 mL	Diabetes Nephritis Hyperthyroidism Early hyperpituitarism Cerebral lesions Infections Pregnancy Uremia	Hyperinsulinism Hypothyroidism Late hyperpituitarism Pernicious vomiting Addison's disease Extensive hepatic damage

**Plasma

Lab Test	Normal Value	Clinical Significance	
		(Increased)	(Decreased)
Icterus index	1 to 6 units	Biliary obstruction Hemolytic anemias	Secondary anemias
Iodine, protein-bound	4.0 to 8.0 μg/100 mL	Hyperthyroidism	Hypothyroidism
Iron	56 to 150 μg/100 ml	Pernicious anemia Aplastic anemia Hemolytic anemia Hepatitis Hemochromatosis	Iron deficiency anemia
Iron binding capacity	150 to 225 μg/100 mL	Iron deficiency anemia	Chronic infectious diseases
Lactic acid*	6 to 16 mg/100 mL	Increased muscular activity Congestive heart failure Hemorrhage Shock	
Lactic dehydrogenase (LDH)	60 to 100 units/mL	Untreated pernicious anemia Myocardial infarction Pulmonary infarction Liver disease	
Leucine aminopeptidase	1 to 3 micromoles/hr/mL	Liver or biliary tract diseases Pancreatic disease Metastatic carcinoma of liver and pancreas Biliary obstruction	

*Whole blood

Lab Test	Normal Value	Clinical Significance	
		(Increased)	(Decreased)
Lipase	0.2 to 1.5 units/mL	Acute and chronic pancreatitis Biliary obstruction Cirrhosis Hepatitis Peptic ulcer	
Lipids (total)	400 to 1000 mg/100 mL	Hypothyroidism Diabetes Nephrosis Glomerulonephritis	Hyperthyroidism
Phospholipids	125 to 300 mg/100 mL	Diabetes Nephritis	
Magnesium	1.8 to 2.2 mEq/L	Ingestion of epsom salts Parathyroidectomy	Chronic alcoholism Toxemia of pregnancy Severe renal disease
Nonprotein nitrogen	20 to 35 mg/100 mL	Acute nephritis Polycystic kidneys Obstructive uropathy Peritonitis Congestive heart failure Pregnancy	

Lab Test	Normal Value	Clinical Significance	
		(Increased)	(Decreased)
Osmolality	285 to 295 milliosmoles/L		Inappropriate secretion of antidiuretic hormone
Oxygen saturation, arterial*	96% to 100%	Polycythemia Anhydremia	Anemia Cardiac decompensation Chronic obstructive lung disease
PCO₂*	35 to 45 mmHg	Respiratory acidosis Metabolic alkalosis	Respiratory alkalosis Metabolic acidosis
pH*	7.35 to 7.45	Vomiting Hyperpnea Fever Intestinal obstruction	Uremia Diabetic acidosis Hemorrhage Nephritis
PO₂*	75 to 100 mmHg	Directly related to oxygen saturation	
Pepsinogen	200 to 425 units/mL		Conditions that decrease gastric acidity Pernicious anemia Achlorhydria
Phenylamine	0 to 2 mg/100 mL	Phenylketonuria Oasthouse urine disease	

*Whole blood

Lab Test	Normal Value	Clinical Significance	
		(Increased)	(Decreased)
Phosphatase, acid	0 to 2 units/mL	Carcinoma of prostate Advanced Paget's disease Hyperparathyroidism	
Phosphatase, alkaline	4 to 17 units/mL	Conditions reflection increased osteoblast activity of bone Rickets Hyperparathyroidism Liver disease	
Phosphorus, inorganic	3.0 to 4.5 mg/100 mL	Chronic nephritis Hypoparathyroidism	Hyperparathyroidism
Potassium	3.5 to 5.0 mEq/L	Addison's disease Oliguria Anuria Tissue breakdown or hemolysis	Diabetic acidosis Diarrhea Vomiting
Protein, total	6 to 8 g/100 mL	Hemoconcentration Shock	Malnutrition Hemorrhage Loss of plasma from burns Proteinuria
Albumin	3.5 to 5 g/100 mL	Multiple myeloma (globulin fraction)	
Globulin	1.5 to 3 g/100 mL	Chronic infections (globulin)	

Lab Test	Normal Value	Clinical Significance	
		(Increased)	(Decreased)
Paper electrophoresis	Percentage of total proteins	Liver disease (globulin)	
Albumin	45% to 60%		
Alpha 1 globulin	2.7% to 6.1%		
Alpha 2 globulin	7.7% to 16.2%		
Beta globulin	10% to 17%		
Gamma globulin	8.7% to 27%		
Sodium	135 to 145 mEq/L	Hemoconcentration	Alkali deficit
		Nephritis	Addison's disease
		Pyloric obstruction	Myxedema
Sulfate	0.5 to 1.5 mg/100 mL	Nephritis	
		Nitrogen retention	
Thymol turbidity	1 to 4.5 units/mL	Liver disease	
		Infectious diseases with antibody production	
Transaminase (serum glutamic oxalacetic transaminase [SGOT])	15 to 45 units/mL	Myocardial infarction	
		Skeletal muscle disease	
		Liver disease	
Transaminase (serum glutamic pyruvic transaminase [SGPT])	5 to 36 units/mL	Same conditions as SGOT	
Urea nitrogen	10 to 20 mg/100 mL	Acute glomerulonephritis	Severe hepatic failure
		Obstructive uropathy	Pregnancy
		Mercury poisoning	
		Nephrotic syndrome	

Lab Test	Normal Value	Clinical Significance	
		(Increased)	(Decreased)
Uric acid	1 to 6 mg/100 mL	Gouty arthritis Acute leukemia Lymphomas treated by chemotherapy Toxemia of pregnancy	
Vitamin A	0.5 to 2.0 units/mL	Hypervitaminosis A	Vitamin A deficiency
Zinc turbidity	2 to 12 units/mL	Same clinical significance as thymol turbidity	

NORMAL VALUES: URINE CHEMISTRY

Lab Test	Normal Value	Clinical Significance	
		(Increased)	(Decreased)
Acetone and acetoacetate	Zero	Uncontrolled diabetes mellitus Starvation	

Lab Test	Normal Value	Clinical Significance	
		(Increased)	(Decreased)
Alpha amino nitrogen	64 to 199 mg/24 hours	Leukemia	
		Diabetes	
		Phenylketonuria	
		Other metabolic diseases	
Ammonia	20 to 70 mEq/L	Diabetes mellitus	
	0.6 g/L	Pernicious vomiting	
		Cirrhosis and other destructive	
		diseases of the liver	
Calcium	<150 mg/24 hours	Hyperparathyroidism	
Catecholamines	Epinephrine: <10 g/24 hours	Pheochromocytoma	
	Norepinephrine: <100 µg/		
	24 hours		
Chorionic	Zero	Pregnancy	
gonadotropin		Chorionepithelioma	
		Hydatidiform mole	
Copper	0 to 100 µg/24 hours	Wilson's disease	
		Cirrhosis of liver	
Coproporphyrin	50 to 200 µg/24 hours	Poliomyelitis	
		Lead poisoning	

Lab Test	Normal Value	Clinical Significance	
		(Increased)	*(Decreased)*
Creatine	<100 mg/24 hours	Muscular dystrophy Fever Carcinoma of the liver Pregnancy	
Creatinine	1 to 2 g/24 hours	Typhoid fever Salmonella infections Tetanus	Muscular atrophy Anemia Advanced degeneration of kidneys Leukemia
Chlorides	9 g/L (as NaCl)		
Bile melanin	Zero	Advanced melanoma Ochronosis	
Creatinine clearance	150 to 180 L/24 hours / 1.73 sq M of body surface		Measures glomerular filtra- tion rate Renal diseases
Cystine	Zero	Cystinuria	
Hemoglobin and myoglobin	Zero	Extensive burns Transfusion of incompatible blood Myoglobin increased in severe crushing injuries to muscle	

Lab Test	Normal Value	Clinical Significance	
		(Increased)	*(Decreased)*
Homogentistic acid	Zero	Alkaptonuria Ochronosis	
5-hydroxindoleacetic acid	Zero	Malignant carcinoid syndrome	
Lead	120 µg or less/24 hours	Lead poisoning	
Phenolphthalein (PSP)	At least 25% excreted in 15 min, 40% by 30 min, 60% by 120 min		Delayed in renal diseases Low in nephritis, cystitis, pyelonephritis, congestive heart failure Primarily measures of renal tubular function
Phenylpyruvic acid	Zero	Phenylketonuria	
Phosphorus, inorganic	Average 1 g/24 hours Varies with intake	Fever Nervous exhaustion Tuberculosis Rickets Chronic lead poisoning	Acute infections Nephritis Cholorosis Pregnancy
Pituitary gonado-tropin	Males: 6 to 24 mouse units/24 hrs Females: 5 to 40 mouse units/24 hrs	Seminoma Teratoma of testis Pregnancy Menopause	

Lab Test	Normal Value	Clinical Significance	
		(Increased)	(Decreased)
Porphobilinogen	Zero	Acute porphyria	
		Liver disease	
Protein	Zero	Nephritis	
		Cardiac failure	
		Mercury poisoning	
		Bence-Jones protein in multiple myeloma	
		Febrile states	
		Hematuria	
		Amyloidosis	
17-Ketosteroids	Males: 10 to 22 mg/24 hours Females: 6 to 18 mg/24 hours	Masculinizing tumors of testes	Addison's disease
17-Hydroxycorticoids	2 to 12 mg/24 hours	Cushing's syndrome	Addison's disease Anterior pituitary hypofunction
Glucose	Zero	Diabetes mellitus	
		Pituitary disorders	
		Intracranial pressure	
		Lesion in floor of fourth ventricle	
Titratable acidity	20 to 40 mEq/24 hours	Metabolic acidosis	Metabolic alkalosis

Lab Test	Normal Value	Clinical Significance	
		(Increased)	(Decreased)
Urea clearance	Over 40 mL blood cleared of urea/min or >60%		Renal diseases
Urobilinogen	Up to 4 mg/24 hours	Liver and biliary tract disease Hemolytic anemias	Complete or nearly complete biliary obstruction Diarrhea Renal insufficiency
Uroporphyrins	Zero	Porphyria	
Vanilmandelic acid	0.7 to 6.8 mg/24 hours	Pheochromocytoma	
D-Xylose absorption	5-hour excretion of 16% to 33% of test dose		Malabsorption syndromes
Urea	25 to 35 g/24 hours	Excessive protein catabolism	Impaired kidney function
Uric acid	0.6 to 1 g/24 hours as urate	Gout (see blood uric acid)	Nephritis (see blood uric acid)

NORMAL VALUES: CEREBROSPINAL FLUID

Lab Test	Normal Value	Clinical Significance (Increased)	(Decreased)
Cell count	0 to 5 mononuclear cells/mm³	Bacterial meningitis Neurosyphilis Anterior poliomyelitis Encephalitis lethargica	
Chloride	100 to 130 mEq/L	Uremia	Acute generalized meningitis Tubercular meningitis
Colloidal gold	0000000000 to 0001222111	Acute meningitis Neurosyphilis	
Glucose	50 to 75 mg/100 mL	Diabetes mellitus Diabetic coma Epidemic encephalitis Uremia	Acute meningitides Tuberculous meningitis Insulin shock
Protein Lumbar Cisternal Ventricular	15 to 45 mg/100 mL 15 to 25 mg/100 mL 5 to 15 mg/100 mL	Acute meningitides Tubercular meningitis Neurosyphilis Poliomyelitis Guillain-Barré syndrome	

NORMAL VALUES: MISCELLANEOUS VALUES

Lab Test	Normal Value	Clinical Significance
Barbiturate	Zero	Coma level approximately 11 mg/100 mL for phenobarbital; most compounds 1.5 mg/100 mL
Bromide	Zero	Toxic level = 17 mEq/L
Carbon monoxide	0% to 2%	Symptoms with over 20% saturation
Dilantin	Zero	Therapeutic level = 1 to 11 mg/100 mL
Ethanol	0% to 0.05%	Maximal level allowable by courts = 0.15%
		Varies by state
		0.3% to 0.4% = marked intoxication
		0.4% to 0.5% = alcoholic stupor
Methanol	Zero	May be fatal in concentrations as low as 10 mg/100 mL
Salicylate	Zero	Therapeutic level = 20 to 25 mg/100 mL
		Toxic level = over 30 mg/100 mL
Sulfonamide	Zero	Therapeutic levels:
		Sulfadiazine 8 to 15 mg/100 mL
		Sulfaguanidine 3 to 5 mg/100 mL
		Sulfamerazine 10 to 15 mg/100 mL
		Sulfanilamide 10 to 15 mg/100 mL

Gastric Analysis	Normal Value	Clinical Significance	
		(Increased)	(Decreased)
Free hydrochloric acid (HCL)	0 to 30 mEq/L	Neuroses	Pernicious anemia
Total acidity	15 to 45 mEq/L	Peptic ulcer	Gastric carcinoma
Combined acid	10 to 15 mEq/L	Zollinger-Ellison syndrome	Chronic atrophic gastritis
			Decreases normally with age

Classification of Fractures

General Fracture Classifications

avulsion: A fracture in which a piece of the bone is torn away from the main bone.

burst: A comminuted fracture associated with pressure along the long axis of the bone, in which bone fragments are displaced centripetally.

comminuted: A fracture that results in a bone broken in three or more fragments.

compact: Condition in which a broken bone pierces the skin and can be viewed.

complicated: The bone is broken and has injured some internal organ (eg, broken rib piercing a lung; vertebral fracture puncturing the spinal cord, etc).

compound (open): A fracture that results in communication between the bone and the external environment. The bone is broken, and there is an external wound leading down to the site of fracture or fragments of bone protruding through the skin.

compression: A fracture resulting from pressure along the long axis of the bone.

depressed: When a piece of the skull is broken and driven inward.

fracture: Defined as any break in the continuity of bone.

greenstick: The bone is partially bent and partially broken, as when a greenstick breaks.

impacted: The bone is broken, and one end is wedged into the interior of the other.

incomplete: The line of fracture does not include the whole bone.

oblique: A fracture in which there is an angulation of the break in the bone.

pathological: A fracture that occurs due to weakened bones by preexisting disease, such as tumors, cysts, osteomyelitis, or osteoporosis.

simple (closed): A fracture in which there is no communication with the exterior. The bone is broken but there is no external wound.

spiral: A fracture due to a torsional (twisting) force that causes fracturing in a spiral-like fashion.

teardrop: Bursting type of fracture (usually in the cervical region) that produces a characteristic anterior-inferior bone chip. The fragment resembles a "teardrop" on x-ray. It is usually associated with compression forces.

transverse: A fracture straight across the bone.

HIP FRACTURE CLASSIFICATIONS

General Definition

femoral neck fracture: Fracture that occurs just inferior to the articular surface of the femoral head and ending just superior to the intertrochanteric region.

hip fracture: Break in the femur in the neck region, trochanter, or upper shaft. Five types exist based on fracture location: subcapital, transcervical, basilar, intertrochanteric, or subtrochanteric. Four classifications exist based on the degree of bone segment displacement: incomplete, complete with no displacement, partially displaced, or completely displaced.

Garden Classifications of Femoral Neck Fractures

type I: An incomplete, impacted fracture in which the bony trabecula of the inferior portion of the femoral neck remains intact.

type II: A complete fracture without displacement of the fracture fragments.

type III: A complete fracture with partial displacement of bony fragments.

type IV: A complete fracture with total displacement of the fragments.

Simple Femoral Neck Fracture Classifications

displaced: A complete fracture in which there is partial or total displacement of the fracture fragments.

nondisplaced: A fracture that is incomplete or complete without displacement of the bony fragments.

intertrochanteric hip fracture: Hip fracture that occurs between the greater and lesser trochanter and is extracapsular (distal to the anatomic limits of the capsule of the hip joint).

Classification of Intertrochanteric Hip Fractures

stable: A fracture in which the posteromedial buttress of the bone is not compromised.

unstable: Discontinuity of the posteromedial integrity of the intertrochanteric area of the femur.

subtrochanteric hip fracture: A fracture occurring below the lesser trochanter involving the proximal portion of the shaft of the femur.

Classification of Subtrochanteric Hip Fractures

stable: Stable fracture pattern characterized by an intact postero-medial cortical buttress.

unstable: A fracture characterized by loss of the posteromedial cortical buttress of the subtrochanteric region of the femur.

Reflexes and Reactions of the Central Nervous System

MYOTATIC REFLEXES (STRETCH)	STIMULUS (S)	RESPONSE (R)
Jaw (trigeminal nerve)	Subject sitting with jaw relaxed and slightly open. Place finger on top of chin; tap downward on top of finger in a direction that causes the jaw to open.	The jaw rebounds.
Biceps (C5 to C6)	Subject sitting with arm flexed and supported. Place thumb over the biceps tendon in the cubital fossa, stretching it slightly. Tap thumb or tap directly on the tendon.	Slight contraction of muscle (elbow flexes) normally occurs.
Triceps (C7 to C8)	Subject sitting with arm supported in abduction, elbow flexed. Palpate triceps tendon just above the olecranon. Tap directly on the tendon.	Slight contraction of muscle (elbow extends) normally occurs.
Hamstrings (L2 to L4)	Subject prone with knee semiflexed and supported. Palpate tendon at the knee. Tap on finger or directly on tendon.	Slight contraction of muscle (knee flexes) normally occurs.
Patellar (L2 to L4)	Subject sitting with knee flexed, foot unsupported. Tap tendon of quadriceps muscle between the patella and tibial tuberosity.	Contraction of muscle (knee extends) normally occurs.

MYOTATIC REFLEXES (STRETCH)	STIMULUS (S)	RESPONSE (R)
Ankle (S1 to S2)	Subject prone with foot over end of table or sitting with knee flexed and foot held in slight dorsiflexion. Tap tendon just above its insertion on the calcaneus. Maintaining slight tension on the gastroc-soleus group improves the response.	Slight contraction of muscle (foot plantarflexes) normally occurs.

Scoring: 0 = no response; 1+ = diminished response; 2+ = normal response; 3+ = exaggerated response; 4+ = clonus.

SUPERFICIAL REFLEXES (CUTANEOUS)	STIMULUS (S)	RESPONSE (R)
Plantar (S1 to S2)	With a large pin or fingertip, stroke the lateral side of the foot, moving from the heel to the base of the little toe and then across the ball of the foot.	Normal response is plantarflexion of the great toe, sometimes the other toes with slight inversion and flexion of the distal foot. Abnormal response, termed a +Babinski, is extension of the great toe with fanning of the four other toes (typically seen in upper motor neuron lesions).
Chaddock	Stroke around lateral ankle and up lateral aspect of foot to the base of the little toe.	Same as for plantar (see above).

SUPERFICIAL REFLEXES (CUTANEOUS)	STIMULUS (S)	RESPONSE (R)
Babinski	Stroke the sole of the foot from heel to base of great toe.	Results in the great toe pointing up and the toes spreading out. Normal in newborns. Abnormal in children and adults.
Abdominal (T7 to T12)	Position subject in supine, relaxed position. Make quick, light stroke with a large pin or fingertip over the skin of the abdominals from the periphery to the umbilicus (test each abdominal quadrant separately).	Localized contraction underlying the stimulus, causing the umbilicus to move toward the quadrant stimulated.
PRIMITIVE/SPINAL REFLEXES	**STIMULUS (S)**	**RESPONSE (R)**
Flexor withdrawal	Noxious stimulus (pinprick) to sole of foot. Tested in supine or sitting position.	Toes extend, foot dorsiflexes, entire leg flexes uncontrollably. Onset: 28 weeks gestation. Integrated: 1 to 2 months of age.
Crossed extension	Noxious stimulus to ball of foot of extremity fixed in extension; tested in supine position.	Opposite lower extremity flexes, then adducts and extends. Onset: 28 weeks gestation. Integrated: 1 to 2 months of age.

Primitive/Spinal Reflexes	Stimulus (S)	Response (R)
Traction	Grasp forearm and pull from supine into sitting position.	Grasp and total flexion of the upper extremity. Onset: 28 weeks gestation. Integrated: 2 to 5 months of age.
Moro	Sudden change in position of head in relation to trunk; drop subject backward from sitting position.	Extension, abduction of upper extremities, hand opening, and crying followed by flexion, adduction of arms across chest. Onset: 28 weeks gestation. Integrated: 5 to 6 months of age.
Startle	Sudden loud or harsh noise.	Sudden extension or abduction of arms, crying. Onset: birth. Integrated: persists.
Grasp	Maintained pressure to palm of hand (palmar grasp) or to ball of foot under toes (plantar grasp).	Maintained flexion of fingers or toes. Onset palmar: birth. Onset plantar: 28 weeks gestation. Integrated palmar: 4 to 6 months. Integrated plantar: 9 months.

TONIC/BRAINSTEM REFLEXES	STIMULUS (S)	RESPONSE (R)
Asymmetrical tonic neck (ATNR)	Rotation of the head to one side.	Flexion of skull limbs, extension of the jaw limbs, "bow and arrow" or "fencing" posture. Onset: birth. Integrated: 4 to 6 months.
Symmetrical tonic neck (STNR)	Flexion or extension of the head.	With head flexion: flexion of arms, extension of legs. With head extension: extension of arms, flexion of legs. Onset: 4 to 6 months. Integrated: 8 to 12 months.
Symmetrical tonic labyrinthine (TLR or STLR)	Prone or supine position.	With prone position: increased flexor tone/flexion of all limbs. With supine: increased extensor tone/extension of all limbs. Onset: birth. Integrated: 6 months.
Positive supporting	Contact to the ball of the foot in upright standing position.	Rigid extension (cocontraction) of the lower extremities. Onset: birth. Integrated: 6 months.

	STIMULUS (S)	RESPONSE (R)
TONIC/BRAINSTEM REFLEXES		
Associated reactions	Resisted voluntary movement in any part of the body.	Involuntary movement in a resting extremity. Onset: birth to 3 months. Integrated: 8 to 9 years of age.
MIDBRAIN/CORTICAL REFLEXES		
Neck righting action on the body (NOB)	Passively turn head to one side; tested in supine.	Body rotates as a whole (log rolls) to align the body to the head. Onset: 4 to 6 months. Integrated: 5 years.
Body righting action on the body (BOB)	Passively rotate upper or lower trunk segment; tested in supine.	Body segment not rotated follows to align the body segments. Onset: 4 to 6 months. Integrated: 5 years.
Labyrinth head righting (LR)	Occlude vision; alter body position by tipping body in all directions.	Head orients to vertical position with mouth horizontal. Onset: birth to 2 months. Integrated: persists.

MIDBRAIN/CORTICAL REFLEXES	STIMULUS (S)	RESPONSE (R)
Optical righting (OR)	Alter body position by tipping body in all directions.	Head orients to vertical position with mouth horizontal. Onset: birth to 2 months. Integrated: persists.
Body righting acting on head (BOH)	Place in prone or supine position.	Head orients to vertical position with mouth horizontal. Onset: birth to 2 months. Integrated: 5 years.
Protective extension (PE)	Displace center of gravity outside the base of support.	Arms or legs extend and abduct to support and protect the body from falling. Onset arms: 4 to 6 months. Onset legs: 6 to 9 months. Integrated: persists.

MIDBRAIN/CORTICAL REFLEXES	STIMULUS (S)	RESPONSE (R)
Equilibrium reactions—tilting (ER)	Displace the center of gravity by tilting or moving the support surface (eg, with a movable object such as an equilibrium board or ball).	Curvature of the trunk toward the upward side along with extension and abduction of the extremities on that side; protective extension on the opposite (downward) side. Onset prone: 6 months. Onset supine: 7 to 8 months. Onset sitting: 7 to 8 months. Onset quadruped: 9 to 12 months. Onset standing: 12 to 21 months. Integrated: persists.

MIDBRAIN/CORTICAL REFLEXES	STIMULUS (S)	RESPONSE (R)
Equilibrium reactions—postural	Apply a displacing force to the body, altering the center of gravity in its relation to the base of support; can also be observed during voluntary activity.	Curvature of the trunk toward the external force with extension and abduction of the extremities on the side to which the force was applied. Onset prone: 6 months. Onset supine: 7 to 8 months. Onset sitting: 7 to 8 months. Onset quadruped: 9 to 12 months. Onset standing: 12 to 21 months. Integrated: persists.

BIBLIOGRAPHY

Bobath B. *Abnormal Postural Reflex Activity Caused by Brain Lesions.* 2nd ed. London, England: William Heinemann Medical Books; 1971.

O'Sullivan SB, Schmitz TJ. *Physical Rehabilitation: Assessment and Treatment.* 2nd ed. Philadelphia, Pa: FA Davis; 1988.

Umphred DA. *Neurological Rehabilitation.* 3rd ed. St. Louis, Mo: Mosby-Year Book; 1995.

Metabolic Equivalent (MET) Values for Activity and Exercise

APPROXIMATE METABOLIC COST OF ACTIVITIES[a,b]

MET Levels	Self-Care Activities	Occupational/Work Activity	Recreational Activity
1.5 to 2.0 METs[c] 4 to 7 mL O$_2$/min/kg 2 to 2.5 kcal/min (70 kg BW)[d] Very light/minimal	Eating Shaving, grooming Getting in and out of bed Standing Walking (1.6 km or 1 mph)	Desk work Typing, writing Auto driving[e]	Standing Walking (1.6 km or 1 mph) Flying,[e] motorcycling[e] Playing cards[e] Knitting, sewing
2 to 3 METs 7 to 11 mL O$_2$/min/kg 2.25 to 4 kcal/min (70 kg BW) Light	Showering in warm water Walking (3.25 km or 2 mph)	Ironing Light woodworking Riding lawn mower Auto repair Radio/TV repair Janitorial work Manual typing Bartending	Walking (3.25 km or 2 mph) Level biking (8 km or 5 mph) Billiards, bowling Skeet,[e] shuffleboard Power golf cart driving Canoeing (4 km or 2.25 mph) Horseback riding (walk) Playing a musical instrument Powerboat driving[e]

MET Levels	*Self-Care Activities*	*Occupational/Work Activity*	*Recreational Activity*
3 to 4 METs 11 to 14 mL O$_2$/min/kg 4 to 5 kcal/min (70 kg BW) Moderate	Dressing, undressing Walking (5 km or 3 mph)	Cleaning windows Making beds Mopping floors, vacuuming Bricklaying, plastering Machine assembly Wheelbarrow (100 kg- or 220 lb load) Trailer truck in traffic Welding (moderate load) Pushing light power mower	Walking (5 km or 3 mph) Biking (10 km or 6 mph) Horseshoe pitching Volleyball (noncompetitive) Golf (pulling bag cart) Archery Sailing (handling small boat) Fly fishing (standing in waders) Horseback riding (sitting to trot) Badminton (social doubles) Energetic musician
4 to 5 METs 14 to 18 mL O$_2$/min/kg 5 to 6 kcal/min (70 kg BW) Heavy	Showering in hot water Walking (5.5 km or 3.5 mph)	Scrubbing floors Hoeing Raking leaves Light carpentry Painting, masonry Hanging wallpaper	Walking (5.5 km or 3.5 mph) Biking (13 km or 8 mph) Table tennis Golf (carrying clubs) Dancing (foxtrot) Badminton (singles) Tennis (doubles) Calisthenics

MET Levels	Self-Care Activities	Occupational/Work Activity	Recreational Activity
5 to 6 METs 18 to 21 mL O$_2$/min/kg 6 to 7 kcal/min (70 kg BW) Very heavy	Walking (6.5 km or 4 mph)	Digging in garden Shoveling light earth	Walking (6.5 km or 4 mph) Biking (16 km or 10 mph) Canoeing (6.5 km or 4 mph) Horseback riding ("posting" or trot) Stream fishing Ice/roller skating (15 km or 9 mph)
6 to 7 METs 21 to 25 mL O$_2$/min/kg 7 to 8 kcal/min (70 kg BW) Very heavy	Walking (8 km or 5 mph)	Snow shoveling 10 min (10 kg or 22 lbs) Manual lawn mowing	Walking (8 km or 5 mph) Biking (17.5 km or 11 mph) Badminton (competitive) Tennis (singles) Folk/square dancing Light downhill skiing Ski touring (4 km or 2.5 mph) Water skiing

MET Levels	Self-Care Activities	Occupational/Work Activity	Recreational Activity
7 to 8 METs 25 to 28 mL O_2/min/kg 8 to 10 kcal/min (70 kg BW)		Digging ditches Carrying 80 kg or 175 lbs Sawing hardwood	Jogging (8 km or 5 mph) Biking (19 km or 12 mph) Horseback riding (gallop) Vigorous downhill skiing Basketball Mountain climbing Ice hockey Canoeing (8 km or 5 mph) Touch football Paddleball
8 to 9 METs 28 to 32 mL O_2/min/kg 10 to 11 kcal/min (70 kg BW)		Shoveling 10 min (14 kg or 31 lbs)	Running (9 km or 5.5 mph) Biking (21 km or 13 mph) Ski touring (6.5 km or 4 mph) Squash/handball (social) Fencing Basketball (vigorous)

MET Levels	Self-Care Activities	Occupational/Work Activity	Recreational Activity

10+ METs
32+ mL O2/min/kg
11+ kcal/min (70 kg BW)
		Shoveling 10 min (16 kg or 35 lbs)	Running
			  6 mph = 10 METs
			  7 mph = 11.5 METs
			  8 mph = 13.5 METs
			  9 mph = 15 METs
			  10 mph = 17 METs
			Ski touring (8+ km or 5+ mph)
			Squash/handball (competitive)

[a]Includes resting metabolic needs.

[b]Source of MET listing: American Heart Association.

[c]1 MET is the energy expenditure at rest, equivalent to approximately 3.5 mL O_2/min/kg.

[d]BW = body weight.

[e]A major increase in metabolic requirements may occur due to excitement, anxiety, or impatience, which are common responses during some activities. The individual's emotional reactivity must be assessed when prescribing or sanctioning certain activities.

Cranial Nerves and Tests for Cranial Nerve Integrity

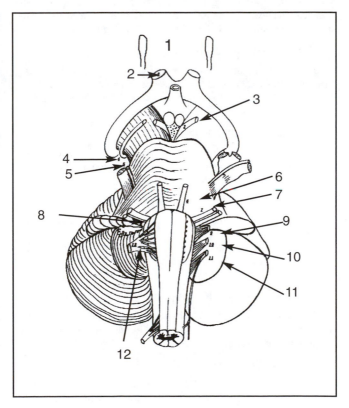

Anterior view of the cerebellum. 1 = olfactory, 2 = optic, 3 = oculomotor, 4 = trochlear, 5 = trigeminal (motor and sensory roots), 6 = abducens, 7 = facial, 8 = vestibulocochlear (acoustic and vestibular), 9 = glossopharyngeal, 10 = vagus, 11 = accessory, 12 = hypoglossal. Modified from: http://www.biomedicale.univ-paris5.fr/anat/anatomie/iconographie/schemas/Dessin/Dessins1/6.GIF. Illustrated by Dr. Dominique Bastian. Reprinted with permission.

CRANIAL NERVE ASSESSMENT

The positioning of the subject for cranial nerve assessment varies according to the nerve being tested. The examiner's action will also vary according to the cranial nerve being tested. The absence, delay, or asymmetry of a response indicates possible involvement of the particular nerve that is being tested.

Cranial Nerve I (Olfactory)

The examiner places an object that has a strong, identifiable odor just under the nasal area of the subject in an attempt to assess his or her ability to perceive the odor. An ammonia capsule is typically used for this test.

Cranial Nerve II (Optic)

The examiner asks the subject to identify objects within view and to clarify what the subject actually sees (eg, letters of the alphabet, numbers, pictures of objects, etc).

Cranial Nerve III (Oculomotor)

The examiner asks the subject to elevate the eyelid and elevate, depress, and adduct the eyes. Voluntary motor control of levator palpebrae; superior, medial, and inferior recti; and the inferior oblique eye muscles is the primary function of the oculomotor nerve.

Cranial Nerve IV (Trochlear)

The examiner asks the subject to elevate the eyes (ie, look up). The trochlear nerve primarily functions in voluntary motor control of the superior oblique eye muscle.

Cranial Nerve V (Trigeminal)

A sensory assessment for integrity of the trigeminal nerve is the ability of the subject to perceive touch along the skin of the face. To test motor function, the examiner asks the subject to perform the motions of elevation, protrusion, retrusion, and lateral deviation of the mandible. The chief function of the trigeminal nerve is the sensation of touch and pain on the skin of the face, mucous membranes of the nose, sinuses, mouth, and anterior tongue. It functions also in voluntary motor control of the muscles of mastication.

Cranial Nerve VI (Abducens)

The examiner asks the subject to abduct the eye (keeping head in one place and looking side-to-side). The chief function of the abducens nerve is voluntary motor control of the lateral rectus muscle of the eye.

Cranial Nerve VII (Facial)

To test sensation of the facial nerve, the examiner assesses the subject's ability to distinguish identifiable tasting substances with the anterior portion of the tongue. Motor function is tested by having the subject elevate, adduct, or depress the eyebrow; close the eyes; flare and constrict the nose; close the mouth; and close and protrude the lips. The primary function of the facial nerve is taste along the anterior portion of the tongue and voluntary motor control of facial muscles.

Cranial Nerve VIII (Vestibulocochlear)

The examiner asks the subject to stand with his or her eyes closed and no support in order to assess the subject's balance. The chief function of the vestibulocochlear nerve is hearing and balance via the ear.

Cranial Nerve IX (Glossopharyngeal)

To test sensation of the glossopharyngeal nerve, the examiner assesses the subject's ability to distinguish identifiable objects and/or substances with the posterior portion of the tongue. To establish motor integrity, the examiner asks the subject to swallow. The primary functions of the glossopharyngeal nerve are the sensation of touch and pain on the posterior portion of the tongue and pharynx, taste on the posterior portion of the tongue, and voluntary motor control of some muscles of the pharynx.

Cranial Nerve X (Vagus)

The examiner assesses the subject's abdominal and thoracic viscera. The chief function of the vagus nerve is sensation of touch and pain of the pharynx, larynx, and bronchi. Autonomic muscle control of the thoracic and abdominal viscera is also a primary function.

Cranial Nerve XI (Accessory)

The examiner asks the subject to elevate (shrug) the shoulders. The primary function of the accessory nerve is voluntary control of the sternocleidomastoid and the trapezius.

Cranial Nerve XII (Hypoglossal)

The examiner asks the subject to protrude the tongue. The primary function of the hypoglossal nerve is voluntary control of the muscles of the tongue.

Bones of the Body

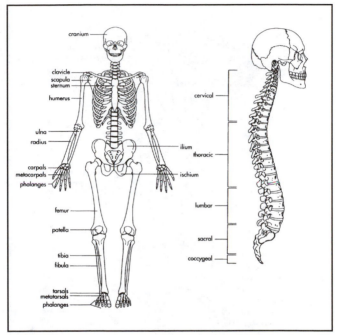

Reprinted with permission from Sladyk K. *OT Student Primer: A Guide to College Success*. Thorofare, NJ: SLACK Incorporated; 1997.

Muscles of the Body

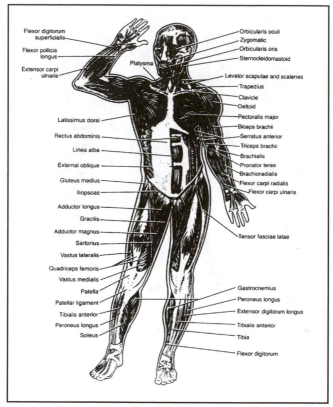

Figure 1. Anterior superficial muscles. Reprinted from *Quick and Easy Terminology*, 2nd ed, Leonard P, © 1995 with permission from Elsevier Science.

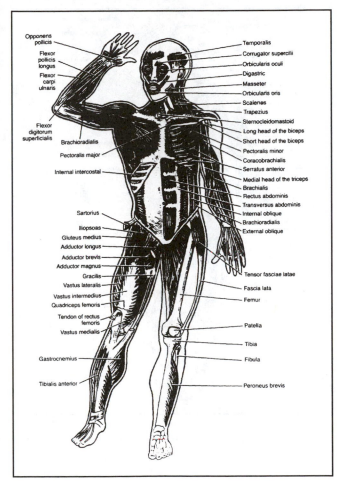

Figure 2. Anterior deep muscles. Reprinted from *Quick and Easy Terminology*, 2nd ed, Leonard P, © 1995 with permission from Elsevier Science.

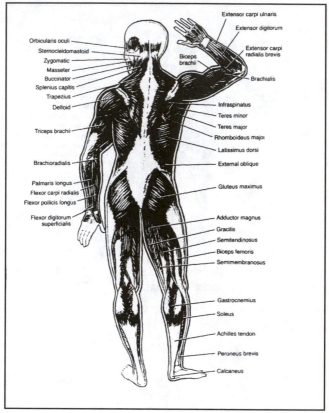

Figure 3. Posterior superficial muscles. Reprinted from *Quick and Easy Terminology*, 2nd ed, Leonard P, © 1995 with permission from Elsevier Science.

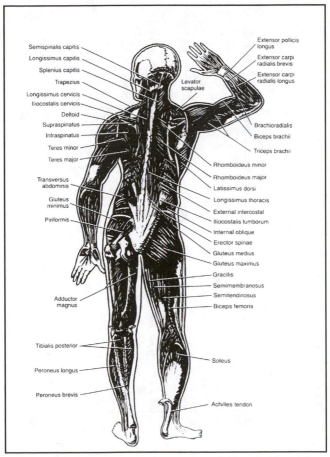

Figure 4. Posterior deep muscles. Reprinted from *Quick and Easy Terminology*, 2nd ed, Leonard P, © 1995 with permission from Elsevier Science.

MUSCLES: ORIGIN/INSERTION/ACTION—INNERVATION—BLOOD SUPPLY

Muscle	Origin	Insertion	Action	Nerve	Artery
NECK					
Sternocleido-mastoid (SCM)	Med or sternal head cranial part of ventral surface of manubrium; lat or clavicular head—sup border & ant surface of med 1/3 clavicle	Lat surface mastoid process & lat 1/2 sup nuchal line of occipital bone	↻ opp side lat ✓same side ✓ forward	Spinal accessory n. C2 & C3 ant rami	Subclavian a.
Platysma	Fascia covering sup part of pectoralis major & deltoid	Some fibers into bone below oblique line, others into skin	Draws lip inf & post	Cervical branch of facial n.	Subclavian a. (branch)
Suprahyoid group					
Digastricus	Post belly: mastoid notch of temporal bone; Ant belly: a depression on inner side of inf border of mandible	Post belly: hyoid bone by fibrous loop; Ant belly: same as post belly	▲ hyoid bone Post: draws backwards Ant: draws forward	Post: facial n. Ant: mylohyoid n.	Lingual a.
Stylohyoideus	Post & lat surface of styloid process	Body of hyoid bone	Draws hyoid sup & post	Facial n. (branch)	Lingual a.

*Please see p. 531 for helpful abbreviations.

Muscle	Origin	Insertion	Action	Nerve	Artery
Mylohyoideus	Whole length of mylohyoid line of mandible	Body of hyoid bone	▲ hyoid & tongue	Mylohyoid n.	Lingual a.
Geniohyoideus	Inf mental spine on inner surface of symphysis menti	Ant surface of hyoid	Draws hyoid & tongue ant	1st cervical n. (through hypoglossal n.)	Lingual a.
Infrahyoid Group					
Sternohyoideus	Post surface of med end of clavicle, post sterno-clav lig & sup & post part of manubrium sterni	Inf border of hyoid bone	Draws hyoid inferiorly	Branch of ansa cervicalis (1st three cervical nerves)	Lingual a. Subclavian a.
Sternothyroideus	Dorsal surface of manubrium sterni (caudal of origin of sternohyoideus)	Oblique line on lamina of thyroid cartilage	Draws thyroid caudally	Branch of ansa cervicalis (1st three cervical nerves)	Lingual a. Subclavian a.
Thyrohyoideus	Oblique line on lamina of thyroid cartilage	Inf border of greater cornu of hyoid bone	Draws hyoid inferiorly Draws thyroid cartilage sup	1st & 2nd cervical n.	Lingual a. Subclavian a.
Omohyoideus	Cranial border of scapula (near or crossing scapular notch)	Caudal border of hyoid bone	Draws hyoid caudally	Branch of ansa cervicalis (1st three cervical nerves)	Subclavian a.

Muscle	Origin	Insertion	Action	Nerve	Artery
Longus Colli	Vertical: ant surface of C5, C6, C7, T1, T2, & T3; Sup: ant tubercles of transverse processes C3, C4, C5; Inf: ant surface of T2 & T3	Vertical: ant surface of C2, C3, C4; Sup: narrow tendon into tubercle on ant arch of atlas; Inf: ant tubercles of transverse processes C5 & C6	✓ of neck ↻ neck (min)	Branches of 2nd to 7th cervical nerves	Subclavian a. (thyrocervical)
Longus Capitus	Four tendinous slips from ant tubercles of transverse processes C3, C4, C5, & C6	Inf surface of the basilar part of occipital bone	Head ✓	Branches from 1st, 2nd, & 3rd cervical nerves	Subclavian a.
Rectus Capitus Anterior	Ant surface of lat mass of the atlas & from root of its transverse process	Inf surface of basilar part of occipital bone	Head ✓	Branch of 1st & 2nd cervical nerves	Subclavian a.
Rectus Capitus Lateralis	Sup surface of transverse process of atlas	Inf surface of jugular process of occipital bone	Lat ✓ head	Branch of 1st & 2nd cervical nerves	Subclavian a.
Scalenus Anterior	Ant tubercles of transverse processes of C3, C4, C5, & C6	Scalene tubercle on inner border of 1st rib & ridge on cranial surface of rib	▲ 1st rib ✓ head ↻ head	Branches of lower cervical nerves	Subclavian a. (thyrocervical)

Muscle	Origin	Insertion	Action	Nerve	Artery
Scalenus Medius	Post tubercles of transverse processes of C2, C3, C4, C5, C6, & C7	Cranial surface of 1st rib between tubercle & subclavian groove	▲1st rib ↙head ↻head	Branches from cervical nerves	Subclavian a. (thyrocervical)
Scalenus Posterior	Post tubercles of transverse processes of C5, C6, & C7	Outer surface of 2nd rib (deep to serratus anterior)	▲2nd rib ↙head ↻head	Ventral primary branches C5, C6 & C7	Subclavian a.
BACK/NECK					
Serratus Posterior Superior	Caudal part of ligamentum nuchae, spinous processes C7, T1, T2, & T3; supraspinal ligament	Four digitations—cranial borders of ribs 2, 3, 4, & 5	Respiratory ▲ribs	Ventral rami T1 to T4	Subclavian a.
Serratus Posterior Inferior	Spinous processes T11, T12, L1, L2, & L3; supraspinal ligament	Four digitations into inf borders last 4 ribs (a little beyond their angles)	Respiratory Draws ribs ▼ & ▶	Ventral rami T9 to T12	Subclavian a.
Splenius Capitis Cervicis	Caudal ½ ligamentum nuchae & spinous processes C7, T1, T2, T3, & sometimes T4	Occipital bone just inf to lat 1/3 of sup nuchal line; into mastoid process of temporal bone	/ head & neck lat ✓same side ↻same side	Lat branches dorsal primary cervical nerves	Subclavian a. (branches)

Muscle	Origin	Insertion	Action	Nerve	Artery
Spinalis Capitis	Usually inseparable from semispinalis capitis		/ spine	Branch dorsal primary spinal nerves	Thoracic aorta (branch)
Semispinalis Capitis	Tips of transverse processes C7, T1, T2, T3, T4, T5, T6, and sometimes T7	Between sup & inf nuchal lines of occipital bone	/ head & neck ↻ opp side	Dorsal rami	Subclavian a. (branches)
Longissimus Capitis	Transverse processes T4 and T5 and cervicis and articular processes C4, C5, C6, and C7	Post margin of mastoid process (deep to splenius capitus and SCM)	/ head ↻ same side ✓ same side	Dorsal primary mid and lower cervical n(s).	Subclavian a. (branches)
Obliquus Capitus Inferior	Arises from apex of spinous process of axis	Inf & dorsal transverse process of atlas	↻ same side	Branch dorsal primary division suboccipital n.	Subclavian a. (branch)
Obliquus Capitus Superior	Tendinous fibers from sup surface transverse process of atlas	Occipital bone between sup & inf nucal lines (lat to semispinalis capitis)	/ head	Branch dorsal primary division suboccipital n.	Subclavian a. (branch)
Rectus Capitis Posterior Major	Spinous process of the axis	Lat part of inf nuchal line of occipital bone and surface immediately inf	/ head ↻ same side	Branch dorsal primary division suboccipital n.	Subclavian a. (branch)

Muscle	Origin	Insertion	Action	Nerve	Artery
Rectus Capitis Posterior Minor	Tendon from tubercle on post arch of atlas	Med part of the inf nuchal line of occipital bone & surface between it and foramen magnum	/ head	Branch dorsal primary division suboccipital n.	Subclavian a. (branch)
Longissimus Cervicis	Long thin tendons from apex transverse processes upper 4 or 5 thoracic vertebrae	Post tubercles of transverse processes of C2 to C6	/ spine lat ✓ ▼ ribs	Dorsal primary branch spinal nerves	Thoracic aorta (branches)
Iliocostalis Cervicis	Angles of the 3rd, 4th, 5th & 6th ribs	Post tubercles of transverse processes of C4, C5, & C6	/ spine lat ✓ ▼ ribs	Dorsal primary branch spinal nerves	Thoracic aorta (branches)
Spinalis Cervicis	Caudal part of ligamentum nuchae, spinous process C7; sometimes T1 and T2	Spinous processes of axis; sometimes spinous process C1 & C2	/ spine	Dorsal primary branch spinal nerves	Thoracic aorta (branch)
Semispinalis Cervicis	Transverse processes of 1st five or six thoracic vertebrae	Cervical spinous processes from axis to C5	/ spine ↻ opp side	Dorsal primary branch spinal nerves	Thoracic aorta (branch)

Muscle	Origin	Insertion	Action	Nerve	Artery
BACK					
Longissimus Thoracis	Arising from erector spinae and post surfaces transverse and accessory processes of lumbar vertebrae and ant layer lumbocostal aponeurosis	Transverse processes of all thoracic vertebrae and lower 9 or 10 ribs between tubercles and angles	/ spine lat ✓ ▶ ribs	Dorsal primary branch spinal nerves	Thoracic aorta (branch)
Iliocostalis Thoracis	Flattened tendons from upper borders of angles of lower 6 ribs (med to iliocostalis lumborum)	Cranial borders of angles of 1st 6 ribs and into dorsum of transverse process C7	/ spine lat ✓ ▶ ribs	Dorsal primary branch spinal nerves	Thoracic aorta (branch)
Spinalis Thoracis	Med continuation of sacrospinalis. Arises from spinous processes of T11, T12, L1, & L2	Spinous processes of upper thoracic vertebrae	/ spine	Dorsal primary branch spinal nerves	Thoracic aorta (branch)
Semispinalis Thoracis	Transverse processes of T6 to T10	Spinous processes of C6, C7, T1, T2, T3, & T4	/ spine ↻ opp side	Dorsal primary branch spinal nerves	Thoracic aorta (branch)
Iliocostalis Lumborum	Flattened tendons from upper portion of erector spinae	Inf borders of angles of last 6 or 7 ribs	/ spine lat ✓ ▶ ribs	Dorsal primary branch spinal nerves	Thoracic aorta (branch)

Muscle	Origin	Insertion	Action	Nerve	Artery
Sacrospinalis (Erector Spinae)	Arises from broad tendon attached to mid crest of sacrum; spinous processes T11 to T12 and lumbar vertebrae; supraspinal ligament to lip of iliac crests and lat crest of sacrum	Splits into longissimus, iliocostalis, spinalis, and semispinalis muscles (see respective muscles)	/ spine ↻ spine ▼ ribs lat ✓	Spinal nerves	Thoracic aorta
Multifidus	Spinous processes of each vertebrae from sacrum to axis. Arises from back of sacrum from aponeurosis of sacrospinalis, from med surface of post sup iliac spine and post sacroiliac ligaments	Each ascends obliquely crossing over 2 to 4 vertebrae and inserted into spinous process of vertebra from last lumbar to axis	/ spine ↻ opp side	Branches of dorsal primary spinal nerves	Thoracic aorta
Rotatores	Transverse process of one vertebra and insert at base of spinous process of vertebrae above from the sacrum to the axis	*Rotatores longi* cross one vertebra in their oblique course. *Rotatores breves* insert in next succeeding vertebra and run horizontal	/ spine ↻ opp side	Branches of dorsal primary spinal nerves	Thoracic aorta

Muscle	Origin	Insertion	Action	Nerve	Artery
Quadratus Lumborum	Sup borders of the transverse processes L2 to L5	Inf border of last rib and transverse process L1 to L4	▼ last rib lat ✓	12th thoracic n. 1st lumbar n.	Iliac circumflex
SHOULDER GIRDLE					
Trapezius	Ext occipital protuberance; med 1/3 sup nuchal line; spinous process C7, T1 to T12	Post border of lat 3rd clavicle; med margin acromion; spine of the scapula	▲ &/shoulder Abd same side ↻ opp side Retraction ▲ ↻ glen fossa ▲ glenoid fossa	Spinal accessory n. C3 & C4 spinal nerves	Suprascapular
Levator Scapulae	Transverse processes C1 to C4	Med border scapula between sup angle and spine	Elevation Protraction / cervical spine Abd same side ↻ same side	Dorsal scapular n. C3 & C4 spinal nerves	Superficial cervical a. Transverse cervical a.
Romboideus Minor	Spinous process of C7 and T1	Med border scapula at level of the spine	Elevation Retraction ▼ ↻ glen fossa	Dorsal scapular n.	Descending scapular a.
Romboideus Major	Spinous process of T2 to T5	Med border scapula between spine and inf angle	Elevation Retraction ▼ ↻ glen fossa	Dorsal scapular n.	Descending scapular a.

Muscle	Origin	Insertion	Action	Nerve	Artery
Latissimus Dorsi	Lumbar aponeurosis; spinous processes of T6 to T12, L1 to L5, & sacral vertebrae	Distal part of intertubercular groove of humerus	/ shoulder; Abd shoulder; Med ↻; Elevation; Retraction	Thoracodorsal n. C6 to C8 spinal nerves	Subscapular a.
Pectoralis Major	Ant surface sternal 1/2 clavicle; ventral surface sternum; aponeurosis of externus abdominis	Crest of greater tubercle of humerus	✓ shoulder; Add shoulder; Med ↻; Protract; ▲▼	Med and lat pectoral n. C5 to C8 spinal nerves; 1st thoracic n.	Thoracoacromial a. obliquus
Pectoralis Minor	Ext surfaces of ribs 3, 4, and 5 near their cartilages	Caracoid process of scapula	Protraction; Depression; ▼ ↻ glen fossa	Med pectoral n.	Thoracoacromial a.
Subclavius	1st rib and its cartilage near their junction	Inf aspect of clavicle in the mid 3rd	Protraction; Depression	Branch from brachial plexus (sup trunk)	Thoracoacromial a.
Serratus Anterior	Ext surfaces of ribs 1 to 9	Ant aspect of med border of scapula from sup to inf angle	Protraction; Depression; ▲ ↻ glen fossa; Med ↻	Long thoracic n.	Lat thoracic a.
Subscapularis	Mid 2/3 subscapular fossa; inf 2/3 groove on axillary	Lesser tubercle of humerus	Med ↻; ✓ /; Abd & add	Subscapular n.	Circumflex scapular a.

Muscle	Origin	Insertion	Action	Nerve	Artery
Supraspinatus	Mid 2/3 supraspinatous fossa	Sub impression of greater tubercle of humerus	Abd Lat ↻ (weak) ✓ (weak)	Suprascapular n.	Supra-scapular
Infraspinatus	Med 2/3 infraspinatus fossa	Mid impression of greater tubercle of humerus	Lat ↻ Abd and add	Suprascapular n.	Supra-scapular
Teres Minor	Dorsal surface of axillary border of scapula	Inf impression of greater tubercle of humerus distal to inf impression	Lat ↻ Add	Branch of axillary n.	Post humeral circumflex a.
Teres Major	Oval area on dorsal surface of inf angle of scapula	Crest of lesser tubercle of humerus	Add / shoulder Med ↻	Lower subscapular n.	Circumflex scapular a.
Deltoideus	Ant border and sup surface of lat 3rd of clavicle; lat margin & sup surface of acromium; inf lip post border scapular spine	Deltoid prominence on mid of lat body of humerus	Abd shoulder ✓ shoulder / shoulder Med & lat ↻	Axillary n. from brachial plexus	Post humeral circumflex a.

SHOULDER/ELBOW

Muscle	Origin	Insertion	Action	Nerve	Artery
Triceps Brachii	Long head: infraglenoid tuberosity of scapula;	Post proximal surface of olecranon	/ elbow / shoulder	Branches radial n. collateral a.	Profunda brachii a.

Muscle	Origin	Insertion	Action	Nerve	Artery
	Lat head: post surface of humerus; Med head: post surface of humerus distal to radial groove		Add shoulder		Inf ulnar
Brachialis	Distal 1/2 of ant aspect of humerus	Tuberosity of ulna; rough depression on ant surface of coronoid process	✓ elbow	Musculocutaneous n. Radial & med n.	Brachial a.
Biceps Brachii	Short head: apex of coracoid process; Long head: supraglenoid tuberosity at sup margin of glenoid	Rough post portion tuberosity of radius	✓ shoulder ✓ elbow Supination	Musculocutaneous n.	Brachial a.
Coracobrachialis	Apex of coracoid process	Impression at med surface & border of humerus	✓ shoulder Add shoulder	Musculocutaneous n.	Brachial a.
FOREARM/WRIST					
Pronator Teres	Humeral head: proximal to med epicondyle of humerus; Ulnar head: med side of coronoid process of ulna	Rough impression at mid of lat surface of radius	Pronation	Median n.	Inf ulnar collateral a.

Muscle	Origin	Insertion	Action	Nerve	Artery
Flexor Carpi Radialis	Med epicondyle of humerus	Base of 2nd metacarpal bone	✓ wrist Radial ✓	Median n.	Radial a.
Palmaris Longus	Med epicondyle of humerus	Palmar aponeurosis	✓ wrist	Median n.	Volar interosseous a.
Flexor Carpi Ulnaris	Humeral head: med epicondyle of humerus; Ulnar head: med margin olecranon; proximal 2/3 dorsal border of ulna	Pisiform bone	✓ wrist Add wrist	Ulnar n.	Ulnar a.
Flexor Digitorum Superficialis	Humeral head: med epicondyle of humerus; Ulnar head: med side of coronoid process; Radial head: oblique line of radius	Divides into 4 tendons which are inserted into the sides of the 2nd phalanx	✓ PIPs ✓ MCPs ✓ wrist	Median n.	Ulnar a.
Flexor Digitorum Profundus	Proximal 3/4 of volar & med surfaces of body of ulnar	Bases of last phalanges	✓ DIPs ✓ PIPs ✓ MCPs ✓ wrist	Palmar interosseous n. from median n. Branch of ulnar n.	Ulnar a. Volar interosseous a.
Flexor Pollicis Longus	Grooved volar surface of body of the radius	Base of distal phalanx of the thumb	✓ IP digit I ✓ MCP digit I ✓ & add wrist	Palmar interosseous n. from median n.	Radial a.

Muscle	Origin	Insertion	Action	Nerve	Artery
Pronator Quadratus	Pronator ridge on distal part of palmar surface of body of ulna; med part of palmar surface of distal 1/4 of ulna	Distal 1/4 of lat border and palmar surface of body of the radius	Pronation	Palmar interosseous from median n.	Ulnar and radial
Brachioradialis	Proximal 2/3 of lat supracondylar ridge of humerus	Lat side of base of styloid process of radius	✓ elbow	Branch of radial n.	Radial a.
Extensor Carpi Radialis Longus	Distal 1/3 lat supracondylar ridge of humerus	Dorsal surface of base of 2nd metacarpal bone—radial side	/ extension Abd wrist	Radial n.	Radial a.
Extensor Carpi Radialis Brevis	Lat epicondyle of humerus	Dorsal surface of base of 3rd metacarpal bone—radial side	/ wrist Abd wrist	Radial n.	Radial a.
Extensor Carpi Ulnaris	Lat epicondyle of humerus	Prominent tubercle on ulnar side of base of metacarpal V	/ wrist Add wrist	Deep radial n.	Ulnar a.
Extensor Digitorum	Lat epicondyle of humerus	2nd & 3rd phalanges of fingers; dorsal surface of distal phalanx	/ PIPs and DIPs / MCPs	Deep radial n.	Ulnar a.
Extensor Digiti Minimi	Common extensor tendon	Expansion of ext digitorum tendon on dorsum of 1st phalanx of little finger	/ wrist / PIPs, DIPs, and MCP digit V	Deep radial n.	Ulnar a.

Muscle	Origin	Insertion	Action	Nerve	Artery
Anconeus	Separate tendon from dorsal part of lat epicondyle of humerus	Side of olecranon; proximal 1/4 of dorsal surface of body of ulna	/ elbow	Radial n.	Ulnar a.
Abductor Pollicis Longus	Lat part of dorsal surface of body of ulna	Radial side of base of 1st metacarpal bone	Abd IP, MCP of digit I Abd wrist	Deep radial n.	Radial a.
Extensor Pollicis Brevis	Dorsal surface of body of radius distal to that muscle and inter-osseous membrane	Base of 1st phalanx of thumb	/ IP, MCP of digit I / wrist	Deep radial n.	Radial a.
Extensor Pollicis Longus	Lat part of mid 1/3 of dorsal surface of body of ulna distal to origin of abductor pollicis longus	Base of last phalanx of thumb	/ IP, MCP of digit I / wrist	Deep radial n.	Radial a.
Extensor Indicis	Dorsal surface of body of ulna below origin of extensor pollicis longus	Joins ulnar side of tendon of extensor digitorum	/ and add of IP, MCP digit II	Deep radial n.	Radial a.
Supinator	Lat epicondyle of humerus from ridge of ulna	Lat edge of radial tuberosity and oblique line of radius and med surface of radius posteriorly	Supination	Deep radial n.	Radial a.

Muscle	Origin	Insertion	Action	Nerve	Artery
HAND					
Abductor Pollicis Brevis	Transverse carpal ligament, tuberosity of scaphoid, ridge of trapezium	Radial side of base of 1st phalanx thumb	Abd thumb	Median n.	Radial a.
Opponens Pollicis	Ridge of trapezium	Length of metacarpal bone of thumb on radial side	Abd thumb ✓ thumb Med ↻	Median n.	Radial a.
Flexor Pollicis Brevis	Distal ridge of trapezium; ulnar side of 1st metacarpal	Radial side of base of proximal phalanx of thumb; ulnar side of base of 1st phalanx	✓ thumb Add thumb	Median & ulnar n.	Radial a.
Adductor Pollicis	Capitale bone, bases of 2nd & 3rd metacarpals	Ulnar side of base of proximal phalanx of thumb	Add thumb	Deep palmar branch of ulnar	Ulnar n.
Palmaris Brevis	Tendinous fasciculi from palmar aponeurosis	Skin on ulnar border of palm of hand	Draws skin midpalm	Ulnar n.	Superficial ulnar a.
Abductor Digiti Minimi	Pisiform bone	Ulnar side of base of 1st phalanx of digit V	Abd digit V ✓ proximal phalanx	Ulnar n.	Ulnar a.
Flexor Digiti Minimi Brevis	Convex surface of hamulus of hamate bone	Ulnar side of base of 1st phalanx of digit V	✓ digit V	Ulnar n.	Ulnar a.

Muscle	Origin	Insertion	Action	Nerve	Artery
Opponens Digiti Minimi	Convexity of hamulus of hamate bone	Length of metacarpal bone of digit V along ulnar margin	Abd digit V ✓ digit V Med ↻ V	Ulnar n.	Ulnar a.
Lumbricals	Originate from the profundus tendons. 1 and 2: radials sides and palmar surfaces of tendons of digits II and III; 3: contiguous sides of mid and ring fingers; 4: contiguous sides of tendons of ring & little finger	Tendinous expansion of extensor digitorum	✓ MCPs / PIPs and DIPs	1 and 2: median n. 3 and 4: ulnar n.	Median a. Ulnar a.
Interosseous Dorsales	Two heads from adjacent sides of metacarpal bone	Bases of 1st phalanx	Abd—midline (digit III)	Deep palmar branch n.	Ulnar a.
Interossei	All from entire length of metacarpal bones	Side of base of 1st phalanx	Add—midline (digit III) ✓ MCPs / PIPs and DIPs	Deep palmar branch n.	Ulnar a.

Muscle	Origin	Insertion	Action	Nerve	Artery
Hip					
Psoas Major (Iliopsoas)	Ventral surface of bases and caudal borders of transverse process of lumbar spine; sides and corresponding intervertebral disks of last thoracic and all lumbar vertebrae	Lesser trochanter of femur	✓ of hip ✓ of spine in lumbar region	2nd and 3rd lumbar n.	Lumbar of iliolumbar a.
Psoas Minor (Iliopsoas)	Vertebral margins of T12 and L1 & corresponding disks	Pectineal line; iliopectineal eminence	✓ of spine in lumbar region	1st & 2nd lumbar n.	Lumbar branch of iliolumbar a.
Iliacus (Iliopsoas)	Upper 2/3 of iliac fossa; iliac crest	Lesser trochanter of femur	✓ at hip	Femoral n. (muscular branches)	Lumbar branch of iliolumbar a.
Tensor Fasciae Latae (TFL)	Ant part of outer lip of iliac crest; ant border of ilium	Lat part of fascia lata at junction of proximal and mid thirds of thigh (proximal end of iliotibial band)	Tenses TFL 3 at hip Abd at hip Int ↻ at hip	Sup gluteal n.	Sup gluteal a.

Muscle	Origin	Insertion	Action	Nerve	Artery
Gluteus Maximus	Post gluteal line; dorsal surface of sacrum and coccyx	Gluteal tuberosity; lat part of TFL at junction of proximal and mid thirds of thigh (proximal end of iliotibial band)	/ at hip; Add at hip; Ext ↻ at hip / lower spine	Inf gluteal n.	Inf gluteal a.
Gluteus Medius	Outer surface of ilium from iliac crest and post gluteal line above to ant gluteal line below	Lat surface of greater trochanter	Abd at hip; Int ↻ at hip	Sup gluteal n.	Sup gluteal a.
Piriformis	Pelvic surface of sacrum between ant sacral foramina and margin of greater sciatic foramen	Upper border of greater trochanter of femur	Ext ↻ at hip; Abd at hip	1st and 2nd sacral n.	Sup gluteal a.
Obturator Internus	Margins of obturator foramen; pelvic surface of hip bone; post and sup obturator foramen	Med surface of greater trochanter	Ext ↻ at hip; Abd at hip	Obturator n. to obturator internus and gemellus sup	Obturator a.; Sup gluteal a.
Gemellus Superior	Outer surface of ischial spine	Med surface of greater trochanter	Ext ↻ at hip	Obturator n. to obturator internus and gemellus sup	Obturator a.; Sup gluteal a.

Muscle	Origin	Insertion	Action	Nerve	Artery
Gemellus Inferior	Upper part of ischial tuberosity	Med surface of greater trochanter	Ext ↻ at hip	Obturator n. to quadratus femoris & gemellus inf	Sup gluteal a.
Quadratus Femoris	Lat margin of ischial tuberosity	Quadrate tubercle of femur; linea quadrata	Add at hip, Ext ↻ at hip	Obturator n. to quadratus femoris & gemellus inf	Sup gluteal a.
Obturator Externus	Outer margin of obturator foramen	Trochanteric fossa of femur	Add at hip, Ext ↻ at hip	Post branch of obturator n.	Obturator a.
HIP/THIGH					
Sartorius	Ant-sup iliac spine; upper half of iliac notch	Upper part of med surface of tibia	✓ at hip, Ext ↻ at hip, ✓ at knee, Abd hip (weak)	Muscular branches of femoral n.	Femoral a.
Quadriceps Femoris Rectus Femoris	Ant-inf iliac spine	Patella by the patellar ligament to the tibial tuberosity	/ at knee, ✓ at hip	Muscular branches of femoral n.	Femoral a.
Vastus Lateralis	Lat aspect of the shaft of the femur	Patella by the patellar ligament to the tibial tuberosity	/ at knee	Muscular branches of femoral n.	Femoral a.
Vastus Medialis	Med aspect of the shaft of the femur	Patella by the patellar ligament to the tibial tuberosity	/ at knee draws patella medially	Muscular branches of femoral n.	Femoral a.

Muscle	Origin	Insertion	Action	Nerve	Artery
Vastus Intermedius	Ant aspect of the shaft of the femur	Patella by the patellar ligament to the tibial tuberosity	/ at knee	Muscular branches of femoral n.	Femoral a.
Gracilis	Lower 1/2 of pubic symphysis; upper 1/2 of pubic arch	Proximal part of med surface of tibia	✓ at knee; Int ↻ at knee; Add at hip	Ant branch of obturator n.	Med femoral circumflex a. (ascending)
Pectineus	Pubic pectineal line and an area of bone ant to it	Line leading from the lesser trochanter to the linea aspera	Add at hip; ✓ at hip; Int ↻ hip	Muscular branches of femoral & obturator n.	Med femoral circumflex a.
Adductor Longus	Ant portion of pubis in angle between crest and symphysis	Mid part of linea aspera	Add at hip; ✓ at hip	Ant branch of obturator n.	Profunda femoris a.
Adductor Brevis	Ext surface of inf ramus of pubis	Proximal part of linea aspera	Add at hip; ✓ at hip	Ant branch of obturator n.	Mid femoral circumflex a.
Adductor Magnus	Pubic arch & ischial tuberosity	Oblique line along entire shaft of the femur	Add at hip; ✓ hip (upper); / hip (lower)	Post branch of obturator & sciatic n.	Profunda femoris & med femoris circumflex a.
Biceps Femoris	Long head: from ischial tuberosity; Short head: lat lip of linea aspera, lat supracondylar line of femur	Head of fibula, lat condyle of tibia, deep fascia on lat side of leg	✓ at knee; / at hip; Ext ↻ knee (semiflexed)	Sciatic n. tibial branch to long head; peroneal branch to short head	Profunda femoris a.

Muscle	Origin	Insertion	Action	Nerve	Artery
Semitendinous	Upper & mid impression of ischial tuberosity (with tendon of the biceps femoris)	Proximal part of ant border & med surface of the tibia	✓ at knee / at hip; Int ↻ knee (semiflexed)	Sciatic n.	Perforating branch profunda femoris a.
Semimembranous	Proximal & lat facet of ischial tuberosity	Med-post surface of med condyle of tibia	✓ at knee / at hip; Int ↻ knee (semiflexed)	Sciatic n.	Perforating branch profunda femoris a.
LEG					
Tibialis Anterior	Lat surface of shaft of tibia; med aspect of fibula; ant interosseous membrane	Med & plantar surface of med cuniform bone; base of 1st metatarsal bone	Dorsiflexion inversion	Deep peroneal n.	Ant tibial a.
Popliteus	Lat condyle of femur	Triangular area on post surface of tibia above ideal line	✓ at knee; Int ↻ at knee	Tibial n. (med & int popliteal)	Post tibial a.
LEG/FOOT					
Extensor Hallucis Longus	Lat surface of shaft of tibia; med aspect of fibula; ant interosseous membrane	Base of distal phalanx of great toe	/ MTP & IP Dorsiflexion	Deep peroneal n. (ant tibial)	Ant tibial a.

Muscle	Origin	Insertion	Action	Nerve	Artery
Extensor Digitorum Longus (EDL)	Lat surface of shaft of tibia; med aspect of fibula; ant interosseous membrane	Dorsal surface of mid and distal phalanges of lat 4 digits	/ IPs digits II to V Dorsiflexion	Deep peroneal n. (ant tibial)	Ant tibial a.
Extensor Digitorum Brevis (EDB)	Proximal and lat surface of calcaneus; lat talocalcaneal ligament	1st tendon dorsal surface of base of proximal phalanx of hallux; other 3 tendons lat sides of tendons of EDL	/ IPs	Deep peroneal n.	Ant tibial a.
Flexor Digitorum Longus	Post surface of shaft of tibia; post aspect of fibula; post interosseous membrane	Plantar surface of base of distal phalanx of lat 4 digits	✓ digits II to V Plantarflexion	Tibial n. (med & int popliteal)	Post tibial a.
Flexor Hallucis Longus	Post surface of shaft of tibia; post aspect of fibula; post interosseous membrane	Base of distal phalanx of hallux	✓ digit I Plantarflexion	Tibial n. (med & int popliteal)	Post tibial a.

Muscle	Origin	Insertion	Action	Nerve	Artery
Tibialis Posterior	Post surface of shaft of tibia; post aspect of fibula; post interosseous membrane	Tuberosity of navicular; plantar surface of cuniform bones; plantar surface of base of 2nd, 3rd and 4th metatarsals, cuboid, sustentaculum tali	Plantarflexion Inversion	Tibial n. (med & int popliteal)	Post tibial a.
Peroneus Tertius	Lat surface of shaft of tibia; med aspect of fibula; ant interosseous membrane	Dorsal surface of base of 5th metatarsal bone	Dorsiflexion Eversion	Deep peroneal n. (ant tibial)	Ant tibial a.
Peroneus Longus	Lat condyle of tibia; head and upper 2/3 of lat surface of fibula	Lat side of med cuniform bone, base of 1st metatarsal bone	Plantarflexion Eversion	Superficial peroneal n. (musculocutaneous)	Peroneal a.
Peroneus Brevis	Lower 2/3 of lat surface of fibula	Lat side of base of 5th metatarsal bone	Plantarflexion Eversion	Superficial peroneal n. (musculocutaneous)	Peroneal a.

Muscle	Origin	Insertion	Action	Nerve	Artery
Gastrocnemius	Med head: med condyle & adjacent part of femur; capsule of knee; Long head: lat condyle and adjacent part of femur; capsule of knee	Calcaneus by the calcaneal tendon	Plantarflexion ✓ at knee	Tibial n. (med popliteal)	Popliteal a.
Soleus	Post surface of head & proximal 1/3 of shaft of fibula; mid 1/3 of med border of tibia	Calcaneus by the calcaneal tendon	Plantarflexion	Tibial n. (med popliteal)	Post tibial a.
Plantaris	Lat supracondylar line of femur	Med side of post part of calcaneus	Plantarflexion	Tibial n. (med popliteal)	Post tibial a.
FOOT					
Quadratus Plantae	Med head: med surface of calcaneus and med border of long plantar ligament; Lat head: lat border of plantar surface of calcaneus and lat border of long plantar ligament	Attached to tendons of flexor digitorum longus	✓ last IP digits II to V	Lat plantar n.	Lat plantar a.

Muscle	Origin	Insertion	Action	Nerve	Artery
Lumbricals (4)	Tendons of flexor digitorum longus	Tendons of EDL & interossei into bases of last phalanges of digits II to V	✓ MP joints / IP joints	Med plantar n. Deep lat plantar n.	Med plantar a.

KEY

✓ flexion
/ extension
↻ rotation
▼ depression, downward, caudal
▲ elevation, upward, cephalic
◆▶ outward, expand
n. = nerve
a. = artery
Lat = lateral
Med = medial
Ext = external
Sup = superior
Ant = anterior

Min = minimal
MTP = metatarsalphalangeal
MCP = metacarpalphalangeal
IP = interphalangeal
PIP = proximal interphalangeal
DIP = distal interphalangeal
Opp = opposite
Abd = abduction
Add = adduction
Mid = middle
Int = internal
Inf = inferior
Post = posterior

Weights and Measures

Linear Measure

1 inch = 2.54 centimeters
12 inches = 1 foot
3 feet = 1 yard (0.9144 meter)
5.5 yards = 1 rod
40 rods = 1 furlong (220 yards)
8 furlongs = 1 statute mile (1760 yards)
5280 feet = 1 statute or land mile
3 miles = 1 league
6076.11549 feet = 1 International Nautical Mile (1852 meters)

Dry Measure

2 pints = 1 quart
8 quarts = 1 peck
4 pecks = 1 bushel (2150.42 cubic inches)

Angular and Circular Measure

60 seconds = 1 minute
60 minutes = 1 degree
90 degrees = 1 right angle = 1 quadrant
180 degrees = 1 straight angle = 2 quadrants
360 degrees = 1 circle = 4 quadrants

Square Measure

144 square inches = 1 square foot
9 square feet = 1 square yard
30.25 square yards = 1 square rod
160 square rods = 1 acre
640 acres = 1 square mile

Troy Weight

24 grains = 1 pennyweight
20 pennyweights = 1 ounce
12 ounces = 1 pound

CUBIC MEASURE

1728 cubic inches = 1 cubic foot
27 cubic feet = 1 cubic yard
2150.42 cubic inches = 1 standard bushel
1 cubic foot = ~4/5th of a bushel
268.8 cubic inches = 1 dry (US) gallon
128 cubic feet = 1 cord (wood)

LIQUID MEASURE

4 gills = 16 ounces = 1 pint
2 pints = 1 quart
4 quarts = 1 gallon (231.0 cubic inches)
31.5 gallons = 1 barrel (US)
2 barrels = 1 hogshead (US)

AVOIRDUPOIS WEIGHT

27.343 grains = 1 dram
16 drams = 1 ounce
16 ounces = 1 pound (0.45359237 kilogram)
100 pounds = 1 hundredweight
20 hundredweights (2000 pounds) = 1 short ton
2240 pounds = 1 long ton

HOUSEHOLD MEASURES AND WEIGHTS

1 teaspoon = 5 mL = 60 grains = 1 dram = 1/8 fluid ounce
1 teaspoon = 1/8 fluid ounce = 1 dram
3 teaspoons = 1 tablespoon
1 tablespoon = 1/2 fluid ounce = 4 drams
16 tablespoons (liquid) = 1 cup
12 tablespoons (dry) = 1 cup
1 cup = 8 fluid ounces = 1/2 pint

APOTHECARIES' WEIGHT

20 grains = 1 scruple
3 scruples = 1 dram
8 drams = 1 ounce
12 ounces = 1 pound

The Metric System

LINEAR MEASURE

1 millimeter = 0.1 centimeter
10 millimeters = 1 centimeter
10 centimeters = 1 decimeter
10 decimeters = 1 meter
10 meters = 1 dekameter
10 dekameters = 1 hectometer
10 hectometers = 1 kilometer

LIQUID MEASURE

1 milliliter = 0.001 liter
10 milliliters = 1 centiliter
10 centiliters = 1 deciliter
10 deciliters = 1 liter
10 liters = 1 dekaliter
10 dekaliters = 1 hectoliter
10 hectoliters = 1 kiloliter

SQUARE MEASURE

1 square millimeter = 0.01 square centimeter
100 square millimeters = 1 square centimeter
100 square centimeters = 1 square decimeter
100 square decimeters = 1 square meter
100 square meters = 1 square dekameter
100 square dekameters = 1 square hectometer
100 square hectometers = 1 square kilometer

WEIGHTS

10 milligrams = 1 centigram
10 centigrams = 1 decigram
10 decigrams = 1 gram
10 grams = 1 dekagram
10 dekagrams = 1 hectogram
10 hectograms = 1 kilogram
100 kilograms = 1 quintal
10 quintals = 1 ton

CUBIC MEASURE

1000 cubic millimeters = 1 cubic centimeter
1000 cubic centimeters = 1 cubic decimeter
1000 cubic decimeters = 1 cubic meter

English and Metric Conversion

LINEAR MEASURE

1 centimeter = 0.3937 inch
1 inch = 2.54 centimeters
1 foot = 0.3048 meter
1 meter = 39.37 inches = 1.0936 yards
1 yard = 0.9144 meter
1 kilometer = 0.621 mile
1 mile = 1.609 kilometers

SQUARE MEASURE

1 square centimeter = 0.1550 square inch
1 square inch = 6.452 square centimeters
1 square foot = 0.0929 square meter
1 square meter = 1.196 square yards
1 square yard = 0.8361 square meter
1 hectare = 2.47 acres
1 acre = 0.4047 hectare
1 square kilometer = 0.386 square mile
1 square mile = 2.59 square kilometers

WEIGHT MEASURE

1 gram = 0.03527 ounce
1 ounce = 28.35 grams
1 kilogram = 2.2046 pounds
1 pound = 0.4536 kilogram
1 metric ton = 0.98421 English ton
1 English ton = 1.016 metric tons

VOLUME MEASURE

1 cubic centimeter = 0.061 cubic inch
1 cubic inch = 16.39 cubic centimeters
1 cubic foot = 0.0283 cubic meter
1 cubic meter = 1.308 cubic yards
1 cubic yard = 0.7646 cubic meter
1 liter = 1.0567 quarts

1 quart dry = 1.101 liters
1 quart liquid = 0.9463 liter
1 gallon = 3.78541 liters
1 peck = 8.810 liters
1 hectoliter = 2.8375 bushels

Symbols

↑	increase
↓	decrease
→	to follow, approaches the limit of
↔	to and from
⇒	implies
⇔	implies and is implied by, is equivalent to
%	percent
°	degree
1°	primary/first degree
2°	secondary/due to/second degree
3°	tertiary/third degree
@	at
α	alpha
β	beta
Δ	delta, change
η	total sample size
N	total population size
χ	mean
μ	micron (former term for micrometer)
π	3.1416, ratio of circumference of a circle to its diameter
√	root, square root, radical
+	plus, excess, positive
−	minus, deficiency, negative
±	plus or minus, indefinite
x	multiplied by
÷	divided by
~	approximately or approximately equal
=	equal to
≠	not equal to
≡	identical to
>	greater than
<	less than
≥	greater than or equal to
≤	less than or equal to
‖	absolute value
Σ	sum
∪	logical sum

∩	logical product
∈	member of a set
∅	empty set, without
∞	infinity, indefinitely great
:	ratio, "is to"
::	equality between ratios, "as"
∴	therefore
...	and so on
∠	angle
∟	right angle
⊥	perpendicular
‖	parallel
w/	with
w/o	without
#	number, pound
/	per
♂	male
♀	female
©	copyright
®	registered
TM	trademark

Prescription Drugs Delineated by Disease and Disorder

DRUGS USED IN NEUROLOGIC DISORDERS

	Generic Name	*Trade Name*
PARKINSON'S DISEASE		
Dopamine precursors	Levodopa	Sinemet*
Anticholinergic drugs	Biperiden	Akineton
	Ethopropazine	Parsidol
	Procyclidine	Kemadrin
Others	Amantadine	Symmetrel
	Bromocriptine	Parlodel
	Selegiline	Eldepryl
SEIZURE DISORDERS		
Barbiturates	Metharbital	Gemonil
	Phenobarbital	Luminal
Benzodiazepines	Clonazepam	Klonopin
	Clorazepate	Tranxene
Hydantoins	Ethotoin	Peganone
	Mephenytoin	Mesantoin
	Phenytoin	Dilantin
Succinimides	Ethosuximide	Zarontin
	Methsuximide	Celontin
Others	Carbamazepine	Tegretol
	Valproic acid	Depakene

*Indicates trade name for levodopa combined with carbidopa, a peripheral decarboxylase inhibitor

DRUGS USED TO TREAT PAIN AND INFLAMMATION

	Generic Name	*Trade Name*
Narcotic analgesics	Codeine	(Many)
	Meperidine	Demerol
	Morphine	Duramorph
	Oxycodone	Percodan
	Propoxyphene	Darvon

	Generic Name	Trade Name
NON-NARCOTIC ANALGESICS		
NSAIDS	Aspirin	(Many)
	Ibuprofen	Advil, Motrin, others
	Piroxicam	Feldene
	Sulindac	Clinoril
Acetaminophen	Acetaminophen	Tylenol, Panadol
CORTICOSTEROIDS		
	Betamethasone	Celestone
	Cortisone	Cortone
	Hydrocortisone	Hydrocortone
	Prednisone	Deltasone
DISEASE-MODIFYING DRUGS*		
Gold compounds	Auranofin	Ridaura
	Aurothioglucose	Solganal
	Gold sodium thiomalate	Myochrysine
Antimalarials	Chloroquine	Aralen
	Hydroxychloro-quine	Palquenil
Others	Penicillamine	Cuprimine, Depen
	Methotrexate	Mexate
	Azathioprine	Imuran

*Drugs used to slow the progression of rheumatoid arthritis.

DRUGS USED IN PSYCHIATRIC DISORDERS

	Generic Name	Trade Name
SEDATIVE-HYPNOTIC AGENTS		
Benzodiazepines	Flurazepam	Dalmane
	Temazepam	Restoril
	Triazolam	Halcion
Barbiturates	Pentobarbital	Nembutal
	Secobarbital	Seconal

	Generic Name	Trade Name
ANXIETY AGENTS		
Benzodiazepines	Chlordiazepoxide	Librium
	Diazepam	Valium
	Lorazepam	Ativan
ANTIDEPRESSANT DRUGS		
Tricyclics	Amitriptyline	Elavil
	Imipramine	Tofranil
MAO inhibitors	Isocarboxazid	Marplan
	Phenelzine	Nardil
Sympathomimetics	Dextroampheta-mine	Dexedrine, others
Second-generation agents	Amoxapine	Asendin
	Maprotiline	Ludiomil
ANTIPSYCHOTIC DRUGS		
Phenothiazines	Chlorpromazine	
	Thioridazine	Mellaril
Thioxanthenes	Chlorprothixene	Taractan
	Thiothixene	Navane
Butyrophenones	Haloperidol	Haldol

DRUGS USED IN CARDIOVASCULAR DISORDERS

Primary Indications	Generic Name	Trade Name
ALPHA-BLOCKERS		
Hypertension	Phenoxybenzamine	Dibenzyline
	Prazosin	Minipress
ANGIOTENSIN-CONVERTING ENZYME INHIBITORS		
Hypertension	Captopril	Capoten
CHF	Enalapril	Vasotec
ANTICOAGULANTS		
Overactive clotting	Heparin	Liquaemin
	Warfarin	Coumadin
BETA-BLOCKERS		
Hypertension	Atenolol	Tenormin
Angina	Metoprolol	Lopressor
Arrhythmias	Nadolol	Corgard
	Propranolol	Inderal

Primary Indications	Generic Name	Trade Name
CALCIUM CHANNEL BLOCKERS		
Hypertension	Diltiazem	Cardizem
Angina	Nifedipine	Procardia
Arrhythmias	Verapamil	Calan, Isoptin
CENTRALLY ACTING SYMPATHOLYTICS		
Hypertension	Clonidine	Catapres
	Methyldopa	Aldomet
DIGITALIS GLYCOSIDES		
CHF	Digoxin	Lanoxin
DIURETICS		
Hypertension	Chlorothiazide	Diuril
CHF	Furosemide	Lasix
	Spironolactone	Aldactone
DRUGS THAT PROLONG REPOLARIZATION		
Arrhythmias	Amiodarone	Cordarone
	Bretylium	Bretylol
ORGANIC NITRATES		
Angina	Nitroglycerin	Nitrostat, others
PRESYNAPTIC ADRENERGIC DEPLETORS		
Hypertension	Guanethidine	Ismelin
	Reserpine	Serpasil, others
SODIUM CHANNEL BLOCKERS		
Arrhythmias	Quinidine	Cardioquin, others
	Lidocaine	Xylocaine, others
VASODILATORS		
Hypertension	Hydralazine	Apresoline
	Minoxidil	Loniten

DRUGS USED IN ENDOCRINE DISORDERS

Primary Indications	Generic Name	Trade Name
ESTROGENS		
Osteoporosis	Conjugated estrogens	Premarin
Severe perimenopausal symptoms	Estradiol	Estrace, others
Some cancers		
Heart disease		
Alzheimer's disease		
INSULIN		
Diabetes mellitus		Iletin, Lente Iletin Humalin, Velosulin, etc
ORAL HYPOGLYCEMIC AGENTS		
Diabetes mellitus	Chlorpropamide	Diabinese
	Glipizide	Glucotrol
	Tolbutamide	Orinase
ANTITHYROID AGENTS		
Hyperthyroidism	Methimazole	Tapazole
	Propylthiouracil	Propyl-Thyracil
THYROID HORMONES		
Hypothyroidism	Levothyroxine	Levothroid, Synthroid
	Liothyronine	Cytomel

DRUGS USED FOR TREATMENT OF INFECTION

	Generic Name	Trade Name
ANTIBACTERIAL DRUGS		
Aminoglycosides	Gentamicin	Garamycin
	Streptomycin	---
Cephalosporins	Cefaclor	Ceclor
	Cephalexin	Keflex
Erythromycins	Erythromycin	E-Mycin, many others

	Generic Name	*Trade Name*
Penicillins	Penicillin G	Bicillin, others
	Penicillin V	V-Cillin K, others
	Amoxicillin	Amoxil, others
	Ampicillin	Amcill, others
Sulfonamides	Sulfadiazine	Silvadene
	Sulfisoxazole	Gantrisin
Tetracyclines	Doxycycline	Vibramycin, others
	Tetracycline	Sumycin, others

DRUGS USED FOR TREATMENT OF INFECTION

	Trade Name	*Principal Indication*
ANTIVIRAL DRUGS		
Acyclovir	Zovirax	*Herpes simplex* infections
Amantadine	Symmetrel	Influenza A
Vidarabine	Vira-A	Herpes virus infections
Zidovudine	Retrovir	HIV infections

CANCER CHEMOTHERAPEUTIC AGENTS

Alkylating Agents

Busulfan (Myleran)
Carmustine (BCNU, BiCNU)
Cyclophosphamide (Cytoxan, Neosar)
Dacarbazine (DTIC-Dome)
Lomustine (CeeNU)
Mechlorethamine (Mustargen)
Melphalan (Alkeran)
Streptozocin (Zanosar)
Thiotepa
Uracil mustard

Antimetabolites

Cytarabine (Cytosar-U)
Floxuridine (FUDR)
Fluorouracil (Adrucil)
Mercaptopurine (Purinethol)
Methotrexate (Mexate)
Thioguanine (Lanvis)

Others

Antineoplastic antibiotics
Hormones
Interferons
Plant alkaloids
Miscellaneous cytotoxic agents

CHF = congestive heart failure, MAO = monoamine oxidase, NSAIDs = non-steroidal anti-inflammatory drugs.

Recommended Daily Dietary Allowances

INFANTS/ CHILDREN	0 TO 2 MO	2 TO 6 MO	6 TO 12 MO	1 TO 2 YR	2 TO 3 YR	3 TO 4 YR	4 TO 6 YR	6 TO 8 YR	8 TO 10 YR
Weight (kg)[a]	4	7	9	12	14	16	19	23	28
Height (cm)[a]	55	63	72	81	91	100	110	121	131
Energy (kg)	kg x 120	kg x 110	kg x 100	1100	1250	1400	1600	2000	2200
Protein (g)	kg x 2.2	kg x 2.0	kg x 1.8	25	25	30	30	35	40
Fat Soluble Vitamins									
Vitamin A (IU)	1500	1500	1500	2000	2000	2500	2500	3500	3500
Vitamin D (IU)	400	400	400	400	400	400	400	400	400
Vitamin E (IU)	5	5	5	10	10	10	10	15	15
Vitamin C (mg)	35	35	35	40	40	40	40	40	40
Folate acid (mg)	0.05	0.05	0.1	0.1	0.2	0.2	0.2	0.2	0.3
Niacin (mg equiv)	5	7	8	8	8	9	11	13	15
Riboflavin (mg)	0.4	0.5	0.6	0.6	0.7	0.8	0.9	1.1	1.2
Thiamine (mg)	0.2	0.4	0.5	0.6	0.6	0.7	0.8	1.0	1.1

[a]Weights and heights represent actual median weights and heights for age groups derived from national data collected by the National Center for Health Statistics.

Infants/Children	0 to 2 mo	2 to 6 mo	6 to 12 mo	1 to 2 yr	2 to 3 yr	3 to 4 yr	4 to 6 yr	6 to 8 yr	8 to 10 yr
Water Soluble Vitamins									
Vitamin B_6 (mg)	0.2	0.3	0.4	0.5	0.6	0.7	0.9	1.0	1.2
Vitamin B_{12} (µg)	1.0	1.5	2.0	2.0	2.5	3.0	4.0	4.0	5.0
Calcium (mg)	400	500	600	700	800	800	800	900	1000
Phosphorus (g)	0.2	0.4	0.5	0.7	0.8	0.8	0.8	0.9	1.0
Iodine (µg)	25	40	45	55	60	70	80	100	110
Iron (mg)	6	10	15	15	15	10	10	10	10
Magnesium (mg)	40	60	70	100	150	200	200	250	250
Zinc (µg)	5	5	5	5	7	8	9	10	11
Selenium (µg)	10	10	10	15	20	25	30	35	40

Males	10 to 12 yr	12 to 14 yr	14 to 18 yr	18 to 22 yr	22 to 35 yr	35 to 55 yr	55 to 75 yr	75+ yr
Weight (kg)[a]	35	43	59	67	70	70	70	70
Height (cm)[a]	140	151	170	175	175	173	171	170
Energy (kg)	2500	2700	3000	2800	1800	2600	2400	2200
Protein (g)	45	50	60	60	65	65	65	65

MALES	10 TO 12 YR	12 TO 14 YR	14 TO 18 YR	18 TO 22 YR	22 TO 35 YR	35 TO 55 YR	55 TO 75 YR	75+ YR
Fat Soluble Vitamins								
Vitamin A (IU)	4500	5000	5000	5000	5000	5000	5000	5000
Vitamin D (IU)	400	400	400	400	400	400	400	400
Vitamin E (IU)	20	20	25	30	30	30	30	30
Vitamin C (mg)	40	45	55	60	60	60	60	60
Folate acid (mg)	0.4	0.4	0.4	0.4	0.4	0.4	0.4	0.4
Niacin (mg equiv)	15	17	18	20	18	18	17	17
Riboflavin (mg)	1.3	1.4	1.5	1.6	1.7	1.7	1.7	1.7
Thiamine (mg)	1.3	1.4	1.5	1.4	1.4	1.3	1.2	1.2
Water Soluble Vitamins								
Vitamin B_6 (mg)	1.2	1.4	1.6	1.8	2.0	2.0	2.0	2.0
Vitamin B_{12} (µg)	5	5	5	5	5	5	5	5
Calcium (mg)	1200	1400	1400	1000	1000	800	800	800
Phosphorus (g)	1.2	1.4	1.4	0.8	0.8	0.8	0.8	0.8
Iodine (µg)	125	135	150	140	140	125	110	100
Iron (mg)	10	18	18	10	10	10	10	10
Magnesium (mg)	250	300	350	400	400	350	350	350
Zinc (µg)	12	12	15	15	15	15	15	15
Selenium (µg)	40	45	50	55	60	60	60	60

FEMALES	10 TO 12 YR	12 TO 14 YR	14 TO 16 YR	16 TO 18 YR	18 TO 22 YR	22 TO 35 YR	35 TO 55 YR	55 TO 75 YR	75+ YR	PREG/LACT[1]
Weight (kg)[a]	35	44	52	54	58	58	58	58	60	--
Height (cm)[a]	142	154	157	160	163	163	160	157	154	--
Energy (kg)	2250	2300	2400	2300	2000	2000	1850	1700	1650	+200/ +1000[2]
Protein (g)	50	50	55	55	55	55	55	55	55	+65/ +75

[1]Values apply during pregnancy and lactation.
[2] + values for pregnant women are added to dietary values indicated for given age group.

Fat Soluble Vitamins

	10 TO 12 YR	12 TO 14 YR	14 TO 16 YR	16 TO 18 YR	18 TO 22 YR	22 TO 35 YR	35 TO 55 YR	55 TO 75 YR	75+ YR	PREG/LACT[1]
Vitamin A (IU)	4500	5000	5000	5000	5000	5000	5000	5000	5000	+100/ +200
Vitamin D (IU)	400	400	400	400	400	400	400	400	400	400
Vitamin E (IU)	20	20	25	25	25	25	25	25	25	30
Vitamin C (mg)	40	45	50	50	55	55	60	100	100	60
Folate acid (mg)	0.4	0.4	0.4	0.4	0.4	0.4	0.4	0.4	0.4	0.8/0.5
Niacin (mg equiv)	15	15	16	15	13	13	13	12	12	15/20
Riboflavin (mg)	1.3	1.4	1.4	1.5	1.5	1.5	1.5	1.5	1.5	1.8/2.0
Thiamine (mg)	1.1	1.2	1.2	1.2	1.0	1.0	1.0	1.0	1.0	+0.1/ +0.5

FEMALES	10 TO 12 YR	12 TO 14 YR	14 TO 16 YR	16 TO 18 YR	18 TO 22 YR	22 TO 35 YR	35 TO 55 YR	55 TO 75 YR	75+ YR	PREG/LACT[1]
Water Soluble Vitamins										
Vitamin B$_6$ (mg)	1.4	1.6	1.8	2.0	2.0	2.0	2.0	2.0	2.0	2.5
Vitamin B$_{12}$ (µg)	5	5	5	5	5	5	5	6	6	8/6
Calcium (mg)	1200	1300	1300	1300	1500	1500	1500	1500	1500	+400/+500
Phosphorus (g)	0.8	1.2	1.3	1.3	1.5	1.5	1.5	1.5	1.5	+0.4/+0.5
Iodine (µg)	110	110	115	120	115	100	100	90	80	125/150
Iron (mg)	10	18	18	18	18	18	18	10	10	18
Magnesium (mg)	300	350	350	350	350	300	300	300	300	450/450
Zinc (µg)	12	12	12	12	15	15	15	15	15	+5
Selenium (µg)	45	45	50	50	55	55	55	55	55	65

Reimbursement Terms and Guidelines for Physical Therapy Claims Review

REIMBURSEMENT TERMS

Medicare

3-day prior hospitalization: A 3-day period of hospitalization is required in order to qualify for a "spell of illness" and to be covered for 100 days under Medicare Part A benefits.

30-day exception rule: If a patient/client is taken off Medicare Part A benefits prior to the completion of 100 days of coverage, he or she can go back on if exacerbation of the condition occurs within 30 days. He or she would resume coverage from the day of discharge (eg, if a patient was discharged from service on day 42, he or she would resume coverage on day 43 within the 30-day period).

30-day transfer rule: A patient/client can be admitted to a skilled nursing facility within a 30-day period following discharge from an acute care facility admission for 3 days and still qualify for a "spell of illness" coverage under Medicare Part A. Reasons for the delay in admission could include nonavailability of appropriate bed space or medical inappropriateness at the time of discharge from the acute care facility.

adjusted average per capita cost (AAPCC): Based on age, sex, institutional status, Medicaid eligibility, disability, and end-stage renal disease status, this is the formula used to estimate the average fee-for-service cost of Medicare benefits for an individual by county of residence.

ambulatory patient group (APG): This is a prospective payment system established by Medicare whereby reimbursement on an outpatient basis is classified by diagnostic category (DRG) and prior use of services in either an in- or outpatient setting.

availability of alternative services: Medicare will cover the more economic care alternative. For instance, if transportation to an outpatient clinic requires an ambulance, it may be more economical from a health delivery viewpoint to provide the needed care in a skilled nursing facility.

average length of stay (ALOS): This is the average length of stay for each inpatient hospitalization.

Balanced Budget Act of 1997: Legislation that established a cost containment program under Medicare. This shifted the reimbursement model from a fee-for-service to a capitation model imposing an upper limit to benefits for clients/patients in skilled nursing facilities under Medicare Part A (resource utilization groups III—RUGS III) and Medicare Part B (fee schedules).

case-mix: A system of payment that measures the intensity of care and services required for each resident in a skilled nursing facility and then translates it into a payment level based on utilization of resources. The adjusted payment system or the amount of payment given to the nursing home for care of a resident is tied to the intensity of resources used (eg, hours of nursing or therapy time needed per day, use of a ventilator, etc).

daily skilled services: Skilled services are required on a daily basis in order to rehabilitate or maintain the "total condition of the patient." This requirement is linked to eligibility.

diagnosis-related groups (DRGs): Established, fixed prices are prospectively set on a cost-per-case basis based on the diagnosis.

eligibility: In order to qualify for Medicare Part A benefits for treatment following an illness, a client/patient must meet the requirements of 3 consecutive days of acute hospital admission (a full 72 hours), be "entitled" to hospital insurance (Medicare Part A), require skilled services on an inpatient basis as a "practical matter," and the physician must certify admission to a skilled nursing facility.

entitlement: In order to qualify for Medicare Part A benefits, a client/patient must have put into the Social Security and Health Care Financing Administration funds under an employer for 40 quarters (one quarter = 3 months).

function-related group (FRG): A prospective payment system based on a client's/patient's diagnosis and level of function.

Health Care Financing Administration (HCFA): Federal agency that administers the Medicare program.

maintenance therapy: Therapy that requires the specialized knowledge and judgment of a qualified professional to establish a maintenance program intended to prevent or minimize deterioration of the patient.

Medicare supplement policy: A health insurance policy that pays certain costs not covered by Medicare, such as coinsurance and deductibles. Also called gap insurance.

prospective payment system: A system of payment for services that uses per diem federal payment rates based on mean skilled nursing facility costs in a base year and updated for inflation to the first effective period of the system.

reconsideration/appeal: If a Medicare claim has been denied coverage by the third-party payer, the claimant has the opportunity to resubmit the claim for reconsideration. The appeal period is 60 days for Part A and 6 months for Part B.

Resource-Based Relative Value Scale: A Medicare weighting system that assigns units of value to each CPT code (procedure) performed by health care providers.

resource utilization groups system (RUGS III): A system of classification associated with the prospective payment system that is utilized in skilled nursing facilities for patients covered by Medicare Part A. Relative cost of patient care is based on the types of services and resources provided.

routine therapy: Routine procedures that are not considered "skilled services," such as the donning of braces or repetitious exercises that are supervised but do not require skilled personnel.

secondary payer: Medicare is not the primary payer when the client/patient is covered by automobile, medical, no-fault, or any liability insurance; has benefits under a spouse's Employer Group Health Plan (EGHP); or is the beneficiary of the Veterans Administration, Workers' Compensation, Federal Black Lung, or other benefits that would cover the condition for which he or she is hospitalized.

skilled services: Requires observation, assessment, and management by skilled personnel and is directly and specifically related to an active written treatment plan.

spell of illness: Provides 100 days of coverage under Part A benefits for each "episode."

waiver of liability: A release of liability of a skilled nursing facility when a client/patient decides to waive his or her Medicare benefits after a "spell of illness."

Medicaid

allowable reserve: Asset limits placed on a client/patient in order to be eligible for Medicaid benefits. A fixed total (which changes with the economic scale of poverty rates) of assets includes income at or below the poverty level and a total dollar value allowable in checking, savings, bonds, stocks, inherited property, cash value of life insurance policies, and other cash assets. Excluded are a house (primary residence), one vehicle (if used for medical transport four times a year), and a personal burial plot.

categorically needy: A category of Social Security income for medical services under Medicaid based on income (eg, poverty) and reserve limits.

medically needy: A category of Social Security income for medical services under Medicaid based on the amount of medical expenses that exceeds the monthly Social Security benefit. A client/patient is eligible for this benefit only if his or her medical bills exceed his or her Social Security income.

piggy-backing: When the client/patient is covered by both Medicare and Medicaid benefits, Medicare picks up 80% of the cost of services and Medicaid covers the remaining 20%.

GENERAL REIMBURSEMENT TERMS

administrative costs: The health care insurer's costs related to administration of services, including such areas as insurance marking, utilization review, quality assurance programs, risk management, medical underwriting, premium collection, claims processing, agent's commissions, and insurer profit.

adverse selection: The tendency for individuals with pre-existing conditions, who are anticipated to utilize more health services, to be enrolled by an insurer in disproportionate numbers and higher deductible plans.

ambulatory care: Health care services provided on an outpatient basis, including in "ambulatory care centers," outpatient departments, physician's offices, and home health care services.

beneficiary: The client/patient who is eligible for health care benefits under a contracted insurance program.

benefit payment schedule: A scheduled list of coverage to be paid by the insurer under any given insurance plan.

capitation: A fixed amount of payment for services based on an upper limit, regardless of the amount of care provided.

cascading coverage: A schedule of payment whereby services are reimbursed initially at 100% with a diminishing rate of the fee schedule based on the number of medical visits or treatments (eg, 100%, 75%, 50%, 25%).

case rate: A flat fee paid for a client's/patient's treatment based on diagnosis or presenting problem.

claims review: The insurer's review of services prior intervention to establish medical necessity and ensure that excessive charges are not being imposed prior to approval for reimbursement.

closed access: A type of managed care system in which services can only be provided by the plan's participating providers.

coinsurance: An agreement between the insurer and the insured that forces the patient/client to pay a certain percentage of the cost of care (eg, 20%) after the deductible has been paid.

common procedural terminology (CPT): A coding system for therapy services that is used to determine provider fee schedule reimbursement.

community rating: Establishing rates for reimbursement based on the geographic area in which those services are provided.

coordination of benefits (COB): This procedure establishes provisions by third-party payers when there is more than one insurance plan covering an individual's health benefits.

cost sharing: Financial arrangements between the consumer and insurer where the consumer pays out-of-pocket for health care or pays a portion of monthly premiums for health care insurance.

cost shifting: Charging one group of clients/patients more in order to offset underpayment by other clients/patients (eg, those covered by Medicare or Medicaid).

deductible: Out-of-pocket expense that must be paid by the insured prior to reimbursement for medical expenses.

enrollee: Any person eligible for benefits from a health insurance plan.

exclusions: Clauses in a health insurance contract that deny coverage for specific services or procedures or select individuals, locations, properties, or risks.

exclusive provider organization (EPO): A managed care organization, similar to a preferred provider organization, in which clients/patients are only allowed to choose medical care from within a network of approved providers.

exclusivity clause: A clause in a health insurance contract that prohibits physicians from contracting with more than one managed care organization.

experience rating: A means for insurance companies to evaluate the risk of an individual or group by looking at the client's/patient's medical history and history of service utilization.

fee disclosure: Medical providers informing clients/patients of fees for services prior to intervention.

fee-for-service (FFS): The traditional payment method whereby patients pay for medical services and then submit expenses to insurers for reimbursement.

fee schedule: A comprehensive listing of fees used by a health care plan to reimburse on a fee-for-service basis.

fiscal intermediary: The agent that has contracted with providers of service to process claims for reimbursement under health care coverage.

flat fee per case: An established fee paid for health care services based on diagnosis or presenting problem.

gatekeeper: A health care provider (eg, physician) responsible for overseeing and coordinating all aspects of an individual's medical care.

group insurance: A health care plan established for a group of individuals (eg, employees in a company).

health maintenance organization (HMO): Health care providers that offer comprehensive health coverage via contracts with health care providers.

indemnify: To make good on a loss.

independent practice association (IPA): An HMO delivery model in which the HMO contracts with a physician organization that in turn contracts with individual physicians.

managed care: A model of medical care that coordinates care by organizing hospitals, doctors, and other providers to enhance the quality of care and the provision for decreasing the cost of delivery of service by preventing duplication of services or medically unnecessary evaluations or interventions.

managed services organization (MSO): An entity that contracts for the provision of management and administrative support services to health care providers.

medical group practice: Health services provided by a group of three or more physicians who share facilities, medical records, equipment, and personnel. The group is formally organized and legally recognized.

medically necessary: Health care services required to preserve and maintain the health status of a beneficiary of an insurance plan.

medical savings account (MSA): An employment-based health insurance in which the least expensive health plans are purchased with high deductibles and the annual difference between the highest price health insurance plan is put into a savings account for the employee.

network model HMO: An HMO that contracts with two or more independent group practices to provide health services.

open enrollment: A time period in which individuals change their enrollment in an insurance plan or transfer between available programs providing health care coverage.

out-of-area benefits: Benefits covered by a health insurance plan when services needed are outside of the HMO's geographical region.

per member per month (PMPM): The average cost of providing services to any member each month.

preadmission review: A review of the claim for inpatient admission before the client/patient is admitted to ensure the medical necessity of admission by the insurer.

preauthorization: Evaluation by the insurer of the need for medical service before it is performed; used as a means of monitoring and controlling utilization of services.

precertification: The prior authorization required by some payers before health benefits are paid.

predetermination: An administrative procedure whereby a health provider submits a treatment plan to a third-party payer before treatment is initiated.

preferred provider organization (PPO): Medical services delivered by a network of providers approved by the insurer.

premium: The amount paid for an insurance plan on an annual basis.

prepayment: Paying for the cost of medical services prior to intervention.

risk adjustment: Adjustment of the rates paid to managed care providers based on demographic factors, such as age, gender, race, ethnicity, medical condition, geographic location, at-risk population (eg, homeless), etc.

risk sharing: A method where insurance premiums are shared by plan sponsors and participants.

third-party payer: The medical insurance agency.

usual, customary, and reasonable (UCR): A reimbursement method whereby a health insurance plan pays a physician's full charge if it is reasonable and does not exceed his or her usual charges and the amount customarily charged for the same service by other physicians in the area.

GUIDELINES FOR PHYSICAL THERAPY CLAIMS REVIEW

Table of Contents

The American Physical Therapy Association (APTA) provides the following guidelines (approved, nonbinding statements of advice) for use by the insurance industry. The intent of the Guidelines is to facilitate review of claims submitted by physical therapists for physical therapy services and to enhance understanding of reimbursement issues related to physical therapy. APTA strongly believes that claims for physical therapy services provided by physical therapists should be reviewed by a licensed physical therapist.

I. Definition of Physical Therapy

Physical therapy, which is the care and services provided by, or under the direction and supervision of, a physical therapist, includes:

1. Examining patients with impairments, functional limitations, and disability or other health-related conditions in order to determine a diagnosis, prognosis, and intervention (see list of examinations in these guidelines);

2. Alleviating impairments and functional limitations by designing, implementing, and modifying therapeutic interventions (see list of interventions under V of these guidelines);

3. Preventing injury, impairments, functional limitations, and disability, including the promotion and maintenance of fitness, health, and quality of life in all age populations; and

4. Engaging in consultation, education, and research.

II. Definition of Physical Therapist

A physical therapist is a graduate of a physical therapist education program that is accredited by the Commission on Accreditation in Physical Therapy Education, a nationally recognized agency; or

An internationally educated client/patient who has the documented equivalent training, education, and experience and who meets any current legal requirements of licensure or registration.

III. Qualifications of Persons Providing Physical Therapy Services

Protection of the public interest requires that physical therapy services be provided only by persons who have successfully completed specialized education in that field and whose practice complies with well-defined regulations.

Physical therapists must be licensed by the jurisdiction in which they practice.

Public laws and regulations and requirements of private organizations should make it clear that the term "physical therapy" is to be applied only to services provided by licensed physical therapists. Selected interventions may be carried out by physical therapist assistants or physical therapy aides, but only under the direction and supervision of licensed physical therapists. Although some aspects of the treatments provided by practitioners in other fields may be similar to physical therapy, they are not physical therapy services and should not be represented or reimbursed as such. To ensure public protection, all non-physical therapist providers using such interventions should meet the same minimal educational preparation standards as physical therapists. Licensure and regulatory requirements should also take these competencies into account. Physical therapy and physical therapy services are not generic terms; they are the use of any intervention, including physical agent modalities/electrotherapy, that is provided by, or under the direction of, a licensed physical therapist.

IV. Roles of the Physical Therapist

The roles of the physical therapist include the following:

Patient Management—Examining patients, identifying potential and existing problems, performing evaluations, establishing a diagnosis, setting forth a prognosis, providing interventions, and modifying treatment to effect the desired outcomes.

Prevention and Wellness (including Health Promotion)—Integrating prevention, wellness, and the promotion of positive health behavior into physical therapy practice to reduce injury, impairment, and disability among patients. Physical therapists also offer preventive and wellness programs designed for the community at large.

Consultation—Providing professional or expert opinion or advice. Consultation includes the application of highly specialized knowledge and skills to identify problems, recommend solutions, or produce some specified result or product in a given amount of time on behalf of a patient or client.

Screening—Determining the need for an examination or consultation by a physical therapist or for referral to another health care practitioner.

Education—Imparting information or skills and instructing by precept, example, and experience so that clients/patients acquire knowledge, master skills, or develop competence.

Critical Inquiry—Applying the principles of scientific methods to read and interpret professional literature; participating in, planning, and conducting research; and analyzing patient care outcomes, new concepts, and findings.

Administration—The skilled process of planning, directing, organizing, and managing human, technical, environmental, and financial resources effectively and efficiently, including the management by client/patient physical therapists of resources for their patients' care as well as the managing of organizational resources.

V. Commonly Used Physical Therapy Examinations and Interventions

Commonly used physical therapy examinations include, but are not limited to, the following:

a. Aerobic capacity or endurance

b. Anthropometric characteristics

c. Arousal, mentation, and cognition

d. Assistive, adaptive, supportive, and protective devices

e. Community or work reintegration

f. Cranial nerve integrity

g. Environmental, home, or work barriers

h. Ergonomics or body mechanics

i. Gait and balance

j. Integumentary integrity

k. Joint integrity and mobility

l. Motor function

m. Muscle performance

n. Neuromotor development and sensory integration

o. Orthotic requirements

p. Pain

q. Posture

r. Prosthetic requirements

s. Range of motion

t. Reflex integrity

u. Self-care and home management

v. Sensory integrity

w. Ventilation, respiration, and circulation

Commonly used physical therapy interventions include, but are not limited to, the following:

a. Therapeutic exercise (including aerobic conditioning)

b. Functional training in self-care and home management (including activities of daily living and instrumental activities of daily living)

c. Functional training in community or work reintegration (including instrumental activities of daily living, work hardening, and work conditioning)

d. Manual therapy techniques (including mobilization and manipulation)

e. Prescription, fabrication, and application of assistive, adaptive, supportive, and protective devices and equipment

f. Airway clearance techniques

g. Debridement and wound care

h. Physical agents and mechanical modalities

i. Electrotherapeutic modalities

j. Patient-related instruction

VI. Synonymous Interventions or Potential Duplications of Services

Physical therapists may bill for interventions that produce similar physiological responses. If billed from the same treatment session, these may represent duplication of service or inappropriate intervention. When this occurs, additional documentation should be requested to substantiate the multiple payment request. The pairs of interventions to which this may apply include:

a. Moist heat (hot pack) and hydrotherapy (whirlpool or Hubbard tank)

b. Microwave and diathermy

c. Moist heat (hot pack) and infrared

d. Massage and soft tissue mobilization

e. Hydrotherapy (whirlpool or Hubbard tank) and pool therapy (aquatic therapy)

VII. Specific Guidelines for Review of Physical Therapy Claims by Physical Therapists

These guidelines may be divided into six categories:

1. General

   a. Was the patient's examination performed by a physical therapist?

   b. For Workers' Compensation, were the physical therapy examination findings and subsequent intervention(s) related to the compensable event?

   c. Was the intervention provided based on the physical therapist's examination?

   d. Did the physical therapy intervention(s) rendered comply with community norms and commonly accepted practice and/or treatment protocols?

   e. Was the frequency of intervention/length of service provided for this episode of care appropriate? Were stated outcomes reached?

   f. Did you, as the claims reviewer, address all the questions and concerns posed by the insurance carrier, medical claims reviewer, or auditing representative?

2. The Referral Process

   a. Was there a referral for physical therapy, if required by state law? Currently, 30 states have eliminated the referral requirement and made physical therapy services directly accessible to the patient.

3. Intervention Records

   a. Was physical therapy intervention provided with document progress or goal attainment?

   b. Did the written report document the results of tests performed?

c. Did the physical therapy documentation follow the American Physical Therapy Association's *Guidelines for Physical Therapy Documentation* and state law where applicable?

d. Were the physical therapy intervention log and docu-mentation consistent with the billing statement?

4. Physical Therapy Modalities

a. Were local modalities, such as ultrasound and electrical stimulation, continued unmodified for more than 2 weeks without evidence of improved condition?

b. Where palliative modalities provide some relief of discomfort but do not necessarily address the source of the problem or contribute to long-term functional gain. Modalities limited to 6 to 8 weeks (normal tissue healing period)?

Palliative modalities are generally appropriate for the acute phase but, even then, must serve an objective purpose.

If palliative modalities are provided without any other service(s) and/or are provided beyond the normal tissue healing period, the physical therapist should be asked to substantiate the treatment plan.

c. If more than three modalities were used daily, was appropriate justification included?

d. Does the intervention schedule "fade," that is, is there a reduction in the visits per week over time?

e. If a medical device was used during intervention, was it FDA-approved and, therefore, reimbursable?

5. Provider Credentials

a. Do services entitled "physical therapy" or "physiotherapy" show evidence of a licensed physical therapist's involvement?

b. If a physical therapist assistant was involved in providing service, was the assistant supervised by a physical therapist in accordance with state laws and regulations?

c. Are the clinical records authenticated by signatures or initials and professional titles?

6. Billing Statements

a. Are fees reasonable for the geographic area?

b. Do the billing dates correspond with intervention notes?

c. Was the patient concurrently billed for the same intervention by another provider?

d. Is the license number of the physical therapist rendering or directing the provision of physical therapy services on all billings for physical therapy?

VIII. Definition and Utilization of the Physical Therapist Assistant

Definition: The physical therapist assistant is an educated health care provider who assists the physical therapist in providing physical therapy. The physical therapist assistant is a graduate of a physical therapist assistant associate degree program accredited by an agency recognized by the Secretary of the United States Department of Education or the Council on Postsecondary Accreditation.

Utilization: The supervising physical therapist is directly responsible for the actions of the physical therapist assistant. The physical therapist assistant performs physical therapy procedures and related tasks that have been selected and delegated by the supervising physical therapist. Where permitted by law, the physical therapist assistant also carries out routine operational functions, including supervising the physical therapy aide and documenting treatment progress. The ability of the physical therapist assistant to perform the selected and delegated tasks is assessed on an ongoing basis by the supervising physical therapist. The physical therapist assistant may modify a specific treatment procedure in accordance with changes in patient status within the scope of the established treatment plan.

APTA Guidelines for Physical Therapy Claims Review; 1997.

Guidelines for Physical Therapy Claims Review reprinted with permission of the American Physical Therapy Association.

Definitions of Complementary/Alternative Therapies

acupuncture: Acupuncture is an Asian system of medicine based on the principle that vital energy flows through a network of meridians in the body. The meridians are mirrored in the foot, ear, and hand. Illness is seen as a state of energy imbalance in particular areas in which there is an excess in some parts and a deficiency in others. Thin needles are inserted superficially on the skin at various locations on the body. These points are located along "channels" of energy, and the insertion of the needles frees the blockage of energy. Heat can be applied by burning (moxibustion), electrical current (electroacupuncture), or pressure (acupressure). Healing is proposed by the restoration of a balance of energy flow called "Qi." Another explanation suggests that, possibly, the stimulation activates endorphin receptors.

Alexander technique: A bodywork technique in which rebalancing of "postural sets" (ie, physical alignment) is taught by mentally focusing on the way correct alignments should look and feel and through verbal and tactile guidance by the practitioner.

applied kinesiology: In complementary/alternative therapies, this is a form of treatment that uses nutrition, physical manipulation, vitamins, diet, and exercise for the purpose of restoring and energizing the body. Weak muscles are proposed to be a source of dysfunctional health.

aromatherapy: A form of herbal medicine that uses various oils from plants. Route of administration can be through absorption in the skin or inhalation. The action of antiviral and antibacterial agents is proposed to aid in healing. The aromatic biochemical structures of certain herbs are thought to act in areas of the brain related to past experiences and emotions (eg, limbic system).

autogenics: A form of biofeedback through which an individual uses mental imaging to decrease pain, relieve muscle tension, facilitate muscle function, reduce blood pressure, or decrease anxiety. A method of mind-body control based on a specific discipline for relaxing parts of the body by means of auto-suggestion, such as in Jacobson's relaxation techniques. Autogenic suggestion also is a major component in hypnosis (*see* biofeedback).

Ayurveda: A major health system that emphasizes a preventive approach to health by focusing on an inner state of harmony and spiritual realization for self-healing. It includes special types of diets, herbs, and mineral parts and changes based on a system of constitutional categories in lifestyle. The use of enemas and purgation is for the purpose of cleansing the body of excess toxins.

biofeedback: A mind-body procedure in which sensors are placed on the body for the purpose of measuring muscle, heart rate, and sweat responses or neural activity. Information is provided by visual, auditory, or body-muscle cell activation for the purpose of teaching the person to either increase or decrease physiologic activity that, when reconstituted, is proposed to improve health problems (ie, pain, anxiety, high blood pressure, and muscle tension or weakness). In some cases, relaxation exercises complement this procedure.

cell therapy: Healthy cellular material from fetuses, embryos, or organs of animals is directly injected into human patients/clients for the purpose of stimulating healing in dysfunctional organs. It may also include blood transfusions or bone marrow transplants.

chiropractic therapy: A system of therapeutics based upon the claim that disease is caused by abnormal function of structure and the nervous system. It attempts to restore normal function of the nerve system by manipulation and treatment of the structures of the human body, especially those of the spinal column.

cognitive therapy: Psychological therapy in which the major focus is on altering and changing irrational beliefs through a type of "Socratic" dialogue and self-evaluation of certain illogical thoughts. Conditioning and learning are important components of this therapy.

craniosacral therapy: A form of gentle manual manipulation used for diagnosis and for making corrections in a system made up of cerebrospinal fluid, cranial and dural membranes, cranial bones, and sacrum. The system is proposed to be dynamic with its own physiologic frequency. Through touch and pressure, tension is proposed to be reduced and cranial rhythms normalized, leading to improvement in health and disease. The individual is seen as an integrated totality where tightness in one area of the craniosacral fascia will affect other areas of the body.

dance therapy: A movement-based therapy that aids in promoting feeling and awareness. The goal is to integrate body, mind, and self-esteem. It uses different parts of the body, such as fingers, wrists, and arms, to respond to music.

diathermy: The use of high-frequency electrical currents as a form of physical therapy and in surgical procedures. The term diathermy, derived from the Greek words "dia" and "therma," literally means "heating through." The three forms of diathermy employed by physical therapists are short-wave, ultrasound, and microwave.

electroencephalographic normalization: A form of biofeedback in which gross neural activity is recorded from the scalp as an electroencephalogram (EEG) to assist in "restoring a balance of health" by training patients/clients to produce more uniform and consistent EEG frequencies throughout certain or all areas of the brain (occipital, frontal, temporal, and parietal).

environmental medicine: A practice of medicine in which the major focus is on cause-and-effect relationships in health. Evaluations are made of such factors as eating and living habits and types of air breathed. Testing in the patient's/client's own environment is performed to determine what precipitators are present that may be related to disease or other health problems. A treatment protocol is developed from this information.

Feldenkrais method: A bodywork technique in which its founder used the integration of physics, judo, and yoga. The practitioner directs sequences of movement using verbal or hands-on techniques or teaches a system of self-directed exercise to treat physical impairments through the learning of new movement patterns.

Hatha yoga: The branch of yoga practice that involves physical exercise, breathing practices, and movement. These exercises are designed to have a salutary effect on posture, flexibility, and strength for the ultimate purpose of preparing the body to remain still for long periods of meditation.

Hellerwork: A bodywork technique that treats and improves proper body alignment through the development of a more complete awareness of the physical body. The goal is to realign fascia for improvement in standing, sitting, and breathing using "body energy," verbal feedback, and changing emotions and attitudes. This practice is based on the osteopathic concept that "structure determines function" and that the physical relationship of the body's tissue (its structure) determines how the body functions, from gross movement to cellular activity.

herbal medicine: Herbs are used to treat various health conditions. Herbal medicine is a major form of treatment for more than 70% of the world's population.

homeopathy: A form of treatment in which substances (minerals, plant extracts, chemicals, or disease-producing germs), which in sufficient doses would produce a set of illness symptoms in healthy individuals, are given in microdoses to produce a "cure" of those same symptoms by activating the individuals own immune system response. The symptom is not thought to be part of the illness, but part of a curative process.

hydrotherapy/aquatherapy: The therapeutic use of water.

hyperbaric oxygen: A therapy in which 100% oxygen is given at or above atmospheric pressure. An increase in oxygen in the tissue is proposed to increase blood circulation, improve healing and health, and influence the course of disease.

hyperthermia: The use of various heating methods (eg, electromagnetic therapy) to produce temperature elevations of a few degrees in cells and tissues, leading to a proposed antitumor effect. This is often used in conjunction with radiotherapy or chemotherapy for cancer treatment.

hypnosis: A trance-like condition, usually induced by a professional, in which the individual is in a state of altered consciousness and responds to suggestion of the hypnotist (eg, used as a modality for smoking cessation and weight loss). This technique influences the subconscious mind through relaxation and suggestion.

imagery: A technique using suggestion and imagery of "pleasant" thoughts or the completion of tasks (eg, athletic, musical, functional) to manage pain or subconsciously accomplish a physical feat.

immunoaugmentative therapy: A cancer treatment that proposes that cancer cells can be arrested by the use of four different blood proteins; this approach is also proposed to restore the immune system. It can be used as an adjunctive therapy.

Jin Shin Jyutsu: A bodywork technique that uses specific "healing points" at the body surface, which are proposed to overlie flowing energy (Qi). The therapist's fingers are used to "redirect, balance, and provide a more efficient energy flow" to and throughout the body.

light therapy: Natural light or light of specified wavelengths is used to treat disease. This may include ultraviolet, colored, or low-intensity laser light. The eye generally is the initial entry point for the light because of its direct connection to the brain.

magnetic therapy: Magnets are placed directly on the skin, stimulating living cells and increasing blood flow by ionic currents that are created from polarities on the magnets. Both acute and chronic health conditions are suggested to be treatable by this procedure.

manual manipulation: A group of therapies with different assumptions and, in part, different areas of treatment. The major focus includes both stimulation and body manipulation, which are proposed to improve health and/or arrest disease. Includes soft tissue manipulation through stroking, kneading, friction, and vibration. Types include massage, adjustment of the spinal column (chiropractic), and tissue and musculoskeletal (osteopathic) manipulation.

meditation: A mind-body therapy by which relaxation is induced by the act of meditating using deep breathing techniques and deep, continual thought and solemn reflection.

Mediterranean diet: A diet that is thought to provide optimal distribution of daily caloric intake of different nutrients and includes 50% to 60% carbohydrates, 30% fats, and 10% proteins. The diet is derived from the eating habits of people in the Mediterranean area, who were shown to have reduced rates of cardiovascular disease.

mind-body therapies: A group of therapies that emphasize using the mind or brain in conjunction with the body to assist the healing process. Mind-body therapies can involve varying degrees of levels of consciousness, including hypnosis, in which selective attention is used to induce a specific altered state (trance) for memory retrieval, relaxation, or suggestion; visual imagery, in which the focus is on a target visual stimulus; yoga, which involves integration of posture and controlled breathing, relaxation, and/or meditation; relaxation, which includes lighter levels of altered states of consciousness through indirect or direct focus; and meditation, in which there is an intentional use of posture, concentration, contemplation, and visualization.

muscle energy technique: A manual therapy with components of both passive mobilization and muscle reeducation. Diagnosis of somatic dysfunction is performed by the practitioner after which the patient/client is guided to provide corrective muscle contraction. This is followed by further testing and correction.

music therapy: The use of music either in an active or passive mode. Proposed to help allow for the expression of feelings, which helps to reduce stress. Other types of "vibratory" sounds can be used mainly to reduce stress, anxiety, and pain.

myofascial release: Techniques used to release fascial tissue restrictions secondary to tonal dysfunction and decrease binding down of the fascia around a muscle. The body is seen as an integrated whole and that fascial tightness in one area will affect all other areas of the body.

Native American therapies: Therapies used by many Native American Indian tribes, including their own healing herbs and ceremonies that use components with a spiritual emphasis.

naturopathy: A major health system that includes practices that emphasize diet, nutrition, homeopathy, acupuncture, herbal medicine, manipulation, and various mind-body therapies. Focal points include self-healing and treatment through changes in lifestyle and emphasis on disease prevention and health.

neuroelectric therapy: Transcranial or cranial neuroelectric stimulation (TENS), once called "electrosleep," originally used in the 1950s for the treatment of insomnia. In a typical TENS session, surface electrodes are placed in the mastoid region (behind the ear) and, similar to electroacupuncture, stimulated using a low-amperage, low-frequency alternating current. It has been suggested that TENS stimulates endogenous neurotransmitters, such as endorphins, that produce symptomatic relief.

nutrition therapy: The use of diet to manage health and prevent disease.

Ornish diet: A life-choice program based on eating a vegetarian diet containing less than 10% fat. The diet is high in complex carbohydrates and fiber. Animal products and oils are avoided.

orthomolecular therapy: A therapeutic approach that uses naturally occurring substances within the body, such as proteins, fats, and water, which promote restoration and/or balance by using vitamins, minerals, or other forms of nutrition to subsequently treat disease and/or promote healing.

Oslo diet: An eating plan that emphasizes increased intake of fish and reduced total fat intake. The diet is combined with regular endurance exercise.

osteopathic therapy: Therapeutic intervention that is based on a school of medicine and surgery employing various methods of diagnosis and treatment, but placing special emphasis on the interrelationship of the musculoskeletal system to all other body systems.

pet therapy: The use of animals for eliciting physical function and changes in behavior.

Pilates: An educational exercise approach using proper body mechanics, movements, truncal and pelvic stabilization, coordinated breathing, and muscle contractions to promote strengthening. Attention is paid to the entire musculoskeletal system.

Piracetam: A pharmacological treatment proposed to be useful in the treatment of dementia. Uses a cyclic relative of the transmitter gamma-aminobutyric acid (GABA).

polarity: The use of touch through applying pressure to patients/clients on the skin surface using the principles of acupuncture where a particular part of the body is related to various meridians or energy channels. Includes techniques such as reflexology and Shiatsu.

prayer: The use of prayer(s) that are offered to "some higher being" or authority for the purpose of healing and/or arresting disease. May be practiced by the individual patient/client, by groups, or by others with or without the patient's/client's knowledge (eg, intercessory).

Pritikin diet: A weight management plan that is based on a vegetarian framework. Meals are low in fat, high in fiber, and high in complex carbohydrates.

Qigong: A form of Chinese exercise-stimulation therapy that proposes to improve health by redirecting mental focus, breathing, coordination, and relaxation. The goal is to "rebalance" the body's own healing capacities by activating proposed electrical or energetic currents that flow along meridians located throughout the body. These meridians, however, do not follow conventional nerve or muscle pathways. In Chinese medical training and practice, this therapy excludes "external Qi," which is energy transmitted from one person to another for the purpose of healing.

Raja yoga: Yoga practice that includes all of the other forms of yoga practice. The practitioner is instructed to follow moral directives, physical exercises, breathing exercises, meditation, devotion, and service to others to facilitate religious awakening.

reconstruction therapy: A nonsurgical therapy for arthritis that involves the injection of nutritional substances into the supporting tissues around an injured joint. The intent is to cause the dilation of blood vessels, which will allow fibroblasts to form around the injury and begin the healing process.

reflexology: A bodywork technique that uses reflex points on the hands and feet. Pressure is applied at points that correspond to various body parts with the intention of eliminating blockages thought to produce pain or disease. The goal is to bring the body into balance.

Reiki: Comes from the Japanese word meaning "universal life force energy." The practitioner serves as a conduit for healing energy directed into the body or energy field of the recipient without physical contact with the body.

relaxation: A therapeutic mode used to loosen muscles and relieve stress incorporating muscle tightening and relaxing and the superficial form of meditation.

restricted environmental stimulation therapy (REST): A procedure that uses a completely sensory-deprived environment for the purpose of increasing physical or mental healing through a nonreactive state.

Rolfing: A bodywork technique that involves the myofascial. The body is realigned by using the hands to apply a deep pressure and friction that allows more sufficient posture, movement, and the "release" of emotions from the body.

ROM dance: A therapeutic mind-body exercise and rest program for individuals with arthritis and other painful or limiting conditions. Slow, flowing, rhythmical movements accompanied by quiet music and a verse with images of water, light, and friendship for visualization. This exercise mode is primarily used to improve flexibility, strength, and endurance and provide a means of relaxation and meditation.

Rosen method: A form of bodywork with the basis of the less a therapist does to intervene in a person's healing process, the better. The therapist serves as a "listener" to the person's spoken words and to the person's body, including breathing, muscle tension, and changes in both.

Shiatsu: A bodywork technique involving finger pressure at specific points on the body mainly for the purpose of balancing "energy" in the body. The major focus is on prevention by keeping the body healthy. The therapy uses more than 600 points on the skin that are proposed to be connected through which energy flows. A Japanese form of acupressure. Also related to the philosophy of reflexology.

soma therapy: A therapeutic intervention based on the osteopathic concept of structure determines function. Soma bodywork includes the balancing of the body with gravity where the physical relationship of the body's tissue (its structure) determines how the body functions, from gross movement to cellular activity.

t'ai chi: An ancient physical art form, originally a martial art in which the defendant uses an attacker's own energy against him- or herself by drawing the attack and side-stepping. It is a technique that uses slow, purposeful motor-physical movements of the body, accompanied by breathing and mental concentration (meditation) for the purpose of control and achieving a more balanced physiologic and psychological state. The Chinese conceived the human mind to be an unlimited dimension and the body as limitless in its physical capacity.

therapeutic riding: A form of animal-assisted (usually a horse) therapy in which either passive or active movements are produced to aid in approximating the human gait. In certain cases physiotherapeutic exercises are performed while riding a horse.

therapeutic touch: A body energy field technique in which hands are passed over the body without actually touching to recreate and change proposed "energy imbalances" for restoring innate healing forces. Verbal interaction between patient/client and therapist helps to maximize effects.

traditional Chinese medicine: An ancient form of medicine that focuses on prevention and secondarily treats disease with an emphasis on maintaining balance through the body by stimulating a constant, smooth-flowing Qi energy. Herbs, acupuncture, massage, diet, and exercise are also used.

Trager psychophysical integration: A bodywork technique in which the practitioner enters a meditative state and guides the patient/client through gentle, light, rhythmic nonintrusive movements. "Mentastics" exercises using self-healing movements are taught to the patient/client. Communicates tactile feelings through the hands of the practitioner to the tissues of the patient/client.

transcranial electrostimulation: Pulsed electrical stimulation of 50 microamperes or less is applied between two electrodes attached to the ear. The stimulation is proposed to activate endogenous opioid activity, which may assist in the treatment of certain health problems, such as substance abuse and physical pain.

12-step program: A program, such as Alcoholics Anonymous, that is based on a series of 12 steps or tasks that participants are asked to complete. As members progress through the 12 steps, they are expected to gain courage to attempt personal change and develop a greater acceptance of themselves. Programs emphasize the group process through the sharing of stories and experiences and through social interactions with other group members. Most 12-step programs incorporate a spiritual component and ask members to turn their lives over to a higher power.

Watsu: Bodywork in which warm water is used for freeing the body integrating stretch and relaxation.

yoga: A blend of physical activity and mental rest that includes gentle stretching and meditation and can include tapping and visceral mobilization. It focuses on abdominal breathing (HARA—the center for yogic breathing).

Resources and Networking

ACCIDENT PREVENTION

American Association of Retired Persons (AARP)
55 Alive/Mature Driving Program, Traffic and Driver Safety Program
601 E Street, NW
Washington, DC 20049
1-202-434-2277 or 1-888-222-7669

National Institute on Aging
Building 31, Room 5C27
31 Center Dr, MSC 2292
Bethesda, MD 20892
1-301-496-1752

National Safety Council
1121 Spring Lake Drive
Itasca, IL 60143-3204
1-630-285-1121

ALCOHOLISM

National Council on Alcoholism
12 W. 21st Street
New York, NY 10010
1-212-645-6770
www.ncadd.org

CANCER

National Cancer Institute
Suite 3036A
6116 Executive Boulevard, MSC 8322
Bethesda, MD 20892-8322

COGNITIVE CHANGES

Alzheimer's Disease and Related Disorders Association
919 N. Michigan Avenue, Suite 1100
Chicago, IL 60611

National Institute for Neurological Disorders and Stroke
NIH Neurological Institute
PO Box 580
Bethesda, MD 20824
1-800-352-9424

DATABASE RESOURCES

Health Resource Inc
1-501-329-5272

MedExpert
1-800-999-1999

Planetree Library
1-415-923-3680

DIABETES

American Diabetes Association (ADA)
2 Park Avenue
New York, NY 10016

Educational/Career Issues
American Association of University Women
1111 16th Street, NW
Washington, DC 20036
1-202-785-7700

American Physical Therapy Association
1111 N. Fairfax Street
Alexandria, VA 22314-9902
1-800-999-2782

National Commission on Working Women
1211 Connecticut Avenue, NW
Suite 400
Washington, DC 20036

EDUCATIONAL MATERIALS

American Association of Retired Persons
1909 K Street, NW
Washington, DC 20049

American Physical Therapy Association
1111 N. Fairfax Street
Alexandria, VA 22314-9902
1-800-999-2782

Department of Health and Human Services
Public Health Service, Agency for Health Care Policy and Research
Executive Office Center
2101 E. Jefferson Street
Suite 501
Rockville, MD 20852

National Institute of Aging
NIA Information Center
2209 Distribution Circle
Silver Spring, MD 20910

Robert Wood Foundation
Consumer Information Center
Pueblo, CO 81009

GENERAL INFORMATION

American Physical Therapy Association
1111 N. Fairfax Street
Alexandria, VA 22314-9902
1-800-999-2782

National Health Information Center
1-800-336-4797

National Organization for Rare Disorders
1-203-744-0100

HEART DISEASE

American Heart Association (AHA)
7272 Greenville Avenue
Dallas, TX 75231
1-214-373-6300

National Heart, Lung, and Blood Institute (NHLBI)
9000 Rockville Pike
Bethesda, MD 20892
1-301-496-4236

HIGH BLOOD PRESSURE

High Blood Pressure Information Center
120/80 National Institutes of Health
Bethesda, MD 20892

HOTLINES

Prostate Hotline
1-800-543-9632

Y-ME National Organization for Breast Cancer
1-800-221-2141

LEGAL ISSUES

American Physical Therapy Association
1111 N. Fairfax Street
Alexandria, VA 22314-9902
1-800-999-2782

National Organization for Victim Assistance (NOVA)
1730 Park Road, NW
Washington, DC 20010
1-800-879-6682

LONG-TERM CARE ISSUES

American Association of Homes for the Aging (AAHA)
1129 20th Street, NW
Washington, DC 20036

National Association of Home Care
228 7th Street, S.E.
Washington, DC 20003
1-202-547-7424

National Citizen's Coalition for Nursing Home Reform
1424 16th Street, NW
Room L2
Washington, DC 20036

MEDICATIONS

American Association of Retired Persons (AARP) Pharmacy Service
PO Box NIA
1 Prince Street
Alexandria, VA 22314

American Pharmaceutical Association
2215 Constitution Avenue, NW
Washington, DC 20037
1-202-628-4410

Food and Drug Administration (FDA)
Division of Regulatory Affairs
Center for Drugs and Biologics
5600 Fisher Lane
Rockville, MD 20857

NUTRITION AND PHYSICAL FITNESS

American Dietetic Association
430 N. Michigan Avenue
Chicago, IL 60611

American Physical Therapy Association
1111 N. Fairfax Street
Alexandria, VA 22314-9902
1-800-999-2782

President's Council on Physical Fitness and Sports
450 5th Street, NW, Suite 7103
Washington, DC 20001

OSTEOARTHRITIS

American Physical Therapy Association
1111 N. Fairfax Street
Alexandria, VA 22314-9902
1-800-999-2782
Arthritis Foundation
1330 W. Peachtree Street
Atlanta, GA 30309
1-404-872-7100

National Institute of Arthritis and Musculoskeletal and Skin Diseases
1 AMS Circle
Bethesda, MD 20892-3675
1-301-496-8188

OSTEOPOROSIS

American Academy of Orthopaedic Surgeons
222 S. Prospect Avenue
Park Ridge, IL 60068

American Physical Therapy Association
1111 N. Fairfax Street
Alexandria, VA 22314-9902
1-800-999-2782

National Institute of Arthritis and Musculoskeletal and Skin Diseases
1 AMS Circle
Bethesda, MD 20892-3675
1-301-496-8188

National Institute on Aging
Public Information Office
Building 31, Room SC27
Bethesda, MD 20892-2292
1-301-496-2947

National Osteoporosis Foundation
1232 22nd Street, NW
Washington, DC 20037-1292
1-202-223-2226

POLITICAL ISSUES

American Physical Therapy Association
1111 N. Fairfax Street
Alexandria, VA 22314-9902
1-800-999-2782

National Coalition on Older Women's Issues (NCOWI)
1120 Connecticut Avenue, NW
Washington, DC 20036
1-202-466-7837

National Council on the Aging (NCOA)
409 3rd Street, SW
Suite 200
Washington, DC 20026
1-202-479-1200

National Organization for Women (NOW)
425 13th Street, NW
Washington, DC 20002

SUPPORT GROUPS

American Self-Help Clearinghouse
1-973-625-7101

National Self-Help Clearinghouse
25 W. 43rd Street
New York, NY 10036

URINARY INCONTINENCE

American Physical Therapy Association
1111 N. Fairfax Street
Alexandria, VA 22314-9902
1-800-999-2782

Continence Restored
785 Park Avenue
New York, NY 10021
1-212-879-313
or
407 Strawberry Hill Avenue
Stamford, CT 06902

HIP (Help for Incontinent People) Organization
PO Box 544
Union, SC 29379

Simon Foundation
PO Box 835X
Wilmette, Il 60091

U.S. Department of Health and Human Services
Public Health Service, Agency for Health Care Policy and Research,
Executive Office Center
2101 E. Jefferson Street
Suite 501
Rockville, MD 20852

American College of Obstetricians and Gynecologists
600 Maryland Avenue, SW
Suite 300 E.
Washington, DC 20024

American Physical Therapy Association
1111 N. Fairfax Street
Alexandria, VA 22314-9902
1-800-999-2782

Center for Climacteric Studies
University of Florida
901 NW 8th Avenue
Suite B1
Gainesville, FL 32601

HERS (Hysterectomy Education Resources)
422 Bryn Mawr Avenue
Bala Cynwood, PA 19004
1-215-667-7757

National Institute on Aging
NIA Information Center
2209 Distribution Circle
Silver Spring, MD 20910

National Women's Health Network
224 Seventh Street, SE
Washington, DC 20024

Notes: Some national organizations are listed in the local yellow pages of
your phonebook, or you can order a printed listing of private and public
sources of information for $17.25 postpaid by writing to: Resource
Information Guide, PO Box 990297, Redding, CA 96099.
Most of the organizations listed above, and the materials they provide, are
accessible on-line via the Internet by typing in the name of the organization
or the subject matter into the "Search" box of your server.

Physical Therapy Organizations

AMERICAN PHYSICAL THERAPY ASSOCIATION (APTA)

The mission of the APTA, the principal membership organization representing and promoting the profession of physical therapy, is to further the profession's role in the prevention, diagnosis, and treatment of movement dysfunction and the enhancement of the physical health and functional abilities of members of the public (see Appendix 12).

American Physical Therapy Association
1111 N. Fairfax Street
Alexandria, VA 22314
Phone: 1-703-684-2782 or 1-800-999-2782
Fax: 1-703-684-7374
www.apta.org

AMERICAN BOARD OF PHYSICAL THERAPY SPECIALTIES

The American Board of Physical Therapy Specialties (ABPTS) offers board certification in seven specialty areas of physical therapy: cardiopulmonary, clinical electrophysiologic, geriatric, neurologic, orthopedic, pediatric, and sports physical therapy.

The purpose of the APTA's Clinical Specialization Program is to assist in the identification and development of appropriate areas of specialty practice in physical therapy, promote the highest possible level of care for individuals seeking physical therapy services in each specialty area, promote development of the science and art underlying each specialty area of practice, provide a reliable and valid method for certification and recertification of individuals who have attained an advanced level of knowledge and skill in each specialty area, and to assist consumers, the health care community, and others in identifying certified clinical specialists in each specialty area. The directory of certified clinical specialists in physical therapy may be viewed via the Internet at www.apta.org under Clinical Specialists. This directory includes listings of certified specialists according to specialty area and is organized by state in alphabetical order. This directory may also be purchased through the APTA Resource catalog, which is available by phone at 1-800-999-2782 ext. 3395, by fax at 1-703-706-3396, or via the APTA's web site at www.apta.org.

Criteria for establishment of a new specialty are established by the ABPTS and guide the development of all new specialty areas. The APTA House of Delegates approves all new specialty areas.

The ABPTS approves certification of clinical specialists in each specialty area. The Specialty Councils define, develop, and modify the requirements for certification and recertification in their specialty areas. The APTA Board of Directors and the Sections of the seven recognized specialty areas provide funding for the specialist certification program, and the APTA Board of Directors serves as an appeal body for certification candidates.

American Board of Physical Therapy Specialties
1111 N. Fairfax Street
Alexandria, VA 22314
Phone: 1-800-999-2782 ext. 8520
Email: spec-cert@apta.org

APTA Specialist Certification Department
Phone: 1-800-999-2782 ext. 3152

COMMISSION ON ACCREDITATION IN PHYSICAL THERAPY EDUCATION

The Commission on Accreditation in Physical Therapy Education (CAPTE) of the APTA is the recognized body that accredits physical therapy education programs and reaffirms the Association's philosophy of opposition to duplication and fragmentation of physical therapy education. The CAPTE grants specialized accreditation status to qualified entry-level education programs for physical therapists and physical therapist assistants. CAPTE is listed as a nationally recognized accrediting agency by the US Department of Education and the Council for Higher Education Accreditation (CHEA).

The Commission is responsible for formulating, revising, adopting, and implementing the evaluative criteria for the accreditation of physical therapist assistant and physical therapist professional education programs. Specialized accreditation is a system for recognizing professional education programs for a level of performance, integrity, and quality that entitles them to the confidence of the educational community and the public they serve. Accreditation status signifies that the program meets established and nationally accepted standards of scope, quality, and relevance.

The CAPTE is comprised of 26 board members representative of the educational community, the physical therapy profession, and the public. Members include physical therapy educators who are basic scientists, curriculum specialists, and academic administrators; physical therapy clinicians and clinical educators; administrators from institutions of higher education; public representatives; and a physician. The wide-ranging experience and expertise of this group in physical therapy education and education in general provide ongoing assurance that the accreditation process of physical therapy education programs is fair, reliable, and effective.

Commission on Accreditation in Physical Therapy Education
1111 N. Fairfax Street
Alexandria, VA 22314
Phone: 1-800-999-2782
Email: capte@apta.org

FEDERATION OF STATE BOARDS OF PHYSICAL THERAPY

The mission of the Federation of State Boards of Physical Therapy (FSBPT) is to serve as a resource to the member boards in their efforts to ensure the protection of the consumer of physical therapy services throughout the United States, its territories, commonwealths, and possessions.

The Federation promotes and protects the health, safety, and welfare of the public by facilitating reasonable uniformity in physical therapy practices. The Federation recommends consistent regulatory practices through the Model Practice Act for Physical Therapy, addresses foreign education equivalency, and collects and disseminates information relevant to the practice of physical therapy.

The Federation administers the National Physical Therapy Examination and continually improves examination methodology and relevance. It also provides educational programs for Member Boards. The principal objectives include strengthening state leadership in policymaking, promoting excellence and continuing competence in the physical therapy profession, and advocating the National Physical Therapy Disciplinary Database.

Federation of State Boards of Physical Therapy
509 Wythe Street
Alexandria, VA 22314
Phone: 1-703-299-3100 or 1-800-200-3031
Fax: 1-703-299-3110 or 1-800-981-3031
www.fsbpt.org

FOUNDATION FOR PHYSICAL THERAPY

The Foundation for Physical Therapy was established in 1979 as a national, independent, nonprofit corporation to support the physical therapy profession's research needs in three areas:

1. Scientific research, to create a solid platform for future clinical research

2. Clinical research, to assess the efficacy of physical therapy intervention and help define best practice

3. Health services research, to assess the effectiveness of physical therapy practice in the emerging health care delivery models for physical therapy

Among the activities of the Foundation to advance its objectives are:

1. Assisting clinicians, researchers, and academicians in their doctoral programs

2. Expanding funding for emerging researchers

3. Supporting clinically relevant research

4. Strengthening the Foundation's capacity to promote the profession's research agenda

This mission of the organization is to advance the physical therapy profession through support for doctoral education and sponsorship of clinically relevant research.

Foundation for Physical Therapy
1111 N. Fairfax Street
Alexandria, VA 22314
Phone: 1-800-875-1378
Email: foundation@apta.org

PHYSICAL THERAPY POLITICAL ACTION COMMITTEE

The Physical Therapy Political Action Committee (PT PAC) of the APTA is a grassroots organization that provides a vital link to APTA's success on Capitol Hill. Through membership donations, this committee is able to move legislative and policy issues through lobbying efforts directed toward policy decision makers. PT PAC sponsors the PTeam grassroots program, which publishes a bimonthly newsletter on legislative activity on Capitol Hill. They also publish three to four Legislative Action Alerts each year on current federal legislative issues. Through the Alerts, members of the APTA are asked to contact members of Congress on particular issues of concern to our patients and the physical therapy profession.

Physical Therapy Political Action Committee
1111 N. Fairfax Street
Alexandria, VA 22314
Phone: 1-703-706-3163
email: ptpac@apta.org

PTeam Grassroots Program
Phone: 1-703-706-3163
Email: michaelmatlack@apta.org

WORLD CONFEDERATION FOR PHYSICAL THERAPY

The World Confederation for Physical Therapy (WCPT) aims to improve the quality of global health through the following methods:

1. Representing physical therapy and physiotherapists internationally through communication and exchange of information and cooperation with international and national organizations

2. Encouraging high standards of physical therapy through research, education, and practice by continuing to organize international congresses every 4 years and other educational meetings, and by encouraging the achievement of appropriate staffing levels

3. Encouraging the development of regions and the communication and exchange of information between the regions and WCPT.

World Confederation for Physical Therapy
4a Abbot's Place
London NW6 4NP
United Kingdom
Phone: +44-171-328-5448
Fax: +44-171-624-7579
Email: 106253.215@compuserve.com

Legislation and Policy Decisions
Affecting Rehabilitation

Americans with Disabilities Act (1990) (ADA): This U.S. federal act protects persons with disabilities from discrimination in employment, transportation, public accommodations, telecommunications, and activities of state and local government.

Architectural Barriers Act (1969): U.S. federal legislation that requires accessibility to certain facilities.

Balanced Budget Act (BBA): Enacted in 1997 in an attempt to balance the national budget of the United States which placed an annual $1500 cap on Medicare recipient benefits for combined physical therapy and speech therapy services under Medicare Part B. The prospective payment system (PPS) fixes the amount that hospitals are reimbursed for the primary diagnosis for each hospital stay. A moratorium was placed on this cap in a legislative decision in November 1999, which was in effect for the years 2000 and 2001.

Civilian Industrial Rehabilitation Act (1920): First U.S. federal legislation to help occupational therapy. It commissioned federal aid for vocational rehabilitation for those disabled by accident or illness in industry.

Community Mental Health Act (1963): Under this act, the National Institute of Mental Health was mandated to establish community mental health centers as part of a national movement to take more responsibility for individuals with mental illness.

Consolidated Omnibus Budget Reconciliation Act of 1985 (COBRA): Federal legislation that requires that all employers with 20 or more employees continue health coverage for up to 18 months after a worker loses benefits due to reduced work hours or loss of employment.

Deficit Reduction Legislation Acts (1984, 1985, 1986): Extended U.S. federal coverage for health and social services through modification of Medicare legislation.

Developmental Disabilities Act Amendments (1984): U.S. federal legislation that ensured that people with developmental disabilities receive necessary services and established a monitoring system.

Developmental Disabilities Services and Facilities Construction Act (1970): U.S. law giving the states broad responsibility for planning and implementing a comprehensive program of services to individuals with developmental delays, epilepsy, cerebral palsy, and other neurological impairments.

Disability Insurance Benefit Program (1956): U.S. federal legislation that provided benefits to qualified workers with disabilities.

Education of All Handicapped Children Act (1975): U.S. federal legislation intended to ensure that children with disabilities receive education in the least restrictive environment.

Education of the Handicapped Act Amendments (1986): Increase in U.S. federal funds for special education and other services provided to preschoolers ages 3 to 5 years.

Employment Retirement Income Security Act (ERISA): A federal act passed by Congress in 1974 that defines requirements and exemptions for self-insuring firms.

Fair Housing Amendment Act (1988): U.S. federal law meant to prohibit discriminatory housing for those with disabilities.

Handicapped Children's Early Education Assistance Act: U.S. federal law in which funds were authorized for the development, evaluation, and dissemination of different projects for persons with disabilities aged birth to 8 years and their families.

Health Maintenance Organization Act of 1973: U.S. federal law that provided for the planning and development of health maintenance organizations; encourages less ambulatory care.

Health Professions Educational Assistance Act: U.S. federal law that provided incentives for medical schools to increase the number of family practice physicians to half of their graduates and also attempted to attract physicians to underserved areas by subsidizing their medical education.

Individuals with Disabilities Act (IDEA): U.S. federal legislation that provides resources to school-aged children with disabilities.

Interim Payment System (IPS): Enacted in 1997 in an attempt to balance the national budget of the United States. The IPS fixes the amount that home care agencies are reimbursed for services for the primary diagnosis.

National Consumer Health Information and Health Promotion Act of 1976: U.S. federal legislation that attempted to set rational goals for health information and education.

National Health Planning and Resource Development Act of 1974: U.S. federal legislation that established regional health systems agencies to assume responsibility for health care planning for community needs and for cost containment.

Older Americans Act: Enacted in 1965 as the major piece of legislation for provision of social and health-related services to older Americans; established federal, state, and local government network for advocacy and service delivery.

Omnibus Budget Reconciliation Act of 1987 (OBRA '87): U.S. federal legislation that recognizes quality of life as most important to nursing home residents. Contains a section of the federal Nursing Home Reform Act, which made sweeping changes in the standards for provision of nursing home care. These mandated changes address such areas as patient care planning, nursing, staffing, nurse's aide training, nurse's aide registry, patient's rights, transfers and discharges, and administrator standards.

Omnibus Reconciliation Act (1981): U.S. federal legislation designed to finance community based services for people with developmental disabilities when that treatment is less expensive than an institution.

Omnibus Social Security Act (1983): U.S. federal legislation that established a prospective payment system based on a fixed price per diagnosis-related group for inpatient services.

Prospective Payment System (PPS): Enacted in 1997 in attempts to balance the national budget of the United States and placed an annual $1500 cap on Medicare recipient benefits for combined physical therapy and speech therapy services under Medicare Part B. The PPS fixes the amount that hospitals are reimbursed for the primary diagnosis for each hospital stay.

Rehabilitation Act (1973): Services were expanded to the severely disabled, affirmative action provided in employment and nondiscrimination in facilities by federal contractors and grantees.

Servicemen's Readjustment Act (GI Bill) of 1944: U.S. federal legislation that provided for the education and training of individuals whose education or career had been interrupted by military service.

Social Security Acts and Amendments (1935): U.S. federal legislation that provided financial support for workers with disabilities and retirement income for the elderly.

Social Security Amendments of 1972: U.S. federal legislation that provided for the establishment of Professional Standard Review Organizations to ensure that federally funded programs were used in an efficient and effective manner.

Tax Equity and Fiscal Responsibility Act (TEFRA) (1982): U.S. federal act that put limits on Medicare and Medicaid reimbursements (including physical and occupational therapy); also limits items such as inpatient hospital costs.

Technology-Related Assistance for Individuals with Disabilities Act of 1988: U.S. federal legislation that requires assistive technology be made available to persons with disabilities to enhance their functional capabilities.

Title VII of the Medicare Prospective Payment Legislation (1983): U.S. federal legislation that provides incentives for cost containment and better management of resources by a reimbursement structure based on client's diagnosis rather than direct cost of care.

Title XVIII and Title XIX of the Social Security Act (1965): U.S. federal legislation that established reimbursement based on reasonable cost for medical services for the elderly and through state grants to the poor.

Vocational Rehabilitation Act and Amendments (1943): U.S. federal legislation that brought about a change to include payment for medical services, thus allowing occupational therapy services (physical therapy services already covered) to be covered as a legitimate service.

Welsh-Clark Act (World War II Disabled Veterans Rehabilitation Act): U.S. federal legislation that provided vocational rehabilitation for veterans of World War II.

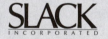